AF813929

The One Health Concept in Asian Contexts

Annisa Utami Rauf • Tri Wibawa
Editors

The One Health Concept in Asian Contexts

Springer

Editors
Annisa Utami Rauf
Department of Health Behavior, Environment, and Social Medicine, Faculty of Medicine, Public Health, and Nursing
Universitas Gadjah Mada
Sleman, Yogyakarta, Indonesia

Tri Wibawa
Department of Microbiology, Faculty of Medicine, Public Health, and Nursing
Universitas Gadjah Mada
Sleman, Yogyakarta, Indonesia

ISBN 978-981-95-9879-3 ISBN 978-981-95-9880-9 (eBook)
https://doi.org/10.1007/978-981-95-9880-9

© The Editor(s) (if applicable) and The Author(s), under exclusive license to Springer Nature Singapore Pte Ltd. 2026

This work is subject to copyright. All rights are solely and exclusively licensed by the Publisher, whether the whole or part of the material is concerned, specifically the rights of translation, reprinting, reuse of illustrations, recitation, broadcasting, reproduction on microfilms or in any other physical way, and transmission or information storage and retrieval, electronic adaptation, computer software, or by similar or dissimilar methodology now known or hereafter developed.
The use of general descriptive names, registered names, trademarks, service marks, etc. in this publication does not imply, even in the absence of a specific statement, that such names are exempt from the relevant protective laws and regulations and therefore free for general use.
The publisher, the authors and the editors are safe to assume that the advice and information in this book are believed to be true and accurate at the date of publication. Neither the publisher nor the authors or the editors give a warranty, expressed or implied, with respect to the material contained herein or for any errors or omissions that may have been made. The publisher remains neutral with regard to jurisdictional claims in published maps and institutional affiliations.

This Springer imprint is published by the registered company Springer Nature Singapore Pte Ltd.
The registered company address is: 152 Beach Road, #21-01/04 Gateway East, Singapore 189721, Singapore

If disposing of this product, please recycle the paper.

Contents

Contributors

Reza Hanifatus Aini Master of Public Health Program, Faculty of Medicine, Public Health, and Nursing, Universitas Gadjah Mada, Yogyakarta, Indonesia

Linda Andriani Department of Epidemiology, Population Biostatistics and Health Promotion, Faculty of Public Health, Universitas Airlangga, Surabaya, Indonesia
Sidoarjo Health Office, East Java, Indonesia

Chaterine Rahel Anggrainy Master of Public Health Program, Faculty of Medicine, Public Health, and Nursing, Universitas Gadjah Mada, Yogyakarta, Indonesia

Miranda Chrisan Anggreni Master of Public Health Program, Faculty of Medicine, Public Health, and Nursing, Universitas Gadjah Mada, Yogyakarta, Indonesia

Neisry Arysta Master of Tropical Medicine Program, Faculty of Medicine, Public Health, and Nursing, Universitas Gadjah Mada, Yogyakarta, Indonesia

Rizka Humardewayanti Asdie Department of Internal Medicine Sub Specialist in Tropical Diseases Infection, Faculty of Medicine, Public Health and Nursing, Universitas Gadjah Mada, Yogyakarta, Indonesia

Annisa Kharismaningtyas Astuti Master of Public Health Program, Faculty of Medicine, Public Health, and Nursing, Universitas Gadjah Mada, Yogyakarta, Indonesia

Ratna Dwi Puji Astuti Department of Environmental Health, Faculty of Public Health, Universitas Airlangga, Surabaya, Indonesia

Ridwan Balatif Department of Microbiology, Faculty of Medicine, Public Health, and Nursing, Universitas Gadjah Mada, Sleman, Yogyakarta, Indonesia

Annisa Nur Balqis Master of Public Health Program, Faculty of Medicine, Public Health, and Nursing, Universitas Gadjah Mada, Yogyakarta, Indonesia

Bagas Suryo Bintoro Department of Health Behavior, Environment, and Social Medicine, Faculty of Medicine, Public Health, and Nursing, Universitas Gadjah Mada, Sleman, Yogyakarta, Indonesia

Annisa Firdaus Winta Damarsya Master of Public Health Program, Faculty of Medicine, Public Health, and Nursing, Universitas Gadjah Mada, Yogyakarta, Indonesia

Denada Jihan Dampi Master of Public Health Program, Faculty of Medicine, Public Health, and Nursing, Universitas Gadjah Mada, Sleman, Indonesia

Marselinus Edwin Widyanto Daniwijaya Department of Microbiology, Faculty of Medicine, Public Health and Nursing, Universitas Gadjah Mada, Yogyakarta, Indonesia

Kharisma Dewi Department of Parasitology, Faculty of Medicine, Public Health, and Nursing, Universitas Gadjah Mada, Yogyakarta, Indonesia

Lita Eliana Master of Tropical Medicine Program, Faculty of Medicine, Public Health, and Nursing, Universitas Gadjah Mada, Yogyakarta, Indonesia

Andang Evrilianto Department of Health Administration and Policy, Faculty of Public Health, University of Indonesia, Depok, Indonesia

Yuliana Fashani Master of Public Health Program, Faculty of Medicine, Public Health, and Nursing, Universitas Gadjah Mada, Yogyakarta, Indonesia

Muhammad Ilham Gibran Doctoral Program in Medical and Health Sciences, Faculty of Medicine, Public Health, and Nursing, Universitas Gadjah Mada, Yogyakarta, Indonesia

Almaasita Yumna Hajar Center of Health Behavior and Promotion, Faculty of Medicine, Public Health and Nursing, Universitas, Gadjah Mada, Yogyakarta, Indonesia

Denis Oxy Handika Master of Public Health Program, Faculty of Medicine, Public Health, and Nursing, Universitas Gadjah Mada, Yogyakarta, Indonesia

Mubasysyir Hasanbasri Department of Biostatistics, Epidemiology, and Population Health, Faculty of Medicine, Public Health, and Nursing, Universitas Gadjah Mada, Yogyakarta, Indonesia

Mukhlish Jamal Musa Holle Faculty of Biology, Universitas Gadjah Mada, Yogyakarta, Indonesia

Vena Jaladara Department of Health Behavior, Environment, and Social Medicine, Faculty of Medicine, Public Health, and Nursing, Universitas Gadjah Mada, Yogyakarta, Indonesia

The Graduate School for the Humanities, Faculty of Arts, University of Groningen, Groningen, Netherlands

Tri Joko Department of Plant Protection, Faculty of Agriculture, Universitas Gadjah Mada, Yogyakarta, Indonesia

Gilbert Renardi Kusila Center for Health Financing Policy and Health Insurance Management (KPMAK), Universitas Gadjah Mada, Yogyakarta, Indonesia

Mustofa Department of Pharmacology and Therapy, Faculty of Medicine, Public Health and Nursing, Universitas Gadjah Mada, Yogyakarta, Indonesia

Rizki Andini Nawawi Department of Clinical Microbiology, Faculty of Medicine, Universitas Sriwijaya, Palembang, Indonesia

Yudhi Ratna Nugraheni Department of Parasitology, Faculty of Veterinary Medicine, Universitas Gadjah Mada, Yogyakarta, Indonesia

One Health Centre of Excellence, Universitas Gadjah Mada, Yogyakarta, Indonesia

Fitri Revita Nurannisa Master of Public Health Program, Faculty of Medicine, Public Health, and Nursing, Universitas Gadjah Mada, Yogyakarta, Indonesia

Sandy Nurvianto Faculty of Forestry, Universitas Gadjah Mada, Yogyakarta, Indonesia

Farida Nur Oktoviani Department of Microbiology, Faculty of Medicine, Public Health and Nursing, Universitas Gadjah Mada, Sleman, Yogyakarta, Indonesia

Thoriq Abi Pramana Master of Public Health Program, Faculty of Medicine, Public Health, and Nursing, Universitas Gadjah Mada, Yogyakarta, Indonesia

Febriani Putri Master of Public Health Program, Faculty of Medicine, Public Health, and Nursing, Universitas Gadjah Mada, Yogyakarta, Indonesia

Khrisdiana Putri Department of Public Health, Faculty of Veterinary Medicine, Universitas Gadjah Mada, Yogyakarta, Indonesia

One Health Centre of Excellence, Universitas Gadjah Mada, Yogyakarta, Indonesia

Qotru A. N. Master of Public Health Program, Faculty of Medicine, Public Health, and Nursing, Universitas Gadjah Mada, Yogyakarta, Indonesia

Vivi Rosalin Rajagukguk Master of Public Health Program, Faculty of Medicine, Public Health, and Nursing, Universitas Gadjah Mada, Sleman, Indonesia

Annisa Utami Rauf Department of Health Behavior, Environment, and Social Medicine, Faculty of Medicine, Public Health, and Nursing, Universitas Gadjah Mada, Sleman, Yogyakarta, Indonesia

Nilna Sa'adatar Rohmah Department of Biostatistics, Epidemiology and Population Health, Faculty of Medicine, Public Health, and Nursing, Universitas Gadjah Mada, Yogyakarta, Indonesia

Nurendah Ratri Azhar Rusprayunita Master of Public Health Program, Faculty of Medicine, Public Health, and Nursing, Universitas Gadjah Mada, Yogyakarta, Indonesia

Salsabila A. F. Department of Health, Faculty of Vocational Studies, Universitas Airlangga, Surabaya, Indonesia

Siti Mei Saroh Master of Public Health Program, Faculty of Medicine, Public Health, and Nursing, Universitas Gadjah Mada, Yogyakarta, Indonesia

Widodo Agus Setianto Department of Communication Sciences, Faculty of Social Sciences & Political Science, Universitas Gadjah Mada, Yogyakarta, Indonesia

Abdul Rahman Siregar Faculty of Biology, Universitas Gadjah Mada, Yogyakarta, Indonesia

Intan Rosenanda Sofiany Master of Public Health Program, Faculty of Medicine, Public Health, and Nursing, Universitas Gadjah Mada, Yogyakarta, Indonesia

Brian Arianto Tanuwidjaja Master of Public Health Program, Faculty of Medicine, Public Health, and Nursing, Universitas Gadjah Mada, Yogyakarta, Indonesia

Auliya Syifaa Urrahman Department of Global Agricultural Sciences, Graduate School of Agricultural and Life Sciences, The University of Tokyo, Tokyo, Japan

Muhamad Imam Utama Department of Biostatistics, Epidemiology and Population Health, Faculty of Medicine, Public Health, and Nursing, Universitas Gadjah Mada, Yogyakarta, Indonesia

Tri Wibawa Department of Microbiology, Faculty of Medicine, Public Health, and Nursing, Universitas Gadjah Mada, Sleman, Yogyakarta, Indonesia

Bayu Satria Wiratama Department of Biostatistics, Epidemiology, and Population Health, Faculty of Medicine, Public Health, and Nursing, Universitas Gadjah Mada, Yogyakarta, Indonesia

Danindra Ario Wiryawan Master of Public Health Program, Faculty of Medicine, Public Health, and Nursing, Universitas Gadjah Mada, Sleman, Indonesia

Chapter 1
Introduction of One Health in Asia

Annisa Utami Rauf, Miranda Chrisan Anggreni, Almaasita Yumna Hajar, and Tri Wibawa

1.1 History and Evolution of the One Health

The historical foundations of the One Health concept can be traced back to the seventeenth and eighteenth centuries, particularly during the *Siècle des Lumières*, when intellectuals began to acknowledge the interdependence of human, animal, and environmental health. Bernardino Ramazzini, in the early 1700s, emphasized the role of environmental exposures in disease development, while Giovanni Maria Lancisi proposed early public health measures to control epizootics. François Quesnay, a central figure of physiocracy, argued that agriculture and livestock were the sources of national wealth, underlining the value of animal health for economic stability. With the support of Henri Léonard Bertin, Claude Bourgelat founded the

A. U. Rauf (✉)
Department of Health Behavior, Environment, and Social Medicine, Faculty of Medicine, Public Health, and Nursing, Universitas Gadjah Mada, Sleman, Yogyakarta, Indonesia
e-mail: annisaur@ugm.ac.id

M. C. Anggreni
Master of Public Health Program, Faculty of Medicine, Public Health, and Nursing, Universitas Gadjah Mada, Yogyakarta, Indonesia
e-mail: mirandachrisananggreni@mail.ugm.ac.id

A. Y. Hajar
Center of Health Behavior and Promotion, Faculty of Medicine, Public Health and Nursing, Universitas Gadjah Mada, Yogyakarta, Indonesia
e-mail: almaasitayumnahajar@mail.ugm.ac.id

T. Wibawa
Department of Microbiology, Faculty of Medicine, Public Health, and Nursing, Universitas Gadjah Mada, Sleman, Yogyakarta, Indonesia
e-mail: twibawa@ugm.ac.id

© The Author(s), under exclusive license to Springer Nature Singapore Pte Ltd. 2026

A. U. Rauf, T. Wibawa (eds.), *The One Health Concept in Asian Contexts*,
https://doi.org/10.1007/978-981-95-9880-9_1

world's first veterinary school in Lyon in 1761, aimed at preventing livestock epidemics. Bourgelat also introduced the concept of *médecine comparée*, asserting that the scientific knowledge gained from veterinary medicine could enrich human medicine, and vice versa (Bourdoiseau, 2023). This integrative approach was later reinforced by Félix Vicq d'Azyr through the establishment of the *Société Royale de Médecine* in 1776, laying early institutional groundwork for what is now known as the One Health paradigm (Mackenzie et al., 2013).

Since the 1800s, parallels between human and animal disease processes were recognized, though the fields remained separate. Rudolf Virchow, who pioneered cellular pathology, championed veterinary science and meat inspection. William Osler, a leader in medical education, taught at a veterinary college and researched animal diseases (Darbellay et al., 2024; Saunders, 2000). Both emphasized the interconnection of human and animal medicine, with Virchow famously stating:

> Between animal and human medicine there are no dividing lines—nor should there be.

There is no universal definition of One Health, as perspectives on health vary. Some focus narrowly on human health, while others value animal health and ecosystem sustainability equally. The core idea of One Health is that human, animal, and environmental health are interdependent. The WHO's 1946 definition of health, which encompasses physical, mental, and social well-being, reflects this interconnectedness by focusing the vital contributions of animals and ecosystems to human health and well-being, even though animals and ecosystems are not explicitly mentioned.

Given the broad scope of the One Health concept, its application extends across diverse geographical regions. Global efforts and emerging cases increasingly demand cross-sectoral collaboration and concern that go beyond the conventional boundaries of the health sector (WHO, 2023b). However, key challenges remain, including fragmented governance, limited intersectoral coordination, unequal resource allocation, and varying levels of awareness and commitment among stakeholders. These barriers often hinder the effective implementation of One Health initiatives, particularly in low- and middle-income countries (Adnyana et al., 2023; Lajaunie et al., 2025).

The renewed prominence of the One Health paradigm in the early twenty-first century reflects a growing global awareness of the intrinsic links among human, animal, and environmental health. In 2007, the One Health Initiative was officially introduced by the United States Centers for Disease Control and Prevention, in partnership with international stakeholders, to promote interdisciplinary collaboration in addressing complex and emerging health threats, particularly zoonotic diseases. The World Health Organization, the Food and Agriculture Organization, and the World Organization for Animal Health (formerly known as OIE) formalized their collaboration through the Tripartite agreement (2010), recognizing the need for coordinated and cross-sectoral responses. The partnership was subsequently expanded to include the United Nations Environment Programme (UNEP), thereby underscoring the essential role of environmental determinants in public health. In

2012, the first-ever One Health Summit was convened in Davos, Switzerland, marking a significant milestone in advancing the global One Health agenda (CDC, 2025). Recently in 2022, WHO, FAO, WOAH, and UNEP signed a Quadripartite Memorandum of Understanding to strengthen their collaboration in implementing the One Health approach. This agreement promotes coordinated action across human, animal, plant, and environmental health to support global and national health systems (Erkyihun & Alemayehu, 2022).

In today's world, accelerating environmental changes have underscored the critical need for integrated health approaches. The One Health framework has gained increasing relevance as climate change, urbanization, and deforestation intensify the interconnectedness among humans, animals, and the environment (Darbellay et al., 2024; Uga & Sapuppo, 2024). These shifts contribute to ecosystem disruption and biodiversity loss, heightening the transmission of pathogens from animals to humans and increasing the likelihood of future pandemics. Strengthening collaboration across sectors, the One Health approach supports early detection, prevention, and coordinated responses to complex global health threats.

1.2 Importance of One Health Approach in Asia

In Asia, where dense populations, rapid urbanization, and close interactions among humans, animals, and the environment are prevalent, the One Health approach holds significant importance. The region has been the epicenter of various emerging infectious diseases, such as SARS, avian influenza, and Nipah virus, underscoring the critical need for integrated monitoring and coordinated response mechanisms. Although countries like China (Liu et al., 2022, 2023), Thailand (Hort et al., 2019), India, and Vietnam (Gómez & Ruger, 2015) have taken notable steps toward implementing One Health strategies, persistent challenges remain, including sectoral fragmentation, unequal resource distribution, and inadequate data sharing. Certain cultural practices and behaviors, such as living in close proximity to livestock enclosures, the consumption of exotic animals, and traditional wet market operations, further elevate the risk of zoonotic disease transmission (Bubpa et al., 2025). An important finding reported by Koren et al. (2024) indicates that the rising consumption of beef in Asia forms part of a broader expansion in meat production, which has been empirically associated with an increased risk of zoonotic disease outbreaks. Evidence from 22 Asian countries between 1996 and 2019 indicates that a one-million-ton increase in meat output, including beef, is correlated with a substantial rise in zoonotic incidences, particularly those caused by influenza viruses (Koren et al., 2024).

The Nipah virus outbreak in Malaysia in the late 1990s and the COVID-19 pandemic are two concrete examples that demonstrate how ecosystem disruption can trigger the emergence of zoonotic diseases with widespread impact (Looi & Chua, 2007). In the case of Nipah, the loss of the natural habitat of fruit bats due to deforestation drove these species closer to livestock areas, facilitating the transmission of the virus from bats to pigs and eventually to humans. Meanwhile, the COVID-19 pandemic, suspected to have originated from wildlife, highlighted the dangers of wildlife trade and unregulated human-animal interactions in densely populated environments. It has been evidenced from the findings that the ongoing consumption of exotic animals, including bats—believed to be the cause of the coronavirus outbreak in Wuhan, China—persists. Moreover, such consumption is familiar and even serves as a form of tourism in Thailand, Myanmar, and Indonesia (Bubpa et al., 2025; Nijman et al., 2023; Xiao et al., 2021).

Given the interconnectedness of health risks across sectors, the One Health approach provides a vital framework for addressing the root causes of emerging zoonotic diseases while also strengthening global health security. One Health enables early detection and more coordinated responses to disease outbreaks by fostering collaboration across the human, animal, and environmental health sectors, reducing the time and resources needed to control the spread (FAO, 2025). This integrated approach is particularly valuable in preventing future pandemics, as it supports joint surveillance systems, promotes responsible land-use planning, and encourages sustainable agricultural practices that minimize human-wildlife conflict. In addition to offering a more cost-efficient approach, One Health strengthens system resilience by targeting broader environmental factors, such as climate change and biodiversity loss, that contribute to the emergence and spread of infectious diseases (One Health High-Level Expert Panel (OHHLEP) et al., 2022). This approach is grounded across local, national, and global levels, enabling the development of more comprehensive and sustainable health solutions (Woods et al., 2018).

Historical outbreaks such as H5N1 avian influenza, SARS, and Nipah virus have not only caused human illness and death but also triggered severe economic disruptions, including the collapse of Malaysia's pig farming industry and significant losses in tourism and agriculture (Smith et al., 2019). Antimicrobial resistance (AMR), fueled by the misuse of antibiotics in both humans and livestock, is projected to cause millions of deaths annually by 2050 and push millions into extreme poverty, with Asia and the Pacific expected to bear a disproportionate burden (Habib et al., 2022). At the same time, the region's food systems face the triple challenge of ensuring adequate nutrition, sustaining livelihoods, and maintaining environmental sustainability, yet policies often favor short-term productivity gains over long-term resilience. The COVID-19 pandemic further exposed these vulnerabilities, straining agri-food supply chains and reversing years of economic progress in low- and middle-income countries (Ben Hassen & El Bilali, 2024). The implementation of the One Health approach in Asia, as underscored by the Asian Development Bank (ADB), presents a strategic opportunity to accelerate post-pandemic recovery (Habib et al., 2022). In the One Health context, ADB supports developing member countries (DMCs) in advancing universal health coverage through improved quality and accessibility of healthcare services, alongside health financing reforms to reduce out-of-pocket costs for vulnerable populations. By leveraging cross-sectoral synergies such as transport for road safety, urban planning for healthy cities, water for safety and sanitation to prevent communicable diseases, and energy for low carbon and pollution-free environments, ADB addresses the interconnected health risks at the human, animal, and environmental interface (ADB, 2018).

Joint monitoring and intervention by the veterinary and human health sectors have played a crucial role in identifying and managing these outbreaks (Musa et al., 2024). Given that approximately 60% of infectious diseases globally originate from animals, including high-impact cases such as avian influenza and COVID-19, advancing a comprehensive One Health framework is crucial (Jones et al., 2008). This approach not only enhances the ability to prevent future outbreaks but also reduces the human and economic toll associated with emerging zoonotic diseases, as supported by previous research findings and data from the ADB (ADB, 2018; Dhama et al., 2022; Habib et al., 2022; Kibenge, 2023).

Antimicrobial resistance (AMR) poses a serious and growing global public health risk. The Review on Antimicrobial Resistance projects that by 2050, antimicrobial resistance could lead to the deaths of 10 million people annually, with Asia accounting for 4,730,000 of those (O'Neill, 2014). AMR occurs when antimicrobial drugs used to eliminate and control the microbes responsible for infectious diseases lose their effectiveness due to genetic and phenotypic changes in the microbes. The consequences of the AMR are as follows: diminishing the effectiveness of treatments for common infections, resulting in longer recovery times, more fatalities, and greater risks of health complications; when treatments are ineffective, patients stay infectious for a longer period, increasing the risk of spreading the disease and resistant microbes to others. This also places a heavier financial strain on healthcare systems, families, and society (WHO, 2023a).

AMR requires a One Health approach based on several key factors. It is well known that humans, animals (including livestock and pets), and the environment share microbes. Antimicrobial-resistant microbes that infect humans can originate from animals or the environment. Overuse and misuse of antimicrobial agents in humans, animals, and agriculture can significantly worsen the problem of AMR, creating a "silent pandemic" (Ahmed et al., 2024). As, for example, Southeast Asia faces a significant threat from the development and transmission of antibiotic resistance in humans. While a risk assessment framework can assist countries in pinpointing the most effective interventions, standalone efforts will not be sufficient. To effectively control antibiotic resistance in Asia and other regions, a holistic strategy based on the One Health approach is essential (Chereau et al., 2017).

The World Health Organization (WHO) and the other Quadripartite partners—the Food and Agriculture Organization of the United Nations (FAO), the United Nations Environment Programme (UNEP), and the World Organization for Animal Health (WOAH)—have supported the global action plan and are working together across sectors to put it into practice (WHO, 2023a). One collaborative initiative in Asia is the Regional Tripartite AMR Project—jointly led by FAO, WHO, and WOAH—titled "Working Together to Fight Antimicrobial Resistance (AMR) in Asia and the Pacific." This project targets several countries, including China, India, Indonesia, Malaysia, the Philippines, Thailand, and Viet Nam, while Japan and the Republic of Korea (ROK) serve as partner countries (FAO, 2022).

1.3 Promoting One Health in Asia

The implementation of the One Health approach in Asia has progressed through collaborative efforts involving government agencies, research institutions, and international organizations (Zhang et al., 2024). Southeast Asia, recognized as a hotspot for emerging infectious diseases, has emphasized operationalizing One Health at the regional level to address zoonotic risks and strengthen preparedness for global health threats (Lâm et al., 2025). In China, One Health principles have been incorporated into national policies; however, significant challenges remain in translating these policies into practical interventions, highlighting the need for a holistic One Health action framework adapted to diverse sociocultural contexts (Gao et al., 2025; Liu et al., 2023). Notable progress has been observed in Singapore, where strong interagency coordination, advanced surveillance systems, and robust institutional frameworks have positioned the country as a leader in One Health implementation (Tan, 2025). Bangladesh and India have also demonstrated the feasibility of advancing One Health despite reliance on donor-driven priorities and limited direct government support, suggesting that meaningful implementation is possible under resource constraints (Dahal et al., 2017).

Despite these advances, multiple challenges hinder the effective implementation of One Health in Asia, including insufficient and unsustainable funding, competing policy priorities, weak surveillance systems, uncertainties surrounding cost-effectiveness, and limited political commitment (Nambiar, 2020; Tiwari et al., 2025). In China, cross-departmental collaboration is constrained by unclear delineation of responsibilities, inadequate intersectoral communication mechanisms, and shortages of trained One Health professionals, underscoring the need for improved coordination and capacity building (Liu et al., 2023). Furthermore, differences in One Health research priorities, shaped by variations in human development indices, reflect potential regional gaps between strategic vision and operational practice (Ahmed et al., 2023). Addressing these barriers will require regionally tailored strategies, enhanced investment in workforce and infrastructure, and sustained political will to ensure that One Health principles are translated into effective, context-specific actions across Asia. In response, numerous institutions and networks have emerged, reflecting growing recognition among governments, academia, and international agencies of the need for integrated, cross-sectoral strategies (Degeling et al., 2015; Sinclair, 2019). This shift marks a commitment to resilience through interdisciplinary cooperation and evidence-based policymaking (Dahal et al., 2017).

Compared to other regions, South Asia records some of the poorest health outcomes globally, second only to sub-Saharan Africa in malnutrition, while Central Europe and the former Soviet Union report poorer health than Latin America, Asia, and Africa (Chin et al., 2017; Witvliet et al., 2012). European and North American countries tend to score higher in One Health governance, reflecting more mature systems, whereas Central Asia benefits from promising intersectoral collaboration driven by shared socioeconomic history and language (Parodi et al., 2011). In research and collaboration, Asia exhibits a core-periphery structure in antimicrobial resistance research networks, with high-income countries leading partnerships, and the One Health approach in the region is increasingly converging with EcoHealth, fostering a holistic understanding of health and addressing emerging infectious diseases (Burns & Stephen, 2015; He et al., 2023; Li et al., 2023; Nguyen-Viet et al., 2015).

Table 1.1 summarizes selected One Health centers and initiatives in Asia, organized by country and focus area. It highlights regional expertise and supports knowledge exchange, cross-border collaboration, and coordinated responses. Over the past decade, these initiatives have expanded rapidly, initially led by academia and now supported by governments, international bodies, and NGOs. Common priorities include antimicrobial resistance, zoonotic surveillance, and capacity building. Regional networks such as SEAOHUN and OHSEA exemplify collective approaches, while several centers are integrating technologies like AI, IoT, and bioinformatics to enhance health monitoring and preparedness.

1.4 Conclusion and Suggestion

The One Health approach represents a vital framework for addressing the interdependencies among human, animal, and environment. While notable progress has been made through diverse regional initiatives and partnerships, advancement continues to be hampered by fragmented governance structures, inadequate financial resources, and the insufficient integration of environmental and structural determinants into health policies. The region's distinct socioecological context, marked by rich biodiversity, culture, and intensive agricultural activities, heightens vulnerability to health risks and offers strong opportunities for cross-border collaboration and coordinated action.

To strengthen its effectiveness, the One Health framework in Asia should be broadened to incorporate climate change adaptation strategies, enhanced environmental governance, and the integration of social equity principles. This will require targeted investment in institutional capacity, including the development of a skilled workforce, improved infrastructure, and advanced disease surveillance systems. Promoting robust interregional cooperation and data-sharing mechanisms is essential for addressing transboundary health threats. Equally important is the engagement of local communities and the inclusion of traditional knowledge to ensure culturally sensitive, sustainable, and impactful interventions. Through these measures, health systems across Asia will be better equipped to respond to emerging and interconnected health challenges with greater resilience and adaptability.

Table 1.1 One Health research and initiatives in Asia

No	Institution/Initiative	Country/region	Year established	Lead institution/affiliation	Type	Main focus areas	Website/source
1	SEAOHUN—Southeast Asia University Network, includes IndoHUN, CAMBOHUN, PhilOHUN, MMOHUN, THOHUN, VOHUN, etc.	Southeast Asia Countries	2011	Regional (multicountry), supported by USAID and Chevron	Academic Network	Workforce development, One Health curriculum, field-based training	https://www.seaohun.org
2	TAOHUN—Taiwan One Health University Network	Taiwan	2019	National Yang Ming Chiao Tung University (NYCU), via RCEP-One Health Center	Academic Network	One Health education, interdisciplinary collaboration, regional epidemic prevention, IoT/AI-driven surveillance, zoonoses, AMR	https://taohun.web.nycu.edu.tw
3	Centre for One Health, Universiti Putra Malaysia (UPM)	Malaysia	2014	Faculty of Veterinary Medicine, UPM	Academic	Veterinary medicine, zoonoses, AMR, food safety	https://vet.upm.edu.my
4	Centre for One Health Education, Advocacy, Research, and Training (COHEART)	India	2013	Kerala Veterinary and Animal Sciences University	Academic	Community-level zoonosis prevention, AMR, education	https://iiphg.edu.in/coherd-new/
5	Eijkman–Oxford Clinical Research Unit (EOCRU)	Indonesia	2008	Eijkman Institute & University of Oxford	Research Collaboration Unit	Pathogen genomics, infectious disease surveillance, zoonotic spillover	https://www.oucru.org/location/oucru-indonesia/

6	Indian Council of Medical Research (ICMR)—National Institute of One Health (NIOH)	India	2021	Indian Council of Medical Research (ICMR)	Government	Disease modeling, veterinary epidemiology, One Health surveillance	https://nioh.org
7	One Health Bangladesh	Bangladesh	2016	IEDCR, DGHS, Ministry of Health	Government Coordination Unit	Interministerial coordination, AMR, zoonotic disease prevention	https://onehealthbd.org/about/
8	One Health Trust India	India	2022	Formerly CDDEP India	Public Research Organization, Think Tank	Data science, AMR, policy development	https://onehealthtrust.org/
9	Onehealth Lab	South Korea	2020	Catholic University of Korea College of Medicine	Academic Research Lab	Communicable diseases, computational epidemiology, modeling, and transmission dynamics of respiratory viruses such as SARS-CoV-2	http://onehealth.or.kr
10	National Taiwan University—One Health Program	Taiwan	2016	NTU College of Public Health	Academic	Food systems, vector-borne diseases, climate-related health risks	https://www.ntu.edu.tw
11	NYCU—Research Center for Epidemic Prevention and One Health	Taiwan	2021	National Yang Ming Chiao Tung University	Research Center	AI and IoT-driven epidemic surveillance, diagnostics	https://enrcep.web.nycu.edu.tw

(continued)

Table 1.1 (continued)

No	Institution/Initiative	Country/region	Year established	Lead institution/affiliation	Type	Main focus areas	Website/source
12	One Health Center of Excellence (OHCE)	Indonesia	2021	Universitas Gadjah Mada (UGM)	Research Center	Training, education, and research capacities of the university network to build the skills, knowledge, and attitude based on One Health	https://ohce.wg.ugm.ac.id/home/
13	One Health Research Center of Excellence for Research and Training	China	2014	School of Public Health, Sun Yat-sen University	Academic/ Research Center	Zoonoses, food safety, environmental health, interdisciplinary training	https://sph.sysu.edu.cn/en/One-Health-Center
14	One Health Research Center (OHRC), Hokkaido University	Japan	2018	Hokkaido University, School of Veterinary Medicine	Academic	Infectome, chem-reactome databases, zoonotic dynamics	https://onehealth.vetmed.hokudai.ac.jp
15	Flying Vets Mongolia–International Council for Game & Wildlife Conservation (CIC) Wildlife One Health	Mongolia	2022	CIC in partnership with World Organisation for Animal Health (WOAH), Ministry of Environment & Tourism, and Wildlife Conservation Society	NGO/ Conservation Initiative	Wildlife & livestock disease surveillance, zoonotic spillover risk, community capacity building, herder livelihoods	https://cic-wildlife.org/one-health-mongolia/
16	World Bank One Health Program in Central Asia	Kazakhstan, Kyrgyzstan, Tajikistan, Uzbekistan, Turkmenistan	2023	World Bank, FAO, WHO, Ministries of Health & Agriculture	Development Program	AMR, food safety systems, pandemic preparedness, infrastructure	https://www.fao.org/one-health/partners/projects/pf-europe-and-central-asia/en

17	Southeast Asian Regional Center for Graduate Study and Research in Agriculture (SEARCA)-UPLB Knowledge Center on Halal & One Health	Philippines	2019	SEARCA, University of the Philippines Los Baños (UPLB)	Academic	Food safety, halal science, interdisciplinary One Health research	https://www.searca.org/
18	OHSEA—One Health Southeast Asia (IRD/CIRAD/CNRS initiative)	Vietnam, Cambodia, Laos, Malaysia	2019	French Research Institutes (IRD, CIRAD, CNRS) and Southeast Asia Universities	International Research	Environmental & zoonotic data platforms, training, policy	https://en.ird.fr/ohsea-one-health-practice-southeast-asia
19	Pak One Health Alliance (POHA)	Pakistan	2014	Independent NGO, Islamabad	Non-profit NGO	Zoonotic disease prevention, AMR, outbreak preparedness, capacity building, community awareness	https://pakonehealth.org
20	One Health Research Panel (OHRP)	Hongkong	2020	City University of Hong Kong	Academic/Research Center	Animal disease surveillance, food safety in supply chains, antimicrobial resistance, outbreak modeling & policy advice	https://www.cityu.edu.hk/ohrp/
21	One Health Madagascar (ZoonOmics Project)	Madagascar	2021	University of Antananarivo in partnership with University of Liverpool & Institut Pasteur de Madagascar	Academic/International Collaboration	Zoonotic disease surveillance, bat-human interface, interdisciplinary training, social science integration	https://zoonomics.org/one-health-in-madagascar/

(continued)

Table 1.1 (continued)

No	Institution/Initiative	Country/region	Year established	Lead institution/affiliation	Type	Main focus areas	Website/source
22	Center of Excellence for Smart Health (KCSH), KAUST	Saudi Arabia	2024	King Abdullah University of Science & Technology	Academic Center of Excellence	One Health (microbiome–ecosystem surveillance, AMR, pandemic preparedness), healthy aging, smart diagnostics & sensing, bioinformatics & computational biology	https://www.kaust.edu.sa/en/research/smart-health/one-health
23	Media One Health Project	Southeast Asia (Vietnam, Cambodia, Laos)	2022	CFI (French Media Development Agency), funded by the French Ministry for Europe and Foreign Affairs	Media/ Development	Science journalism, public awareness on AMR and zoonoses, One Health communication training	https://cfi.fr/en/project/media-one-health
24	The Joint Programming Initiative on Antimicrobial Resistance (JPIAMR) Membership	South Korea	2016	Ministry of Health and Welfare, Ministry of Science and ICT	Government/ International Research Network	AMR surveillance, research coordination, One Health collaboration, diagnostics, therapeutics, stewardship	https://jpiamr.eu

Competing Interests The authors have no competing interests to declare that are relevant to the content of this manuscript.

References

ADB. (2018). *Strategy 2030 achieving a prosperous, inclusive, resilient, and sustainable Asia and the Pacific*. https://www.adb.org/sites/default/files/institutional-document/435391/strategy-2030-main-document.pdf

Adnyana, I. M., Utomo, B., Eljatin, D. S., & Sudaryati, N. L. (2023). One Health approach and zoonotic diseases in Indonesia: Urgency of implementation and challenges. *Narra J, 3*(3), 10.52225/narra.v3i3.257.

Ahmed, T., Tahir, M. F., Boden, L., & Kingston, T. (2023). Future directions for One Health research: Regional and sectoral gaps. *One Health, 17*, 100584. https://doi.org/10.1016/j.onehlt.2023.100584

Ahmed, S. K., Hussein, S., Qurbani, K., Ibrahim, R. H., Fareeq, A., Mahmood, K. A., & Mohamed, M. G. (2024). Antimicrobial resistance: Impacts, challenges, and future prospects. *Journal of Medicine, Surgery, and Public Health, 2*, 100081. https://doi.org/10.1016/j.glmedi.2024.100081

Ben Hassen, T., & El Bilali, H. (2024). Three years into the pandemic: Insights of the COVID-19 impacts on food security and nutrition in low and middle-income countries. *Heliyon, 10*(7), e28946. https://doi.org/10.1016/j.heliyon.2024.e28946

Bourdoiseau, G. (2023). Origine de la notion de «Une seule santé». *Bulletin de l'Académie Nationale de Médecine, 207*(9), 1270–1275. https://doi.org/10.1016/j.banm.2023.04.020

Bubpa, N., Suwannarong, K., Thammasutti, K., Ponlap, T., Thongkan, W., Boonyakawee, P., Kanthawee, P., Suwannarong, K., & Chanchai, W. (2025). Cultural practices, healthcare-seeking behaviors, and wildlife interface: Zoonotic disease risks among the Phu Thai Ethnic Group in Thailand. *Veterinary World*, 624–635. https://doi.org/10.14202/vetworld.2025.624-635

Burns, T. E., & Stephen, C. (2015). Finding a place for systems-based, collaborative research in emerging disease research in Asia. *EcoHealth, 12*(4), 672–684. https://doi.org/10.1007/s10393-015-1072-x

CDC. (2025). *One Health history*. One Health. https://www.cdc.gov/one-health/about/one-health-history.html

Chereau, F., Opatowski, L., Tourdjman, M., & Vong, S. (2017). Risk assessment for antibiotic resistance in South East Asia. *BMJ*, j3393. https://doi.org/10.1136/bmj.j3393

Chin, B., Rani, M., & Bonu, S. (2017). South Asia, Health systems of. In *International encyclopedia of public health* (pp. 1–9). Elsevier. https://doi.org/10.1016/B978-0-12-803678-5.00422-7

Dahal, R., Upadhyay, A., & Ewald, B. (2017). One Health in South Asia and its challenges in implementation from stakeholder perspective. *Veterinary Record, 181*(23), 626–626. https://doi.org/10.1136/vr.104189

Darbellay, F., Russell, W. C., & James, H. S. (2024). One Health. In *Elgar encyclopedia of interdisciplinarity and transdisciplinarity* (pp. 357–361). Edward Elgar Publishing. https://doi.org/10.4337/9781035317967.ch78

Degeling, C., Johnson, J., Kerridge, I., Wilson, A., Ward, M., Stewart, C., & Gilbert, G. (2015). Implementing a One Health approach to emerging infectious disease: Reflections on the socio-political, ethical and legal dimensions. *BMC Public Health, 15*(1), 1307. https://doi.org/10.1186/s12889-015-2617-1

Dhama, K., Chandran, D., Chakraborty, S., Yatoo, M. I., Islam, M. A., Bhattacharya, M., Chakraborty, C., Harapan, H., & Chaicumpa, W. (2022). Zoonotic concerns of Marburg virus: Current knowledge and counteracting strategies including One Health approach to limit

animal-human interface: An update. *International Journal of Surgery, 106*, 106941. https://doi.org/10.1016/j.ijsu.2022.106941
Erkyihun, G. A., & Alemayehu, M. B. (2022). One Health approach for the control of zoonotic diseases. *Zoonoses, 2*(1), 10.15212/zoonoses-2022-0037.
FAO. (2022). *Regional Tripartite AMR Project (FAO, WHO and WOAH) "Working together to fight Antimicrobial Resistance"*. https://www.fao.org/antimicrobial-resistance/projects/ongoing/project-11/en/
FAO. (2025). *Food and Agriculture Organization of the United Nations One Health: A collaborative approach to preventing the next pandemic*. https://www.fao.org/one-health/highlights/preventing-the-next-pandemic/en#:~:text=The%20power%20of%20collaboration,response%20when%20an%20outbreak%20occurs
Gao, Y., Li, C., Zhou, Q., & Hao, M. (2025). The application of One Health concept in China and its practice and innovation in cross-sector cooperation. *Public Health in Practice, 9*, 100574. https://doi.org/10.1016/j.puhip.2024.100574
Gómez, E. J., & Ruger, J. P. (2015). The global and domestic politics of health policy in emerging nations. *Journal of Health Politics, Policy and Law, 40*(1), 3–11. https://doi.org/10.1215/03616878-2854256
Habib, N., Parry, J., Elfving, R., & Dunn, B. (2022). *Practical actions to operationalize the One Health Approach in The Asian Development Bank* (ADB East Asia working paper series). https://doi.org/10.22617/WPS220202-2
He, S., Shrestha, P., Henry, A. D., & Legido-Quigley, H. (2023). Leveraging collaborative research networks against antimicrobial resistance in Asia. *Frontiers in Public Health, 11*, 1191036. https://doi.org/10.3389/fpubh.2023.1191036
Hort, K., Sommanustweechai, A., Adisasmito, W., & Gleeson, L. (2019). Stewardship of health security: The challenges of applying the One Health approach. *Public Administration and Development, 39*(1), 23–33. https://doi.org/10.1002/pad.1826
Jones, K. E., Patel, N. G., Levy, M. A., Storeygard, A., Balk, D., Gittleman, J. L., & Daszak, P. (2008). Global trends in emerging infectious diseases. *Nature, 451*(7181), 990–993. https://doi.org/10.1038/nature06536
Kibenge, F. S. B. (2023). Continuous surveillance and viral discovery in animals and humans are a core component of a one-health approach to address recent viral reverse zoonoses. *Journal of the American Veterinary Medical Association, 261*(6), 789–797. https://doi.org/10.2460/javma.23.03.0148
Koren, O., Steinberg, J., & Hagar, A. (2024). Meat production and zoonotic disease outbreaks in Asia. *Australian Journal of Agricultural and Resource Economics, 68*(3), 567–586. https://doi.org/10.1111/1467-8489.12576
Lajaunie, C., Morand, S., & Hinjoy, S. (2025). Southeast Asia at the heart of the implementation of the One Health approach. *Discover Public Health, 22*(1). https://doi.org/10.1186/s12982-025-00720-5
Lâm, S., Dang-Xuan, S., Unger, F., Meeyam, T., Pham-Duc, P., Wacharapluesadee, S., & Nguyen-Viet, H. (2025). Operationalizing regional One Health initiatives in Southeast Asia: Ways forward. *One Health, 20*, 101034. https://doi.org/10.1016/j.onehlt.2025.101034
Li, O. Y., Wang, X., Yang, K., Liu, D., & Shi, H. (2023). The approaching pilot for One Health governance index. *Infectious Diseases of Poverty, 12*(1), 16. https://doi.org/10.1186/s40249-023-01067-2
Liu, Y., He, Z.-Q., & Wang, D. (2022). One Health approach to improve the malaria elimination programme in Henan Province. In *Advances in parasitology* (Vol. 116, pp. 153–186). Elsevier. https://doi.org/10.1016/bs.apar.2022.02.001
Liu, J.-S., Li, X.-C., Zhang, Q.-Y., Han, L.-F., Xia, S., Kassegne, K., Zhu, Y.-Z., Yin, K., Hu, Q.-Q., Xiu, L.-S., Wang, X.-C., Li, O. Y., Li, M., Zhou, Z.-B., Dong, K., He, L., Wang, S.-X., Yang, X.-C., Zhang, Y., et al. (2023). China's application of the One Health approach in addressing public health threats at the human-animal-environment interface: Advances and challenges. *One Health, 17*, 100607. https://doi.org/10.1016/j.onehlt.2023.100607

Looi, L.-M., & Chua, K.-B. (2007). *Lessons from the Nipah virus outbreak in Malaysia. 2*. English.
Mackenzie, J. S., Jeggo, M., Daszak, P., & Richt, J. A. (Eds.). (2013). *One Health: The human-animal-environment interfaces in emerging infectious diseases: The concept and examples of a One Health Approach* (Vol. 365). Springer. https://doi.org/10.1007/978-3-642-36889-9
Musa, E., Nia, Z. M., Bragazzi, N. L., Leung, D., Lee, N., & Kong, J. D. (2024). Avian influenza: Lessons from past outbreaks and an inventory of data sources, mathematical and AI models, and early warning systems for forecasting and hotspot detection to tackle ongoing outbreaks. *Healthcare, 12*(19), 1959. https://doi.org/10.3390/healthcare12191959
Nambiar, P. (2020). India to envision One Health movement for confronting emerging health threats: From concept to approach toward institutionalization. *International Journal of One Health, 6*(2), 165–176. https://doi.org/10.14202/IJOH.2020.165-176
Nguyen-Viet, H., Doria, S., Tung, D. X., Mallee, H., Wilcox, B. A., & Grace, D. (2015). Ecohealth research in Southeast Asia: Past, present and the way forward. *Infectious Diseases of Poverty, 4*(1), 5. https://doi.org/10.1186/2049-9957-4-5
Nijman, V., Nekaris, K. A. I., Shepherd, C. R., Vigne, L., Ardiansyah, A., Imron, M. A., Ni, Q., Hedger, K., Campera, M., & Morcatty, T. Q. (2023). Potential mammalian vector-borne diseases in live and wet markets in Indonesia and Myanmar. *Microbiology Research, 14*(1), 116–131. https://doi.org/10.3390/microbiolres14010011
O'Neill, J. (2014). *Antimicrobial resistance: Tackling a crisis for the health and wealth of nations*. https://amr-review.org/sites/default/files/AMR%20Review%20Paper%20-%20Tackling%20a%20crisis%20for%20the%20health%20and%20wealth%20of%20nations_1.pdf
One Health High-Level Expert Panel (OHHLEP), Adisasmito, W. B., Almuhairi, S., Behravesh, C. B., Bilivogui, P., Bukachi, S. A., Casas, N., Cediel Becerra, N., Charron, D. F., Chaudhary, A., Ciacci Zanella, J. R., Cunningham, A. A., Dar, O., Debnath, N., Dungu, B., Farag, E., Gao, G. F., Hayman, D. T. S., Khaitsa, M., et al. (2022). One Health: A new definition for a sustainable and healthy future. *PLoS Pathogens, 18*(6), e1010537. https://doi.org/10.1371/journal.ppat.1010537
Parodi, P., Schmid, G., & Ward, D. (2011). One health in central Asia. A situational analysis informing the future. *Giornale Italiano Di Medicina Tropicale*, 3–4.
Saunders, L. Z. (2000). Virchow's contributions to veterinary medicine: Celebrated then, forgotten now. *Veterinary Pathology, 37*(3), 199–207. https://doi.org/10.1354/vp.37-3-199
Sinclair, J. R. (2019). Importance of a One Health approach in advancing global health security and the Sustainable Development Goals. *Revue Scientifique et Technique de l'OIE, 38*(1), 145–154. https://doi.org/10.20506/rst.38.1.2949
Smith, K. M., Machalaba, C. C., Seifman, R., Feferholtz, Y., & Karesh, W. B. (2019). Infectious disease and economics: The case for considering multi-sectoral impacts. *One Health, 7*, 100080. https://doi.org/10.1016/j.onehlt.2018.100080
Tan, H. Y. (2025). Overview of Singapore's One Health Strategy. *Zoonotic Diseases, 5*(1), 2. https://doi.org/10.3390/zoonoticdis5010002
Tiwari, H. K., Tan, D. K. Y., Chinda, C., My, D. N. T., Hoang, H. T. T., Keonam, K., Huong, L. Q., Chanvatanak, L., Virak, M., Tram, N. T., Soulinthone, N., Phuc, P. D., Nguyen, T. T. H., Tra, V. T. T., & Beardsley, J. (2025). Challenges and opportunities for AMR research in the ASEAN following the One Health approach. *One Health, 20*, 101001. https://doi.org/10.1016/j.onehlt.2025.101001
Uga, E., & Sapuppo, A. (2024). One Health, Global Health and Child Wellbeing: An integrated approach. *SALUTE E SOCIETÀ, 23*(3), 54–67. https://doi.org/10.3280/ses2024-003004
WHO. (2023a). *Antimicrobial resistance*. https://www.who.int/news-room/fact-sheets/detail/antimicrobial-resistance
WHO. (2023b). *One health*. One Health. https://www.who.int/news-room/fact-sheets/detail/one-health
Witvliet, M. I., Kunst, A. E., Stronks, K., & Arah, O. A. (2012). Variations between world regions in individual health: A multilevel analysis of the role of socio-economic factors. *European Journal of Public Health, 22*(2), 284–289. https://doi.org/10.1093/eurpub/ckr001

Woods, A., Bresalier, M., Cassidy, A., & Mason Dentinger, R. (2018). *Animals and the shaping of modern medicine*. Springer. https://doi.org/10.1007/978-3-319-64337-3

Xiao, X., Newman, C., Buesching, C. D., Macdonald, D. W., & Zhou, Z.-M. (2021). Animal sales from Wuhan wet markets immediately prior to the COVID-19 pandemic. *Scientific Reports, 11*(1), 11898. https://doi.org/10.1038/s41598-021-91470-2

Zhang, X.-X., Lederman, Z., Han, L.-F., Schurer, J. M., Xiao, L.-H., Zhang, Z.-B., Chen, Q.-L., Pfeiffer, D., Ward, M. P., Sripa, B., Gabriël, S., Dhama, K., Acharya, K. P., Robertson, L. J., Deem, S. L., Aenishaenslin, C., Dantas-Torres, F., Otranto, D., Grace, D., et al. (2024). Towards an actionable One Health approach. *Infectious Diseases of Poverty, 13*(1), 28. https://doi.org/10.1186/s40249-024-01198-0

Chapter 2
Zoonotic Diseases

Khrisdiana Putri, Yudhi Ratna Nugraheni, Rizka Humardewayanti Asdie, and Farida Nur Oktoviani

2.1 Overview of Zoonotic Disease Transmission

The term "zoonosis" was first coined by Rudolf Virchow to describe diseases transmitted from animals to humans (Chomel, 2014). Early on, the concept of a "one medicine" approach was initiated, emphasizing multidisciplinary collaboration to better understand these diseases. The idea was later expanded to include environmental factors, leading to the broader concept of One Health (Ray & Bhattacharya, 2024).

K. Putri (✉)
Department of Public Health, Faculty of Veterinary Medicine, Universitas Gadjah Mada, Yogyakarta, Indonesia

One Health Centre of Excellence, Universitas Gadjah Mada, Yogyakarta, Indonesia
e-mail: khrisdiana@ugm.ac.id

Y. R. Nugraheni
Department of Parasitology, Faculty of Veterinary Medicine, Universitas Gadjah Mada, Yogyakarta, Indonesia

One Health Centre of Excellence, Universitas Gadjah Mada, Yogyakarta, Indonesia
e-mail: yudhi.ratna.n@mail.ugm.ac.id

R. H. Asdie
Department of Internal Medicine Sub Specialist in Tropical Diseases Infection, Faculty of Medicine, Public Health and Nursing, Universitas Gadjah Mada, Yogyakarta, Indonesia
e-mail: rizka_asdie@ugm.ac.id

F. N. Oktoviani
Department of Microbiology, Faculty of Medicine, Public Health and Nursing, Universitas Gadjah Mada, Sleman, Yogyakarta, Indonesia
e-mail: farida.nur.o@mail.ugm.ac.id

© The Author(s), under exclusive license to Springer Nature Singapore Pte Ltd. 2026

A. U. Rauf, T. Wibawa (eds.), *The One Health Concept in Asian Contexts*,
https://doi.org/10.1007/978-981-95-9880-9_2

The World Health Organization (WHO) formally defined zoonoses in 1951 as "diseases and infections that are naturally transmitted between vertebrate animals and man." This term is widely used today as it is more convenient than specific phrases like anthropozoonosies (animal to human) and zooanthroponosis (human to animal). However, the WHO's definition has some specific limitations. It is suggested that the definition should include the term "infestation" to properly cover parasitic diseases and pertain to agents that can proliferate in an animal host. The definition specifically excludes diseases caused by animal venom or toxins, allergic reactions, or pathogens that are simply transmitted by animals or animal products through contamination (such as contaminated food) (Chomel, 2014).

The conversion nomadic hunter-gatherer to an agrarian life caused a major transformation in the dynamics of infectious diseases. The rise in human population density and the intensification of food animal production created a perfect storm for disease transmission. These societal developments, coupled with the expansion of trade networks, facilitated the jump of zoonotic pathogens from animals to humans. Furthermore, modern factors like global travel and environmental changes continue to exacerbate this risk, underscoring the ongoing challenge of zoonotic spillover (Lindahl et al., 2015). Zoonotic transmission is a cornerstone mechanism in the emergence of human infectious diseases. Human activities like hunting, the bushmeat trade, and the exotic pet trade significantly heighten the risk of cross-species transmission, particularly in rural areas. The adaptation process of a pathogen to a new host often begins with a cross-species event, where the infection is initially limited to the animal population (Fig. 2.1). This is followed by a spillover event,

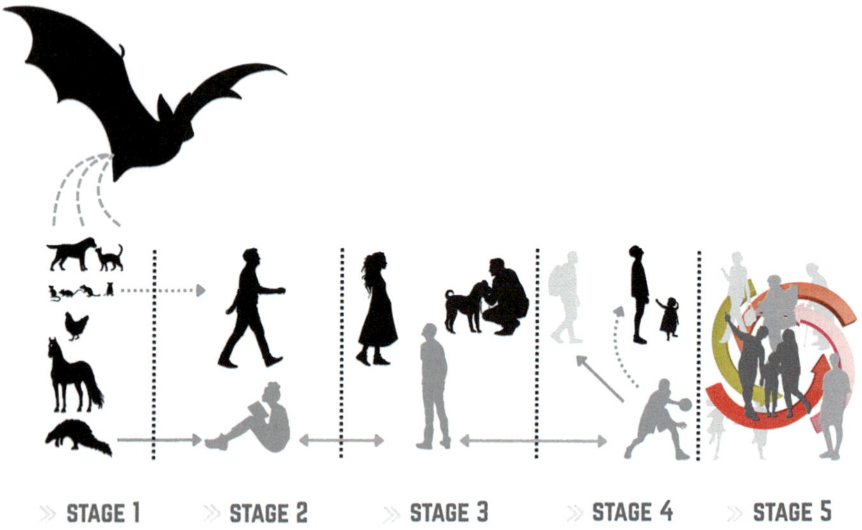

Fig. 2.1 Stages of zoonotic spillover and adaptation in human populations. (Adapted from Wolfe et al., 2007)

where the pathogen jumps to a human host without subsequent sustained spread between people. The subsequent stages of a successful spillover event are an important part of the disease emergence process. Over time, repeated spillover events or host adaptation can lead to limited human-to-human transmission, where the pathogen can spread between a small number of people. This may then progress to sustained human-to-human transmission, where the pathogen no longer needs an animal host to continue spreading. Ultimately, the pathogen may become an exclusively human infection, completely adapted to its new human host and no longer circulating in the original animal reservoir (Bengis et al., 2004; Stout et al., 2021; Wolfe et al., 2007).

The precise origins of many established human diseases remain a subject of extensive scientific debate. While determining a disease's origin is crucial for understanding its emergence, it also highlights a complex nexus between human behaviors and the lodgment of zoonotic agents. Emerging health threats at the human-animal interface require innovative strategies to improve vigilance. Proactive measures—such as robust international hazard identification, effective risk communication, and sound risk management—are critical for mitigating the impact of future disease emergence (Bengis et al., 2004; Keenan et al., 2024; Wolfe et al., 2007).

2.2 Classification

Zoonotic diseases are classified based on the agent type, transmission direction, lifecycle, and ecosystem category (Chomel, 2014). However, research has proposed new frameworks that combine these different classification systems into a single, more systematic method to better understand and manage diseases at the human-wildlife interface (Fig. 2.2). This is a crucial step for improving surveillance and public health policy, as wildlife contribute significantly to the rise of new infectious diseases (Chomel, 2014; Keenan et al., 2024).

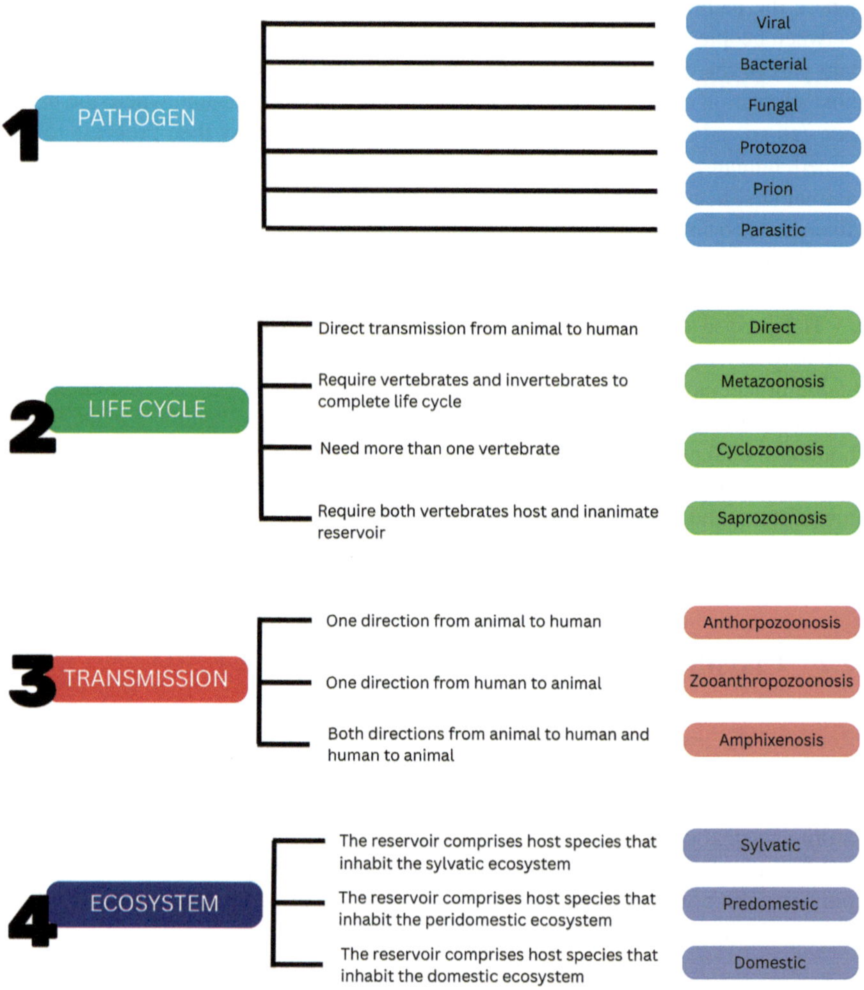

Fig. 2.2 The new framework of zoonotic pathogens is characterized by including wildlife using four classification categories: (1) pathogen category (bacterial, viral, protozoan, parasitic, fungal, or prion); (2) transmission route (anthropozoonosis, zooanthropozoonosis, or amphixenosis); (3) course (direct, metazoonosis, saprozoonosis, or cyclozoonosis); and (4) type of ecosystem (sylvatic, peridomestic, and/or domestic). For the first three categories, each pathogen is assigned to a single classification group, whereas in the ecosystem category, pathogens may be associated with multiple environments. (Adapted from Keenan et al., 2024, licensed under CC-BY 4.0)

2.3 Prevalent Zoonotic Diseases in Indonesia

2.3.1 *Rabies*

2.3.1.1 Overview of the Disease

Rabies virus (RABV) is an RNA virus of the genus *Lyssavirus*, family *Rhabdoviridae*, and order *Mononegavirales*. Since 2021, the International Committee of Taxonomy Virus: ICTV has renamed it to "Lyssavirus rabies" (Walker et al., 2022). The name "rabies" originates from the Latin word *rabere*, connotating "to be mad," which reflects the characteristic behavioral changes in infected animals. While it is endemic on every continent except Antarctica, rabies has a close to 100% case fatality rate once onset manifests (CDC, 2012). However, rabies is 100% preventable by application of vaccine (WOAH, 2023).

Rabies is a neglected tropical disease (NTD), a designation by the World Health Organization (WHO, 2024) that underscores its disproportionate impact on impoverished populations. The persistence of rabies, like other NTDs, is fundamentally rooted in the neglect of disease control programs and insufficient public health awareness. This neglect manifests as limited access to essential medical interventions, such as vaccines and post-exposure prophylaxis (PEP), which are pivotal for preventing human fatalities. Consequently, rabies continues to be a considerable global public health concern, although over 29 million people globally have received annual human rabies vaccine, but it is estimated there are 59,000 deaths annually (WHO, 2024).

2.3.1.2 Clinical Signs in Animal and Human

The rabies virus is a neurotropic virus that primarily targets the central nervous system (CNS) of all mammals. This targeting leads to the progressive degeneration of the brain and spinal cord, culminating in fatal encephalitis (WHO, 2024; WOAH, 2023). Following inoculation, typically through an animal bite, the virus propagates in the peripheral tissues near the site of the bite. After this initial replication, it spreads to the peripheral nerves. The virus then travels along the spinal cord to reach the CNS. Once in the brain, it spreads outwards, or centrifugally, along the nerves to other organs. The spread to the salivary glands is crucial for the infection of new hosts (Gnanadurai et al., 2013).

Early symptoms in animals often include common lethargy, fever, vomiting, and anorexia. As the disease progresses, the signs become more severe and neurological in nature. These can include cerebral dysfunction, ataxia, paralysis, difficulty breathing and swallowing, hypersalivation, atypical behavior, aggressivity, and possible self-mutilation. The incubation time for rabies is widely divergent and depends on factors like viral entry area and load. However, once clinical symptoms appear, the disease is almost always fatal after coma and cardiac arrest (Gnanadurai et al.,

2013; Muller & Freuling, 2020; WOAH, 2023). Rabies in dogs can appear in two forms: "furious" and "dumb." In the "furious" form, dogs become highly aggressive and may attack without warning. In the "dumb" form, they become paralyzed and lethargic. A key symptom of both forms is a sudden and dramatic change in personality, such as a friendly dog becoming aggressive or an unfriendly one becoming unusually friendly and withdrawn. It is often found in the stomachs during necropsy of infected dogs, and ruminants contain foreign objects like wood, stones, or even their own feces (Muller & Freuling, 2020).

Like in dogs, rabies virus infection in humans is primarily categorized into furious and the paralytic form. Paralytic rabies presents a major obstacle to effective public health surveillance, contributing to an underestimation of the true disease burden. Its clinical presentation is characterized by a less dramatic, non-aggressive progression. The hallmark of this form is a progressive, flaccid paralysis that can be easily mistaken for other neurological conditions. Due to the insidious onset and the absence of the classic behavioral changes associated with furious rabies, paralytic cases are frequently misdiagnosed. This diagnostic ambiguity, particularly in the initial stages, leads to a delay in appropriate medical intervention and hinders accurate case reporting, thus obscuring the true epidemiological scope of the disease (Ina et al., 2016; Susilawathi et al., 2012; WHO, 2024).

2.3.1.3 Situation in Indonesia

The first animal rabies case in Indonesia was officially documented in 1884, with the first human case appearing a decade later. Rabies is included within the significant priority zoonotic disease list in Indonesia due to its severe public health and the economic impact. The disease carries a high fatality rate, with an average of 142 human deaths per year reported in the country (Hukmi et al., 2019). The primary epidemiological characteristic of rabies in Indonesia is that domestic dogs serve as the main reservoir for the virus, mediating its spread. Phylogenetic analysis of the nucleoprotein (N) gene reveals that the rabies virus lineage circulating in Indonesia is part of a broader Asian clade, with a high degree of genetic relatedness to strains from China. This suggests that the virus was likely introduced into Indonesia through the human-mediated movement of dogs from China, rather than from a wildlife reservoir (Susetya et al., 2008). Rabies eradication efforts in the Indonesian archipelago have faced significant challenges, leading to persistent endemicity in many regions and continued geographic expansion. Key factors contributing to these failures include logistical constraints, sociocultural and behavioral factors, and resource limitations. The inefficacy of these control measures is demonstrated by the recurrent spread of rabies to previously disease-free islands, including Flores (1997), Bali (2008), Nias (2010), and Kisar (2012). Furthermore, the absence of a confirmed sylvatic rabies reservoir (i.e., in wild animal populations) in Indonesia suggests that the trans-island dissemination of the virus is a direct consequence of human-mediated inter-island movement and trafficking of dogs. This highlights the critical role of human activity in the propagation of the disease's primary reservoir host (Hukmi et al., 2019; Dibia et al., 2015).

Out of Indonesia's 38 provinces, 26 are classified as rabies-endemic, while 12 remain rabies-free. The provinces free from the disease include Jakarta, Central Java, East Java, Yogyakarta, Riau Islands, Bangka Belitung Islands, and all six provinces in Papua. According to the 2024 monthly zoonosis report, there were 185,359 cases of animal bites suspected of rabies transmission and 122 human deaths from the disease. The high incidence continues into 2025, with 13,453 suspected cases and 25 human deaths recorded from January through March 7 (Surat Edaran Kementrian Kesehatan Republik Indonesia No. HK.02.02/C/508/2025 Tentang Kewaspadaan Terhadap Kasus Rabies). These statistics underscore the persistent public health threat posed by rabies and highlight the need for continued vigilance and effective disease control measures.

2.3.1.4 Treatment, Prevention, and Intervention

Immediate and proper management of an animal bite is critical for preventing rabies. The initial first aid for all bites is to thoroughly wash the wound with soap and running water. Following first aid, immediate medical attention is required to determine the need for post-exposure prophylaxis (PEP), which includes rabies vaccination and immunoglobulin. The decisions regarding PEP are based on the rabies status of the biting animal (Ertll, 2020; WHO, 2024; WOAH, 2023). Wild animals should be euthanized and their brain tissue submitted for laboratory testing to confirm the presence of the rabies virus. Domestic animals like dogs and cats should be restrain and observed for 10 days. If the animal remains healthy throughout this period, it is considered non-rabid, and PEP may be discontinued. If the biting animal cannot be located or is unavailable for testing, the risk of rabies exposure is assumed to be high, and the full course of PEP is initiated immediately (Hukmi et al., 2019).

Mass dog vaccination remains the most effective and humane approach to rabies control, as supported by the World Health Organization (WHO). Despite this, dog culling is often used as a first-response measure during rabies outbreaks, particularly in low- and middle-income countries (LMICs) (Suseno et al., 2019). However, culling can be ineffective and inhumane, especially when conducted without proper multisectoral coordination and oversight of free-roaming dog populations. Its ineffectiveness is further compounded by a lack of knowledge among dog owners, who often replace culled animals with new, unvaccinated dogs. This cycle of culling and replacement creates a constant supply of susceptible hosts, ultimately hindering rabies elimination efforts (Acharya et al., 2022; Aréchiga Ceballos et al., 2014; Suseno et al., 2019). Sustained rabies control hinges on achieving and maintaining a herd immunity threshold of at least 70% through periodic mass dog vaccination (Ertll, 2020; Muller & Freuling, 2020). However, this effort is logistically challenging, particularly concerning the free-roaming canine population. The capture of these animals for initial vaccination demands specialized skills and resources. A further operational hurdle is encountered during revaccination campaigns, as previously vaccinated dogs often develop trap-shyness or heightened wariness, making their recapture for subsequent booster shots increasingly difficult (Widyastuti et al., 2015). The experimental oral rabies vaccine (ORV), SPBN-GASGAS, has demonstrated potential for application in Indonesia's free-roaming canine populations. This efficacy is supported by the development of a bait formulation that exhibited high palatability among indigenous dogs, a critical factor for successful widespread deployment (Husein et al., 2023; Megawati Saputra et al., 2023).

2.3.2 Avian Influenza

2.3.2.1 Overview of the Disease

Avian influenza is caused by influenza A viruses, which belong to the genus *Alphainfluenzavirus* within the family *Orthomyxoviridae* (Walker et al., 2022). The family name *Orthomyxoviridae* originates from Greek roots: *myxa*, meaning "mucus," and *orthos*, meaning "straight" or "correct." This name likely refers to the virus's affinity for mucin glycoproteins on cell surfaces and was historically used to differentiate it from paramyxoviruses. The term "influenza" has a different etymological origin, coming from the medieval Italian form of the Latin word *influentia*, meaning "influence." This term reflects the historical belief that epidemics were caused by celestial or supernatural "influences" rather than a biological agent (Barthold et al., 2011).

Influenza A viruses are subtyped based on two major surface glycoproteins: hemagglutinin (HA) and neuraminidase (NA). These proteins are crucial for the virus's lifecycle; HA enables the virus to attach to and enter host cells, while NA allows newly formed viral particles to be released from the infected cell surface. There are currently 19 known HA subtypes (H1–H19) and 11 known NA subtypes (N1–N11). The potential for influenza viruses to reassort leads to numerous combinations of hemagglutinin (HA) and neuraminidase (NA) proteins, many of which have been detected in their natural reservoirs. While most HA and NA subtypes are identified in avian hosts, H17 and H18, along with NA subtypes N10 and N11, have only been isolated from bats (Barthold et al., 2011; WOAH, 2021). The latest described H19 subtype was first identified in 2008 from a Common Pochard (*Aythya ferina*) in Kazakhstan (Fereidouni et al., 2023). A subsequent study by Karakus, U., et al. (2024) demonstrated that, unlike most influenza A viruses which bind to sialic acid (Sia) as their canonical receptor for host cell entry, the H19 hemagglutinin (HA) protein utilizes major histocompatibility complex class II (MHC-II). This novel mechanism of cell entry suggests a broader and more complex interaction with the host's immune system, potentially expanding our understanding of viral tropism and host range (Karakus et al., 2024).

Influenza A viruses have a vast host range, with a primary natural reservoir in wild aquatic birds. However, they can infect a different range of other species, including humans, horses, swine, and, less commonly, marine mammals and dogs. In domestic poultry, two subtypes of influenza A viruses—H5 and H7—are of significant economic concern. These subtypes can produce highly pathogenic avian influenza (HPAI), which causes severe clinical disease and high mortality rates in poultry, leading to devastating economic losses. While many H5 and H7 viruses are initially low pathogenic, they can mutate into HPAI strains after circulating in poultry. Human infections with influenza A viruses from avian or other animal hosts are sporadic and often result from direct contact with infected animals or contaminated environments (Barthold et al., 2011; Spackman, 2014; WOAH, 2021). Among the subtypes that have been documented to cause human infection are H5, H6, H7, H9, and H10. Historically, H5N1 and H7N9 have accounted for most human cases and have a high case-fatality rate. Other subtypes, such as H6N1, H10N3, H10N7, and H10N8, have also been reported to cause rare human infections, although these are typically detected in small, localized populations (CDC, 2024).

2.3.2.2 Clinical Signs in Animal and Human

The clinical presentation of avian influenza virus (AIV) infection in birds is variable and depends on several factors, including the host species, age, and the pathogenicity of the viral strain. The clinical presentation of avian influenza virus (AIV) infection in birds is highly variable and depends on several factors, including the host species, age, and the pathogenicity of the viral strain (WOAH, 2021). The pathogenicity of influenza A viruses is fundamentally determined by the cleavage site of the hemagglutinin (HA) protein. The HA protein is first synthesized as a single polypeptide precursor, HA0, which is then proteolytically cleaved into two subunits, HA1 and HA2, to become biologically active and infectious. The amino acid sequence at this cleavage site dictates which host proteases can perform this critical step, thereby controlling the virus's ability to spread throughout the host (Barthold et al., 2011; Kalil & Thomas, 2019; Wibowo et al., 2006). The hemagglutinin (HA) glycoprotein mediates viral entry by binding to sialic acid residues on host cells and facilitating membrane fusion. HA is synthesized as a precursor (HA0), which assembles into homotrimers in the endoplasmic reticulum and requires proteolytic cleavage to become fusogenic. Cleavage of HA0 into HA1 and HA2 subunits exposes the hydrophobic fusion peptide at the HA2 N-terminus, a critical step for membrane fusion in the acidic environment of endosomes. Host proteases perform this cleavage, as avian influenza virus (AIV) genomes do not encode proteases. In low pathogenic AIVs (LPAIVs), HA contains a single amino acid cleavage site recognized by trypsin-like proteases with restricted tissue expression, limiting viral propagation in the respiratory and gastrointestinal tracts. In contrast, highly pathogenic AIVs (HPAIVs) possess a multibasic cleavage site (MBCS) cleaved by ubiquitously expressed subtilisin-like proteases such as furin, enabling systemic spread. The MBCS is the primary virulence determinant of HPAIVs in terrestrial poultry, as confirmed by reverse genetics studies (de Bruin et al., 2022; Horimoto & Kawaoka, 1994).

Low pathogenic avian influenza (LPAI) strains typically cause either no clinical signs or mild symptoms in poultry. Infections are often localized to the respiratory or gastrointestinal tracts. Symptoms, when present, may include mild respiratory signs: sneezing, coughing, and nasal discharge, reduced feed and water consumption, decreased egg production, lethargy and depression. In wild birds, LPAI viruses often cause no apparent illness, allowing them to act as natural reservoirs for the virus. However, highly pathogenic avian influenza (HPAI) strains cause severe systemic disease in poultry. HPAI can lead to sudden death with little to no prior symptoms, severe systemic signs: swelling of the head, eyelids, comb, and wattles, neurological signs: tremors, lack of coordination, and paralysis, hemorrhaging on the shanks and feet, diarrhea, and a significant drop in egg production. The infection is recognized by very high mortality rates up to 100% within a few days in domestic poultry (Barthold et al., 2011; Charostad et al., 2023; Kalil & Thomas, 2019; WOAH, 2021). These clinical signs—including cyanotic wattles, brain congestion, hemorrhages in the feet and proventriculus, and hemorrhages and adhesions between ovarian follicles—are consistent with the findings reported by researchers in Indonesia. Additional pathological observations include edema and swelling of the kidney, as well as lesions in the abdominal fat and pectoral muscles (Putri et al., 2020b).

In humans, clinical symptoms of influenza A virus infection, ranging from conjunctivitis (Belser et al., 2018) to severe pneumonia (Thompson et al., 2006), are influenced by the virus's binding preference for α-2,6-linked sialic acid receptors; however, the severity of the disease is ultimately determined by the individual's immune response, with an excessive inflammatory reaction contributing significantly to cellular damage, particularly within the alveoli in postmortem examination (Zhuang et al., 2017).

2.3.2.3 Situation in Indonesia

Since its emergence in 2003, highly pathogenic avian influenza (HPAI) has been a persistent challenge for Indonesia's poultry industry. The initial H5N1 outbreak spread rapidly across most provinces, causing the death of over 10 million poultry before its abatement in late 2008. A subsequent outbreak report from Gorontalo in April 2011 left only one province free of the disease. Indonesia is still an endemic area, with 110,812 cases spreading over 23 provinces (WOAH, 2021). Phylogenetic analysis of Indonesian H5N1 clade 2.1 viruses indicates a direct ancestor-descendant link to genotype Z viruses isolated in China's Hunan province in 2002, suggesting a single introduction event. However, the exact transmission route from Hunan to Indonesia remains unclear (Takano et al., 2009; Wibawa et al., 2011).

Until 2008, all Indonesian H5N1 isolates belonged to clade 2.1, which was further divided into three sublineages: 2.1.1, 2.1.2, and 2.1.3. Despite the endemic nature of clade 2.1.3 viruses, a significant shift occurred. In September 2012, a new H5 subtype emerged in duck farms in Central Java, causing high mortality. Phylogenetic analysis revealed that the HA genes of these duck isolates were not related to the established Indonesian clade 2.1 viruses but were closely related to clade 2.3.2.1 viruses, which had recently been found in Vietnam, China, and Hong Kong (Lam et al., 2008; Takano et al., 2009; Wibawa et al., 2011). Since late 2021, Indonesia has observed a notable shift in circulating avian influenza viruses. A new strain, HPAI H5N1 clade 2.3.2.1c, was identified in a duck farm in Sidenreng, South Sulawesi (Mutisari et al., 2021). Additionally, low pathogenic avian influenza (LPAI) subtypes H9N2 and H11N9 were also detected in the region (Wibawa, 2022). More recently, a new introduction of HPAI H5N1 clade 2.3.4.4b has been reported in broiler duck farms in South Kalimantan. This particular strain is genetically similar to viruses that have been circulating in East Asia during 2021 and 2022, indicating a separate, limited introduction of a distinct viral lineage into the country (Angeliya, 2024).

2.3.2.4 Treatment, Prevention, and Intervention

For severe cases of avian influenza in humans, treatment involves the administration of antivirals, alongside supportive care with broad-spectrum antibiotics for potential secondary bacterial infections and/or corticosteroids to manage excessive inflammatory responses. The majority of hospitalized patients require intensive care, including mechanical ventilation for respiratory failure, due to complications such as multiorgan failure and hypotension, which can develop within 48 h of admission. Oseltamivir is the recommended antiviral for reducing viral load, and early administration is associated with improved clinical outcomes. However, some patients may still experience fatal outcomes despite early treatment, particularly in cases where the pharyngeal viral load cannot be effectively reduced. This lack of viral clearance suggests that host factors or viral resistance may contribute to disease progression even with appropriate antiviral therapy (Writing Committee of the Second World Health Organization Consultation on Clinical Aspects of Human Infection with Avian Influenza A (H5N1) Virus, 2008). In 2005, WHO confirmed the first fatal human case of avian influenza in Indonesia, which was linked to handling infected birds (Parry, 2005). The 200th case was confirmed in 2017 in Klungkung, Bali, leading to speculation that Bali is a utopian hub for influenza reassortment (Putri et al., 2020b). Although raising backyard chicken remains a part of Indonesian culture, which facilitates exposure to sick birds, washing hands after handling them is still considered an effective way to prevent infection (Rehman et al., 2023).

Since 2005, the Indonesian government has implemented a multifaceted approach to control HPAI H5N1, focusing on mass vaccination of poultry flocks, enhanced biosecurity measures on farms, active disease surveillance, stamping-out policies, applied extensively in newly infected areas and more limitedly in endemic regions, and public awareness campaigns (Swayne, 2012; Wibawa et al., 2011; WOAH, 2009). The International Alliance for Biological Standardization (IABS) and the World Organization for Animal Health (WOAH) in 2024 recommend vaccination as a tool for disease control, complementing biosecurity, movement restrictions, and culling. While vaccination is a crucial preventive tool, it does not provide sterilizing immunity, meaning vaccinated birds can still become infected and shed infectious virus without showing clinical signs. Accordingly, the meeting highlighted the importance of using RT-qPCR to detect asymptomatic infections in vaccinated flocks, which can lead to trade barriers (Sajjadi et al., 2025). This makes it difficult to distinguish between vaccinated and naturally infected animals, a challenge addressed by Differentiating Infected from Vaccinated Animals (DIVA) strategies. One proposed DIVA approach involved using sentinel naive chickens in West Java (Bouma et al., 2008). However, this method has not gained widespread acceptance in Indonesia due to the risk of these birds becoming infected before or during their placement, thereby potentially introducing the virus into a flock. Due to the challenges with sentinel-based DIVA, alternative strategies have been developed using specific viral proteins as markers in chickens. These marker proteins allow for serological differentiation between a vaccine-induced immune response and a response to a wild-type infection. Examples of these alternative markers include Non-structural protein 1 (NS1) (Avellaneda et al., 2010), Matrix protein 2 ectodomain (M2e) (Hadifar et al., 2014; Hemmatzadeh et al., 2013; Tarigan et al., 2015; Wibowo et al., 2017), and Hemagglutinin 2 (HA2) (Li et al., 2022; Putri et al., 2018, 2020a). These molecular approaches aim to improve the effectiveness of vaccination campaigns by accurately monitoring the circulation of the wild-type virus. Ultimately, the IABS meeting also emphasized the need for vaccine antigen matching to circulating field strains and scientifically standardized surveillance to support fair trade (Sajjadi et al., 2025).

2.3.3 *Plasmodium Knowlesi*

2.3.3.1 Overview of the Disease

Plasmodium knowlesi is the zoonotic blood parasite that causes knowlesi malaria, a disease that mostly affects pig-tailed macaques (*Macaca nemestrina*) and long-tailed macaques (*Macaca fascicularis*). It is a main cause of human malaria in Southeast Asia (van de Straat et al., 2022). The disease has a wide distribution in Southeast Asian countries, particularly East Malaysia, where the two states are Sabah and Sarawak (Zaw & Lin, 2019). Infections mainly occur in forested areas where monkeys and humans coexist, with the assumption that humans are incidentally infected when attacked by an *Anopheles* mosquito which has fed on an infected macaque reservoir host (Anstey et al., 2021).

2.3.3.2 Clinical Signs of Plasmodium Knowlesi

Clinical signs observed in animals, particularly in long-tailed macaques (*Macaca fascicularis*) as the primary hosts, are like those in humans. *Plasmodium knowlesi* has a very rapid erythrocytic cycle, occurring every 24 h, which can cause hyperparasitemic infections in humans (Singh & Daneshvar, 2010, 2013). Laboratory tests in cases of *P. knowlesi* infection typically show thrombocytopenia and moderate to severe hemolytic anemia (Peterson et al., 2021). Furthermore, the infection can cause serious complications like kidney failure and respiratory distress, which may also occur in the natural host (Lee et al., 2009).

The clinical manifestations of *P. knowlesi* malaria are generally mild, with approximately 10% of cases progressing to severe disease and only 1–2% resulting in fatal outcomes. The incubation period for *P. knowlesi* typically ranges from 8 to 12 days, with a reported variability of 3 to 27 days (Anstey et al., 2021; Milam & Kusch, 1938). Due to the rapid 24-h asexual replication cycle of the parasite, patients often experience daily fever, known as quotidian fever. This febrile pattern usually begins with chills lasting 4–5 days and is accompanied by symptoms such as headache, muscle and joint pain, fatigue, decreased appetite, respiratory discomfort, and digestive disturbances (Singh & Daneshvar, 2010). The most common symptoms include fever (100%), chills, headache (89–94%), myalgia (47–88%), nausea and vomiting (24–34%), cough (35–56%), and abdominal pain (23–52%) (Anstey et al., 2021). In addition, increased body temperature, tachycardia, and tachypnea are frequently observed.

Laboratory findings commonly reveal thrombocytopenia, a hallmark indicator of *P. knowlesi* infection (Daneshvar et al., 2009). Severe malaria due to *P. knowlesi* is characterized by parasitemia exceeding 35,000 parasites/μL, bilirubin levels above 43 μmol/L, serum creatinine greater than 256 μmol/L, and platelet counts below 45,000/μL (Kurniawan et al., 2020). High parasite burdens are often associated with clinical complications such as vomiting and shortness of breath. Although the severe manifestations of *P. knowlesi* malaria are similar to those caused by *P. falciparum*, a key distinguishing feature is that *P. knowlesi* does not induce coma, making this an important consideration in diagnosis and treatment (Anstey et al., 2021).

2.3.3.3 Plasmodium Knowlesi Situation in Indonesia

The malaria parasites affecting non-human primates present an increasing obstacle to the eradication of malaria in areas where human populations coexist closely with these primates. *P. knowlesi*, *P. cynomolgi*, and *P. inui* have been reported as zoonotic malaria cases in South and Southeast Asia, as well as *P. brazilianum* and *P. simium* in Latin America (Brasil et al., 2017; Chaves et al., 2022; Ta et al., 2014). These parasites are inherently present in both Old and New World monkeys, with a particular prevalence among macaque species. In Indonesia, this emerging threat is linked to the distribution of non-human primates and the malaria parasites they carry, as well as environmental changes such as deforestation and land-use transformation. These ecological disruptions increase the frequency of human-primate interactions and create opportunities for cross-species transmission of malaria parasites (Lempang et al., 2022). Although Indonesia is rich in primate biodiversity, studies on malaria parasites in non-human primates remain limited. In Indonesia, there have been 545 *P. knowlesi* cases reported, primarily in the provinces of Aceh and North Sumatra, with 95% of these occurrences taking place in the last 4 years (Bin Said et al., 2022). DNA from dried blood spot testing of 110 primates of the genus *Macaca* revealed that 50% were positive for *P. cynomolgi*, *P. coatneyi*, *P. inui*, and *P. knowlesi*, while blood smear microscopic examination was 42% (Permana et al., 2023).

Plasmodium knowlesi, which was previously underrecognized in Indonesia, is now emerging as a significant public health threat, particularly in light of the impending relocation of the national capital to East Kalimantan, Borneo. Between 2010 and 2021, there were 545 documented cases of human *P. knowlesi* infections in Indonesia, with over 95% of these cases reported after 2017, primarily concentrated in the provinces of Aceh and North Sumatra (Bin Said et al., 2022). The substantial rise in reported cases can be attributed to advancements in diagnostic capacity, particularly the implementation of a molecular approach that accurately differentiates *P. knowlesi* from morphologically similar species such as *P. falciparum* and *P. malariae*, which are often misidentified through microscopy (Barber et al., 2013). Enhanced training in recognizing subtle morphological differences improves microscopy, but definitive diagnosis still requires molecular confirmation.

The development of Nusantara, Indonesia's new capital in East Kalimantan, raises significant environmental and health concerns. As large areas of forest are cleared and infrastructure is built, people will be in closer contact with macaques and certain types of mosquitoes known to transmit diseases. These macaques and mosquitoes are already present in Borneo (Bin Said et al., 2022). This proximity increases the risk of a specific form of malaria called *P. knowlesi*, which can be transmitted from animals to humans. Currently, Indonesia's strategy to eliminate malaria does not adequately address this zoonotic risk, highlighting the urgent need for improved monitoring and collaboration among various sectors. This coordinated effort is essential to safeguard public health and reduce the likelihood of disease transmission in the new capital area.

2.3.3.4 Treatment of Plasmodium Knowlesi

Most human *P. knowlesi* infections are uncomplicated and exhibit low parasite densities and mild symptoms resembling *P. vivax* or *P. falciparum* malaria, with severely elevated parasitemia (Anstey et al., 2021). Treatment should be initiated promptly upon confirmation of diagnosis. The recommended treatment regimen is an oral artemisinin combination therapy (ACT). Chloroquine is effective against *P. knowlesi*, but artemisinin-based combination therapies (ACTs) lead to faster clearance of the parasite. However, administering chloroquine to patients diagnosed with *P. knowlesi* malaria poses a risk of misdiagnosing cases of *P. vivax* or *P. falciparum* malaria. In regions where *P. vivax* and *P. falciparum* are commonly resistant to chloroquine, its use as an antimalarial treatment is not recommended (Antony & Parija, 2016). In severe cases with parasitemia exceeding 20,000 parasites per mL, intravenous artesunate is the preferred treatment. It should be administered for a minimum of three doses at a rate of 2.4 mg/kg, given 12 h apart (Centers for Disease Control and Prevention, 2024).

2.3.3.5 Prevention or Intervention of Plasmodium Knowlesi

The global prevention of P. knowlesi can be effectively addressed through the management of infectious diseases within the "One Health" framework, aimed at achieving optimal health outcomes for both people and animals (Scott, 2020). A key strategy for prevention involves vector control methods, which encompass Indoor Residual Spraying (IRS), Outdoor Residual Spraying (ORS), Insecticide-Treated Nets (ITNs), and Larval Source Management (LSM). Currently, no cases of insecticide resistance have been reported among the vectors of *P. knowlesi* (Alam et al., 2017; Scott, 2020). However, given that *P. knowlesi* is predominantly transmitted by mosquitoes that bite outdoors, it is crucial to choose insecticides specifically effective against these outdoor vectors. The application of insecticide-treated nets is one of the main ways to protect people against *Anopheles* mosquito bites (Centers for Disease Control and Prevention, 2022). Furthermore, while less frequently employed, LSM is equally essential; it addresses mosquito breeding sites with methods including habitat change, habitat manipulation, biological control, and larvicide (Mohammad et al., 2022).

Competing Interests The authors have no competing interests to declare that are relevant to the content of this manuscript.

References

Acharya, K. P., Chand, R., Huettmann, F., & Ghimire, T. R. (2022). Rabies elimination: Is it feasible without considering wildlife? *Journal of Tropical Medicine, 2022*. Hindawi Limited. https://doi.org/10.1155/2022/5942693

Alam, M. Z., Niaz Arifin, S. M., Al-Amin, H. M., Alam, M. S., & Rahman, M. S. (2017). A spatial agent-based model of Anopheles vagus for malaria epidemiology: Examining the impact of vector control interventions. *Malaria Journal, 16*(1), 432. https://doi.org/10.1186/s12936-017-2075-6

Angeliya, L. (2024). *National prevention and control measures for avian disease*. https://rr-asia.woah.org/app/uploads/2024/08/S1.M17_Indonesia.pdf

Anstey, N. M., Grigg, M. J., Rajahram, G. S., Cooper, D. J., William, T., Kho, S., & Barber, B. E. (2021). Knowlesi malaria: Human risk factors, clinical spectrum, and pathophysiology. *Advances in Parasitology, 113*. https://doi.org/10.1016/bs.apar.2021.08.001

Antony, H. A., & Parija, S. C. (2016). Antimalarial drug resistance: An overview. *Tropical Parasitology*, *6*(1). https://journals.lww.com/tpar/fulltext/2016/06010/antimalarial_drug_resistance__an_overview.5.aspx

Aréchiga Ceballos, N., Karunaratna, D., & Aguilar Setién, A. (2014). Control of canine rabies in developing countries: Key features and animal welfare implications. *Revue scientifique et technique/ Office international des épizooties*, *33*(1).

Avellaneda, G., Mundt, E., Lee, C.-W., Jadhao, S., & Suarez, D. L. (2010). Differentiation of infected and vaccinated animals (DIVA) using the NS1 protein of avian influenza virus. *Avian Diseases, 54*(s1), 278–286. https://doi.org/10.1637/8644-020409-Reg.1

Barber, B. E., William, T., Grigg, M. J., Yeo, T. W., & Anstey, N. M. (2013). Limitations of microscopy to differentiate Plasmodium species in a region co-endemic for Plasmodium falciparum, Plasmodium vivax and Plasmodium knowlesi. *Malaria Journal, 12*(1). https://doi.org/10.1186/1475-2875-12-8

Barthold, S. W., Bowen, R. A., Hedrick, R. P., Knowles Donald, P., Lairmore, M. D., Parrish, C. R., Saif, L. J., & Swayne, D. E. (2011). Orthomyxoviridae. In J. MacLachlan & E. J. Dubovi (Eds.), *Fenner's veterinary virology* (pp. 353–370). Elsevier. https://doi.org/10.1016/B978-0-12-375158-4.00021-3

Belser, J. A., Lash, R. R., Garg, S., Tumpey, T. M., & Maines, T. R. (2018). The eyes have it: Influenza virus infection beyond the respiratory tract. *The Lancet Infectious Diseases, 18*(7), e220–e227. Lancet Publishing Group. https://doi.org/10.1016/S1473-3099(18)30102-6

Bengis, R. G., Leighton, F. A., Fischer, J. R., Artois, M., Mörner, T., & Tate, C. M. (2004). The role of wildlife in emerging and re-emerging zoonoses. *OIE Revue Scientifique et Technique, 23*(2), 497–511. https://doi.org/10.20506/rst.23.2.1498

Bin Said, I., Kouakou, Y. I., Omorou, R., Bienvenu, A. L., Ahmed, K., Culleton, R., & Picot, S. (2022). Systematic review of Plasmodium knowlesi in Indonesia: A risk of emergence in the context of capital relocation to Borneo? *Parasites and Vectors, 15*(1). https://doi.org/10.1186/s13071-022-05375-8

Bouma, A., Muljono, A. T., Jatikusumah, A., Nell, A. J., Mudjiartiningsih, S., Dharmayanti, I., Siregar, E. S., Claassen, I., Koch, G., & Stegeman, J. A. (2008). Field trial for assessment of avian influenza vaccination effectiveness in Indonesia. *Revue Scientifique et Technique de l'OIE, 27*(3), 633–642. https://doi.org/10.20506/rst.27.3.1823

Brasil, P., Zalis, M. G., de Pina-Costa, A., Siqueira, A. M., Júnior, C. B., Silva, S., Areas, A. L. L., Pelajo-Machado, M., de Alvarenga, D. A. M., da Silva Santelli, A. C. F., Albuquerque, H. G., Cravo, P., Santos de Abreu, F. V., Peterka, C. L., Zanini, G. M., Suárez Mutis, M. C., Pissinatti, A., Lourenço-de-Oliveira, R., de Brito, C. F. A., et al. (2017). Outbreak of human malaria caused by Plasmodium simium in the Atlantic Forest in Rio de Janeiro: A molecular epidemiological investigation. *The Lancet Global Health, 5*(10). https://doi.org/10.1016/S2214-109X(17)30333-9

CDC. (2012). Etymologia: Rabies. *Emerging Infectious Diseases, 18*(7), 1169–1169. https://doi.org/10.3201/eid1807.ET1807

Centers for Disease Control and Prevention. (2022, April 2). *Insecticide-treated nets (ITNs). U.S.* Department of Health & Human Services. Public Health. https://www.cdc.gov/malaria/php/public-health-strategy/insecticide-treated-nets.html

Centers for Disease Control and Prevention. (2024, March 27). *Treatment of severe malaria clinical guidance: Malaria diagnosis & treatment in the U.S.* Health Care Providers.

Charostad, J., Rezaei Zadeh Rukerd, M., Mahmoudvand, S., Bashash, D., Hashemi, S. M. A., Nakhaie, M., & Zandi, K. (2023). A comprehensive review of highly pathogenic avian influenza (HPAI) H5N1: An imminent threat at doorstep. *Travel Medicine and Infectious Disease, 55*. Elsevier Inc. https://doi.org/10.1016/j.tmaid.2023.102638

Chaves, A., Dolz, G., Ibarra-Cerdeña, C. N., Núñez, G., Ortiz-Malavasi, E. E., Bernal-Valle, S., & Gutiérrez-Espeleta, G. A. (2022). Presence and potential distribution of malaria-infected New World primates of Costa Rica. *Malaria Journal, 21*(1). https://doi.org/10.1186/s12936-021-04036-y

Chomel, B. B. (2014). Zoonoses☆. In *Reference module in biomedical sciences*. Elsevier. https://doi.org/10.1016/B978-0-12-801238-3.02426-0

Daneshvar, C., Davis, T. M. E., Cox-Singh, J., Rafa'ee, M. Z., Zakaria, S. K., Divis, P. C. S., & Singh, B. (2009). Clinical and laboratory features of human Plasmodium knowlesi infection. *Clinical Infectious Diseases, 49*(6). https://doi.org/10.1086/605439

de Bruin, A. C. M., Funk, M., Spronken, M. I., Gultyaev, A. P., Fouchier, R. A. M., & Richard, M. (2022). Hemagglutinin subtype specificity and mechanisms of highly pathogenic avian influenza virus genesis. *Viruses, 14*(7). MDPI. https://doi.org/10.3390/v14071566

Dibia, I. N., Sumiarto, B., Susetya, H., Putra, A. A. G., Scott-Orr, H., & Mahardika, G. N. (2015). Phylogeography of the current rabies viruses in Indonesia. *Journal of Veterinary Science, 16*(4), 459–466. https://doi.org/10.4142/jvs.2015.16.4.459

Ertll, H. J. (2020). *Rabies and rabies vaccines*. Springer. https://doi.org/10.1007/978-3-030-21084-7

Fereidouni, S., Starick, E., Karamendin, K., Di Genova, C., Scott, S. D., Khan, Y., Harder, T., & Kydyrmanov, A. (2023). Genetic characterization of a new candidate hemagglutinin subtype of influenza A viruses. *Emerging Microbes & Infections, 12*(2). https://doi.org/10.1080/22221751.2023.2225645

Gnanadurai, C. W., Lyon, David, C., Jackson, A. C., & Fu, Z. F. (2013). Mononegaviruses of veterinary importance volume I: Pathobiology and molecular diagnosis. In M. Munir (Ed.), *Mononegaviruses of veterinary importance* (1st ed., Vol. 1).

Hadifar, F., Ignjatovic, J., Tarigan, S., Indriani, R., Ebrahimie, E., Hasan, N. H., McWhorter, A., Putland, S., Ownagh, A., & Hemmatzadeh, F. (2014). Multimeric recombinant M2e protein-based ELISA: A significant improvement in differentiating avian influenza infected chickens from vaccinated ones. *PLoS ONE, 9*(10), e108420. https://doi.org/10.1371/journal.pone.0108420

Hemmatzadeh, F., Sumarningsih, S., Tarigan, S., Indriani, R., Dharmayanti, N. L. P. I., Ebrahimie, E., & Igniatovic, J. (2013). Recombinant M2e protein-based ELISA: A novel and inexpensive approach for differentiating avian influenza infected chickens from vaccinated ones. *PLoS ONE, 8*(2), e56801. https://doi.org/10.1371/journal.pone.0056801

Horimoto, T., & Kawaoka, Y. (1994). Reverse genetics provides direct evidence for a correlation of hemagglutinin cleavability and virulence of an avian influenza A virus. *Journal of Virology, 68*(5). https://journals.asm.org/journal/jvi

Hukmi, A., Wicaksono, A., Ermawanto, Ernawati, Rasa, F.S.T., Mardiatmi, Azhar, M., Suseno, P. P., Pujiatmoko, Ekowati, R. V., Butarbutar, R. M., Nurtanto, S., Kurniawan, W. E., & Yupiana, Y. (2019). *Masterplan Nasional Pemberantasan Rabies di Indonesia*.

Husein, W. F., Saputra, I. L. M., Suseno, P. P., Arthawan, I. M., Prayoga, I. M. A., Daryono, J., Vos, A., Wicaksono, A., Schoonman, L., Weaver, J., & Zainuddin, N. (2023). Assessing bait acceptance of local dogs, oral rabies vaccination success and human contact risk in Bali, Indonesia. *One Health & Implementation Research, 3*(2), 16–29. https://doi.org/10.20517/ohir.2022.32

Ina, A., Detha, R., Feny, & Bili, A. L. (2016). *The important zoonoses in East Nusa Tenggara*.

Kalil, A. C., & Thomas, P. G. (2019). Influenza virus-related critical illness: Pathophysiology and epidemiology. *Critical Care, 23*(1). https://doi.org/10.1186/s13054-019-2539-x

Karakus, U., Mena, I., Kottur, J., El Zahed, S. S., Seoane, R., Yildiz, S., Chen, L., Plancarte, M., Lindsay, L. A., Halpin, R., Stockwell, T. B., Wentworth, D. E., Boons, G. J., Krammer, F., Stertz, S., Boyce, W., de Vries, R. P., Aggarwal, A. K., & García-Sastre, A. (2024). H19 influenza A virus exhibits species-specific MHC class II receptor usage. *Cell Host & Microbe, 32*(7), 1089–1102.e10. https://doi.org/10.1016/j.chom.2024.05.018

Keenan, S., Niedziela, D., Morera-Pujol, V., Franklin, D., Murphy, K. J., Ciuti, S., & McMahon, B. J. (2024). Zoonotic disease classification in wildlife: A theoretical framework for researchers. *Mammal Review, 54*(1), 63–77. Wiley. https://doi.org/10.1111/mam.12329

Kurniawan, B., Suwandi, J. F., Mustofa, S., & Hayati, S. J. (2020). A review: Plasmodium knowlesi. *Jurnal Kedokteran Dan Kesehatan: Publikasi Ilmiah Fakultas Kedokteran Universitas Sriwijaya, 7*(2), 106–111. https://doi.org/10.32539/jkk.v7i2.139

Lam, T. T. Y., Hon, C. C., Pybus, O. G., Kosakovsky Pond, S. L., Wong, R. T. Y., Yip, C. W., Zeng, F., & Leung, F. C. C. (2008). Evolutionary and transmission dynamics of reassortant H5N1 influenza virus in Indonesia. *PLoS Pathogens, 4*(8). https://doi.org/10.1371/journal.ppat.1000130

Lee, K. S., Cox-Singh, J., Brooke, G., Matusop, A., & Singh, B. (2009). Plasmodium knowlesi from archival blood films: Further evidence that human infections are widely distributed and

not newly emergent in Malaysian Borneo. *International Journal for Parasitology, 39*(10). https://doi.org/10.1016/j.ijpara.2009.03.003
Lempang, M. E. P., Dewayanti, F. K., Syahrani, L., Permana, D. H., Malaka, R., Asih, P. B. S., & Syafruddin, D. (2022). Primate malaria: An emerging challenge of zoonotic malaria in Indonesia. *One Health, 14*. https://doi.org/10.1016/j.onehlt.2022.100389
Li, G., Feng, J., Quan, K., Sun, Z., Yin, Y., Yin, Y., Chen, S., Qin, T., Peng, D., & Liu, X. (2022). Generation of an avian influenza DIVA vaccine with a H3-peptide replacement located at HA2 against both highly and low pathogenic H7N9 virus. *Virulence, 13*(1), 530–541. https://doi.org/10.1080/21505594.2022.2040190
Lindahl, J. F., Grace, D., & Strand, T. (2015). The consequences of human actions on risks for infectious diseases: A review. *Infection Ecology and Epidemiology, 5*(1). Taylor and Francis Ltd. https://doi.org/10.3402/IEE.V5.30048
Megawati Saputra, I. L., Suwarno, S., Husein, W. F., Suseno, P. P., Prayoga, I. M. A., Vos, A., Arthawan, I. M., Schoonman, L., Weaver, J., & Zainuddin, N. (2023). Immunogenicity of oral rabies vaccine strain SPBN GASGAS in local dogs in Bali, Indonesia. *Viruses, 15*(6). https://doi.org/10.3390/v15061405
Milam, D. F., & Kusch, E. (1938). Observations on plasmodium knowlesi malaria in general paresis. *Southern Medical Journal, 31*(8). https://doi.org/10.1097/00007611-193808000-00027
Mohammad, A. H., Naserrudin, N. A., Syed Abdul Rahim, S. S., Jelip, J., Atil, A., Sazali, M. F., Muyou, A. J., Kunasagran, P. D., Ahmad Kamarudin, N., Azhar, Z. I., Dapari, R., Jeffree, M. S., & Hassan, M. R. (2022). Narrative review of the control and prevention of knowlesi malaria. *Tropical Medicine and Infectious Disease, 7*(8). https://doi.org/10.3390/tropicalmed7080178
Muller, T., & Freuling, C. M. (2020). Rabies in terrestrial animal. In A. R. Fooks & A. C. Jackson (Eds.), *Rabies, scientific basis of the disease and its management* (4th ed.). Academic.
Mutisari, D., Muflihanah, M., Wibawa, H., Hendrawati, F., Putra, H. H., Sulistyo, K. P., Ahmad, A., Sjahril, R., Mubin, R. H., Sari, D. K., & Massi, M. N. (2021). Phylogenetic analysis of HPAI H5N1 virus from duck swab specimens in Indonesia. *Journal of Advanced Veterinary and Animal Research, 8*(2), 346–354. https://doi.org/10.5455/javar.2021.h521
Parry, J. (2005). WHO confirms four human cases of avian flu in Indonesia. *BMJ, 331*(7520), 796.3. https://doi.org/10.1136/bmj.331.7520.796-b
Permana, D. H., Hasmiwati, Suryandari, D. A., Rozi, I. E., Syahrani, L., Setiadi, W., Irawati, N., Rizaldi, Wangsamuda, S., Yusuf, Y., Irdayanti, Aswad, H., Asih, P. B. S., & Syafruddin, D. (2023). The potential for zoonotic malaria transmission in five areas of Indonesia inhabited by non-human primates. *Parasites and Vectors, 16*(1). https://doi.org/10.1186/s13071-023-05880-4
Peterson, M. S., Joyner, C. J., Brady, J. A., Wood, J. S., Cabrera-Mora, M., Saney, C. L., Fonseca, L. L., Cheng, W. T., Jiang, J., Lapp, S. A., Soderberg, S. R., Nural, M. V., Humphrey, J. C., Hankus, A., Machiah, D., Karpuzoglu, E., DeBarry, J. D., Anderson, M., HPIC-Consortium, Tirouvanziam, R., Kissinger, J. C., Moreno, A., Gumber, S., Voit, E. O., Gutiérrez, J. B., Cordy, R. J., & Galinski, M. R. (2021). Clinical recovery of Macaca fascicularis infected with Plasmodium knowlesi. *Malaria Journal, 20*(1). https://doi.org/10.1186/s12936-021-03925-6
Putri, K., Wawegama, N., Ignjatovic, J., & Noormohammadi, A. H. (2018). Characterisation of the antigenic epitopes in the subunit 2 haemagglutinin of avian influenza virus H5N1. *Archives of Virology, 163*(8), 2199–2212. https://doi.org/10.1007/s00705-018-3896-5
Putri, K., Wibowo, M. H., Tarigan, S., Wawegama, N., Ignjatovic, J., & Noormohammadi, A. H. (2020a). Analysis of antibody response to an epitope in the haemagglutinin subunit 2 of avian influenza virus H5N1 for differentiation of infected and vaccinated chickens. *Avian Pathology, 49*(2), 161–170. https://doi.org/10.1080/03079457.2019.1694635
Putri, K., Widyarini, S., Sugiyono, & Asmara, W. (2020b). The thrift of avian influenza in Indonesia. In *Viruses and viral infections in developing countries*. IntechOpen. https://doi.org/10.5772/intechopen.85105

Ray, A. S., & Bhattacharya, K. (2024). An overview on the zoonotic aspects of COVID-19. *Proceedings of the National Academy of Sciences India Section B—Biological Sciences, 94*(1), 9–13. Springer. https://doi.org/10.1007/s40011-023-01445-8

Rehman, S., Effendi, M. H., Witaningruma, A. M., Nnabuikeb, U. E., Bilal, M., Abbas, A., Abbas, R. Z., & Hussain, K. (2023). Avian influenza (H5N1) virus, epidemiology and its effects on backyard poultry in Indonesia: A review. *F1000Research, 11*, 1321. https://doi.org/10.12688/f1000research.125878.2

Sajjadi, N. C., Abolnik, C., Baldinelli, F., Brown, I., Cameron, A., de Wit, S., Dhingra, M., Espeisse, O., Guerrin, J. L., Harder, T., Ho, J., Chua, T. H., Hussein, K., Lyons, N., Monne, I., Okamuro, Y., Pacheco, D. T., Pavade, G., Poncon, N., et al. (2025). Vaccination and surveillance for high pathogenicity avian influenza in poultry—Current situation and perspectives. *Biologicals, 91*. https://doi.org/10.1016/j.biologicals.2025.101840

Scott, J. (2020). Proposed integrated control of zoonotic Plasmodium knowlesi in Southeast Asia using themes of One Health. *Tropical Medicine and Infectious Disease, 5*(4). https://doi.org/10.3390/tropicalmed5040175

Singh, B., & Daneshvar, C. (2010). Plasmodium knowlesi malaria in Malaysia. *SARAWAK, 65*(3), 224–230.

Singh, B., & Daneshvar, C. (2013). Human infections and detection of Plasmodium knowlesi. *Clinical Microbiology Reviews*. https://doi.org/10.1128/CMR.00079-12

Spackman, E. (2014). A brief introduction to Avian influenza virus. In E. Spackman (Ed.), *Animal influenza virus*. Humana Press. http://www.springer.com/series/7651

Stout, A. E., Guo, Q., Millet, J. K., & Whittaker, G. R. (2021). Viral and host attributes underlying the origins of zoonotic coronaviruses in bats. *Comparative Medicine, 71*(5), 442–450. American Association for Laboratory Animal Science. https://doi.org/10.30802/AALAS-CM-21-000027

Suseno, P. P., Ryava, K., Brum, E., De Balogh, K., Diarmita, I. K., Husein, W. F., Mcgrane, J., Rasa, F. S. T., Schoonman, L., Crafter, S., Sumantra, I. P., & Hampson, K. (2019). Lessons for rabies control and elimination programmes: A decade of One Health experience from Bali, Indonesia. *Revue Scientifique et Technique (International Office of Epizootics), 38*(1), 213–224. https://doi.org/10.20506/rst.38.1.2954

Susetya, H., Sugiyama, M., Inagaki, A., Ito, N., Mudiarto, G., & Minamoto, N. (2008). Molecular epidemiology of rabies in Indonesia. *Virus Research, 135*(1), 144–149. https://doi.org/10.1016/j.virusres.2008.03.001

Susilawathi, N. M., Darwinata, A. E., Dwija, I. B. N. P., Budayanti, N. S., Wirasandhi, G. A. K., Subrata, K., Susilarini, N. K., Sudewi, R. A. A., Wignall, F. S., & Mahardika, G. N. K. (2012). Epidemiological and clinical features of human rabies cases in Bali 2008–2010. *BMC Infectious Diseases, 12*. https://doi.org/10.1186/1471-2334-12-81

Swayne, D. E. (2012). Impact of vaccines and vaccination on global control of Avian influenza. *Avian Diseases, 56*(4s1), 818–828. https://doi.org/10.1637/10183-041012-Review.1

Ta, T. H., Hisam, S., Lanza, M., Jiram, A. I., Ismail, N., & Rubio, J. M. (2014). First case of a naturally acquired human infection with Plasmodium cynomolgi. *Malaria Journal, 13*(1). https://doi.org/10.1186/1475-2875-13-68

Takano, R., Nidom, C. A., Kiso, M., Muramoto, Y., Yamada, S., Sakai-Tagawa, Y., Macken, C., & Kawaoka, Y. (2009). Phylogenetic characterization of H5N1 avian influenza viruses isolated in Indonesia from 2003–2007. *Virology, 390*(1), 13–21. https://doi.org/10.1016/j.virol.2009.04.024

Tarigan, S., Indriani, R., Durr, P. A., & Ignjatovic, J. (2015). Characterization of the M2e antibody response following highly pathogenic H5N1 avian influenza virus infection and reliability of M2e ELISA for identifying infected among vaccinated chickens. *Avian Pathology, 44*(4), 259–268. https://doi.org/10.1080/03079457.2015.1042428

Thompson, C. I., Barclay, W. S., Zambon, M. C., & Pickles, R. J. (2006). Infection of human airway epithelium by human and avian strains of influenza A virus. *Journal of Virology, 80*(16), 8060–8068. https://doi.org/10.1128/jvi.00384-06

van de Straat, B., Sebayang, B., Grigg, M. J., Staunton, K., Garjito, T. A., Vythilingam, I., Russell, T. L., & Burkot, T. R. (2022). Zoonotic malaria transmission and land use change in Southeast Asia: what is known about the vectors. *Malaria Journal, 21*(1). https://doi.org/10.1186/s12936-022-04129-2

Walker, P. J., Siddell, S. G., Lefkowitz, E. J., Mushegian, A. R., Adriaenssens, E. M., Alfenas-Zerbini, P., Dempsey, D. M., Dutilh, B. E., García, M. L., Curtis Hendrickson, R., Junglen, S., Krupovic, M., Kuhn, J. H., Lambert, A. J., Łobocka, M., Oksanen, H. M., Orton, R. J., Robertson, D. L., Rubino, L., et al. (2022). Recent changes to virus taxonomy ratified by the International Committee on Taxonomy of Viruses (2022). *Archives of Virology, 167*(11), 2429–2440. https://doi.org/10.1007/s00705-022-05516-5

WHO. (2024, June 5). *Rabies*. https://www.who.int/News-Room/Fact-Sheets/Detail/Rabies

Wibawa, H. (2022). *Avian influenza disease update, control strategy, and poultry vaccination in Indonesia*. https://rr-asia.woah.org/app/uploads/2022/12/3-c-avian-disease-update_indonesia_hendra.pdf

Wibawa, H., Henning, J., Wong, F., Selleck, P., Junaidi, A., Bingham, J., Daniels, P., & Meers, J. (2011). A molecular and antigenic survey of H5N1 highly pathogenic avian influenza virus isolates from smallholder duck farms in Central Java, Indonesia during 2007–2008. *Virology Journal, 8*. https://doi.org/10.1186/1743-422X-8-425

Wibowo, M. H., Susetya, H., Untari, T., Putri, K., Tabbu, C. R., & Asmara, W. (2006). Molecular study on the pathogenicity of AVian influenza virus. *Indonesian Journal Of Biotechnology, 11*(2), 901–907.

Wibowo, M. H., Tarigan, S., Sumarningsih, Artanto, S., Indriani, R., Anggoro, D., Putra, C. P., Idris, S., Untari, T., Asmara, W., Tabbu, C. R., & Ignjatovic, J. (2017). Use of M2e ELISAs for longitudinal surveillance of commercial poultry in Indonesia vaccinated against highly pathogenic avian influenza. *Journal of Virological Methods, 249*, 181–188. https://doi.org/10.1016/j.jviromet.2017.08.014

Widyastuti, M. D. W., Bardosh, K. L., Sunandar, B. C., Basuno, E., Jatikusumah, A., Arief, R. A., Putra, A. A. G., Rukmantara, A., Estoepangestie, A. T. S., Willyanto, I., Natakesuma, I. K. G., Sumantra, I. P., Grace, D., Unger, F., & Gilbert, J. (2015). On dogs, people, and a rabies epidemic: Results from a sociocultural study in Bali, Indonesia. *Infectious Diseases of Poverty, 4*(1). https://doi.org/10.1186/s40249-015-0061-1

WOAH. (2009). AVIAN INFLUENZA. In *OIE terrestrial manual*. World Organization of Animal Health.

WOAH. (2021). Avian influenza. In *WOAH terrestrial manual*. https://www.woah.org/fileadmin/Home/eng/Health_standards/tahm/3.03.04_AI.pdf

WOAH. (2023). Rabies. In *WOAH terrestrial manual* (Vol. 1). WOAH. https://ictv.global/report/chapter/rhabdoviridae/rhabdoviridae/lyssavirus

Wolfe, N. D., Dunavan, C. P., & Diamond, J. (2007). Origins of major human infectious diseases. *Nature, 447*(7142), 279–283. Nature Publishing Group. https://doi.org/10.1038/nature05775

Writing Committee of the Second World Health Organization Consultation on Clinical Aspects of Human Infection with Avian Influenza A (H5N1) Virus. (2008). Avian Influenza A (H5N1) infection in humans. *New England Journal of Medicine, 353*(13), 1374–1385. https://doi.org/10.1056/NEJMra052211

Zaw, M. T., & Lin, Z. (2019). Human Plasmodium knowlesi infections in South-East Asian countries. *Journal of Microbiology, Immunology and Infection, 52*(5). https://doi.org/10.1016/j.jmii.2019.05.012

Zhuang, J., Zang, N., Ye, C., & Xu, F. (2017). *Lethal avian influenza A (H5N1) virus induces ataxic breathing in mice with apoptosis of pre-Botzinger complex neurons expressing neurokinin-1 receptor*. https://doi.org/10.1152/ajplung.00145.2017.-Lethal

Chapter 3
Global Health Governance

Thoriq Abi Pramana, Gilbert Renardi Kusila, Denis Oxy Handika, Brian Arianto Tanuwidjaja, Bayu Satria Wiratama, Widodo Agus Setianto, and Bagas Suryo Bintoro

3.1 International Health Regulations in Asia

The International Health Regulations (IHRs) trace their roots to the mid-nineteenth century, originating from International Sanitary Conventions aimed at preventing disease spread while minimizing disruptions to trade and travel. Over time, the IHR evolved to address the limitations of earlier frameworks, which covered only a few diseases such as cholera, yellow fever, and plague. The revised IHR (2005) expanded both the scope and speed of response by requiring countries to detect, assess, and

T. A. Pramana (✉) · D. O. Handika · B. A. Tanuwidjaja
Master of Public Health Program, Faculty of Medicine, Public Health, and Nursing, Universitas Gadjah Mada, Yogyakarta, Indonesia
e-mail: thoriqabipramana@mail.ugm.ac.id; denisoxyhandika@mail.ugm.ac.id; brian.arianto0903@mail.ugm.ac.id

G. R. Kusila
Center for Health Financing Policy and Health Insurance Management (KPMAK), Universitas Gadjah Mada, Yogyakarta, Indonesia
e-mail: gilbert.renardi.k@mail.ugm.ac.id

B. S. Wiratama
Department of Biostatistics, Epidemiology, and Population Health, Faculty of Medicine, Public Health, and Nursing, Universitas Gadjah Mada, Yogyakarta, Indonesia
e-mail: bayu.satria@ugm.ac.id

W. A. Setianto
Department of Communication Sciences, Faculty of Social Sciences & Political Science, Universitas Gadjah Mada, Yogyakarta, Indonesia
e-mail: widas@ugm.ac.id

B. S. Bintoro
Department of Health Behavior, Environment, and Social Medicine, Faculty of Medicine, Public Health, and Nursing, Universitas Gadjah Mada, Sleman, Yogyakarta, Indonesia
e-mail: bagas.suryo.b@ugm.ac.id

© The Author(s), under exclusive license to Springer Nature Singapore Pte Ltd. 2026

A. U. Rauf, T. Wibawa (eds.), *The One Health Concept in Asian Contexts*,
https://doi.org/10.1007/978-981-95-9880-9_3

report potential Public Health Emergencies of International Concern (PHEIC) within 24 hours (Fidler, 2005; Sah et al., 2022). This marked a shift toward a broader understanding of health security that intersects with governance, equity, and cross-sector collaboration, principles that are central to the One Health approach.

The IHR (2005) outlines core capacities for preparedness and response, later refined into 15 capacities in the Self-Assessment Annual Reporting (SPAR) tool. These include laboratory and surveillance systems, zoonotic disease control, food safety, and risk communication that align directly with One Health priorities. By explicitly including zoonotic threats and environmental health factors, the IHR framework acknowledges that health risks often emerge at the interface of humans, animals, and ecosystems (Broberg, 2020; Buzgan & Güner, 2020; Gostin & Katz, 2016). Integrating these dimensions into national capacities strengthens resilience against future pandemics.

As a legally binding agreement among 196 States Parties, the IHR provides a mechanism for coordinated action against health threats, many of which are zoonotic in origin, such as avian influenza, Ebola, and COVID-19. The World Health Organization (WHO)'s authority to declare a PHEIC enables rapid mobilization of multisectoral responses involving public health, veterinary services, and environmental management. However, the COVID-19 pandemic exposed critical weaknesses, including delayed reporting, inadequate enforcement, and insufficient integration of non-health sectors in decision-making processes (Guetiya Wadoum et al., 2021; Ratzan et al., 2020).

Reforms to strengthen the IHR increasingly emphasize the One Health perspective, advocating for faster reporting, mandatory sharing of pathogen genetic data, and stronger coordination between human, animal, and environmental health sectors (Mayank & Saxena, 2024; The Lancet Global Health, 2022). Aligning IHR implementation with One Health and Universal Health Coverage agendas can build more inclusive, well-resourced, and responsive systems. Such integration not only enhances outbreak preparedness but also addresses the broader ecological and social drivers of emerging diseases, supporting sustainable global health security (Pagotto & Eccleston-Turner, 2024).

3.1.1 Implementation Challenges and Gaps

There are various problems concerning the implementation of the International Health Regulations (IHRs) both globally and in Asia. These include insufficient financial and technical resources, a lack of enforcement procedures, and insufficient international cooperation. Uncoordinated government departments and a lack of defined emergency response facilities are among the issues encountered at points of entry, such as airports. Developing countries face challenges in combining enforcement with government authority and human rights. They also have inadequate surveillance and reporting infrastructure. The COVID-19 pandemic has shown additional limits in IHR implementation, underlining the need for adjustment to improve global health security (Sturtevant et al., 2007).

The challenges of transparency and reporting in Asia during the early phase of COVID-19 were significant, impacting the effectiveness of the International Health Regulations (IHRs). The initial outbreak in Wuhan highlighted operational deficiencies in the IHR, particularly regarding timely information sharing and compliance among member states. Countries like China initially controlled the flow of information, delaying the WHO's ability to declare a public health emergency. This lack of transparency hindered a coordinated global response, as countries struggled to report accurate data and share critical information.

Furthermore, the IHR's cumbersome processes for evaluating outbreaks led to delays in international alerts, undermining timely interventions. The IHR urges states to notify the WHO regarding potential public health emergencies using a decision procedure, which can be complicated and time-consuming. The self-assessment method for core competencies differs substantially among countries, resulting in inconsistent reporting and delays in notifying the WHO (Fischer & Katz, 2013). While the early phase of COVID-19 revealed significant transparency and reporting issues, it also underscored the necessity for improved international cooperation and regulatory frameworks to better manage future health crises.

3.1.2 International Health Regulations

While the International Health Regulations (IHRs) serve as the main legal instrument for managing cross-border public health threats, they lack explicit mechanisms for implementing the One Health approach (De La Rocque et al., 2021). One Health acknowledges the interconnectedness of human, animal, and environmental health and is essential for preventing, detecting, and responding to zoonotic diseases, antimicrobial resistance (AMR), and climate-sensitive health risks (Adnyana et al., 2023). The COVID-19 pandemic highlighted the boundaries of the current IHR framework in dealing with zoonotic epidemics. Although countries are required to build core capacities, the IHR (2005) does not obligate multisectoral coordination, resulting in fragmented surveillance and response systems, particularly in low- and middle-income countries (Santalucia et al., 2025).

In Asia, countries like Indonesia, Thailand, and Vietnam have established national One Health coordination mechanisms. However, these often operate in silos, separated from IHR implementation. Recent studies indicate that most countries have not fully integrated animal and environmental health systems into their national health security plans (Adnyana et al., 2023; Morris & Wang, 2024).

Efforts by the Quadripartite (WHO, FAO, WOAH, and UNEP) to institutionalize One Health are ongoing, including the One Health Joint Plan of Action (2022–2026) (WHO, 2022b). Yet, a legal gap remains between international frameworks and operational practices. Without revisions to the IHR to include mandates for intersectoral coordination, One Health implementation will remain inconsistent (De La Rocque et al., 2021). Critical question: *Is the IHR sufficiently adaptable to support One Health in Asia?* Experts argue that a reformed IHR must include provisions for intersectoral early warning systems, data sharing protocols, and integrated workforce capacity across human, veterinary, and environmental sectors (Carlson & Phelan, 2022; Negri & Eccleston-Turner, 2022).

The COVID-19 pandemic has accelerated global efforts to reform the International Health Regulations (IHRs). Since 2022, WHO Member States have been negotiating targeted amendments to address weaknesses in early detection, equity, and compliance, alongside the drafting of a new pandemic agreement to complement and strengthen the IHR (Santalucia et al., 2025). Proposed reforms include stronger reporting obligations, improved access to medical countermeasures, and greater international support for countries with limited capacities, though negotiations remain sensitive on sovereignty and transparency (Burci & Negri, 2022; Eccleston-Turner et al., 2023).

In the Asia-Pacific, countries have approached the reform agenda with cautious but increasing engagement. Several ASEAN Member States advocate for a balanced approach that strengthens global health governance while ensuring fairness for low- and middle-income countries (Caballero-Anthony, 2018; Cook, 2021). Key priorities include international financial and technical assistance, equitable access to health technologies during emergencies, and stronger regional cooperation through ASEAN and other platforms. Asia's experience with outbreaks such as SARS, H5N1, MERS, and COVID-19 underscores the need for coordinated, multisectoral strategies. However, disparities in national capacities and fragmented governance hinder a unified regional position. Regional organizations such as ASEAN, ADB, and WHO-SEARO can bridge these gaps by harmonizing priorities, building capacity, and fostering health diplomacy rooted in the One Health approach (Durrance-Bagale et al., 2022).

The IHRs (2005) remain central to global health governance, but adapting them to Asia's unique challenges, where zoonotic diseases, environmental degradation, and inequities converge, requires urgent integration of One Health principles. This includes legal frameworks for multisectoral coordination, interoperable surveillance systems that integrate human, animal, and environmental health data, and equitable resource allocation, technical support, and access to emergency tools for low-capacity countries. With the right reforms, Asia can transition from being primarily at risk to becoming a global leader in embedding equity, One Health, and resilience into the evolving IHR system.

3.2 Global Health Funding Mechanisms and Challenges

3.2.1 Asia's Health Landscape

The Asia-Pacific region counts more than half of the global population with the recent International Monetary Fund (2025) data showing 4.47 billion people living in the region, of which 75% of them living in East and South Asia (International

Monetary Fund, 2022). Countries such as India, Mongolia, Kirgiz Republic, and Tajikistan experience >6% gross domestic product (GDP) growth in 2025 compared to the similar period in 2025, while more countries have marked >4% GDP growth. With its growth, some health indicators have also improved. Nevertheless, the challenge in health financing remains as national health spending as a share of GDP does not always align with higher UHC Index scores (Barcellona et al., 2023). Inequality persists across the region: In 2021, life expectancy ranged from 66 years in Myanmar to 79 years in Thailand, while maternal mortality was estimated at 178 per 100,000 live births in Indonesia compared to only 7.3 in Singapore (World Health Organization, 2023). Nevertheless, Southeast Asia has shown an increased commitment to UHC and health financing reform (Barcellona et al., 2023).

Bangladesh, the most densely populated country in the world, has been cut by half from 4.5 in 1990 to 2.2 births per woman in 2022. Their poverty headcount has dropped from 41% of total population in 2000 to 8% in 2023. Their life expectancy has reached 75, outnumbering its neighboring countries. The government of Bangladesh initiated a health financing scheme called Shasthyo Surokhsha Karmasuchi, which was piloted in 2017 as a result of the government Health Care Financing Strategy in 2012 aiming to achieve Universal Health Coverage (UHC) by 2032 and has covered 96,432 households (Hasan et al., 2022). Still, after the expansion of the program, the out-of-pocket (OOP) expenditure among the population remains high. It peaked during the COVID-19 pandemic and only slightly reduced to 72.53% of total health expenditures in 2022, which equals US$44.31. On the contrary, the government portion in health spending showed a declining trend from 21.23% of the health expenditure in 2017 to only 6.48% in 2022 (World Bank, 2022).

Indonesia, the most archipelagic country, has total health expenditure amounted to approximately Rp 614.5 trillion (about US$375.5 billion), with public funding contributing 57.4%, while out-of-pocket (OOP) spending accounted for 28.6% of total health expenditure—showing a gradual reduction from 30.6% in 2022 (World Health Organization, 2025). Government health spending stood at just 2.9% of GDP, underscoring the limited yet essential role of public funding in national healthcare (World Health Organization, 2025). Meanwhile, Indonesia's national health insurance system, Jaminan Kesehatan Nasional (JKN), targets for 98% overall participation in NHI to support UHC's goals regarding financial protection and equitable accessibility to healthcare (Indonesia, 2020). As of June 30, 2024, JKN membership coverage had reached 273.5 million people, equivalent to 96.83% of Indonesia's total population in the second semester of 2024 (DJSN, 2024). Misnaniarti et al. (2025) reported lower coverage as of 2023, about 72.5% of the adult (>15 yo) population was enrolled, while initiatives remain underway to reach those in remote and underserved regions.

Thailand presents another interesting issue. It is considered a global model for achieving UHC. Introduced in 2001, their Universal Coverage Scheme (UCS) allocates per capita budget, which mainly derived from tax-based financing (Tangcharoensathien et al., 2020). Each citizen entitled to one of the three UCSs based on their eligibility criteria. The first is the Civil Servant Medical Benefit Scheme, whose funding derived from general tax revenue. It has covered 7% of the population, including the retired public servants and their dependents. The other UCS called the Social Security Scheme is mandatory for private sector employees, and the scheme has covered 18% of Thailand population. The 30 Baht UCS covered the rest of the population (74%) regardless of their socioeconomic status and is funded almost fully by the government. The scheme requires 30 Baht (US$ 1) copayment for certain healthcare facility visits and utilizes the primary care as the gatekeeper before referring to the higher level of care (Tangcharoensathien et al., 2020). *Nevertheless, Thailand is now an "aged society" with 14.7% population aged ≥65 years and a median age of over 40* (Sakamoto, 2025). Some media even mentioned that Thailand is getting old before getting rich (The Economist, 2023). The country must address the rising costs of eldercare and chronic diseases. The government-based financing becomes a long-term concern when the productive age decreases, which will increase the demographic dependency ratio.

Across Asia, countries face a double burden of disease. Noncommunicable diseases (NCDs) such as diabetes, cardiovascular disease, and cancer now account for more deaths than the infectious ones. At the same time, infectious diseases such as dengue, tuberculosis, and hepatitis continue to burden health systems. These overlapping burdens often drive households into poverty due to high out-of-pocket payments and loss of income, which further emphasize the needs of health financing collaboration.

3.2.2 The Path to UHC: Financing Innovations and Partnerships

Innovative financing strategies and strategic partnerships have emerged as critical tools as UHC is recognized as a foundational goal for improving population health.

Domestic resource mobilization remains the backbone of sustainable UHC. The Philippines and Indonesia are two countries that have implemented sin-tax reforms to fund their UCS. In the Philippines, the Sin Tax Reform Act of 2012 and its 2020 expansion increased excise taxes on cigarettes, alcoholic beverages, and sugary drinks, with a portion of the revenue earmarked for the Philippine Health Insurance Corporation (PhilHealth) (Obermann et al., 2018). Similarly, Indonesia passed a tobacco excise reform that resulted in the Tobacco Excise Sharing Fund (DBHCHT) between the central and regional governments to fund several priority programs. According to the 2017 Minister of Health Decree (PMK), at least 50% of the allocated budget was required to support the National Health Insurance program (JKN). However, the updated PMK in 2020 no longer specifies a dedicated portion for JKN. Instead, it only mandates that 25% of the funds be used for general healthcare improvements (Ahsan et al., 2024). The main advantage of using sin taxes is the dual benefit of reducing consumption of harmful products while generating health financing. However, challenges remain: Sin-tax revenues may fluctuate due to declining consumption, and enforcement can be weak in regions with high illicit trade. Additionally, over-reliance on sin tax can be regressive, disproportionately affecting lower income populations who are more likely to consume taxed products

Social impact bond (SIB) is another financing mechanism where private investors fund social programs upfront and are repaid by governments or donors only if the program achieves measurable results (Katz et al., 2018; Mishra & Dash, 2023). This outcome-based approach shifts financial risk away from governments and incentivizes effective service delivery. The funding process involves three main actors: investors who provide initial capital, service providers who implement the program, and outcome funders (usually governments or foundations) who repay the investors if the agreed outcomes are met. High-income countries like South Korea, Japan, and the United Arab Emirates have adopted SIBs to improve various areas such as health care, education, and employment (Mishra & Dash, 2023).

India piloted the first maternal and newborn SIB, called Utkrisht Impact Bond in Rajasthan. The UBS Optimus Foundation acted as the investor, the program was implemented by Population Services International (PSI) and its local partner HLFPP, while the outcome funders like USAID and Merck for Mothers repaid the investors with a return based on the outcome (Bärnreuther, 2025; Mishra & Dash, 2023). Although SIBs may seem like an innovative approach, they have several major drawbacks, such as restricting program scope over time and being highly speculative due to investor concerns. Furthermore, initiating such programs can be costly and complex to design, with high legal and administrative fees, and they often result in policy fragmentation (Katz et al., 2018).

Risk pooling is another UCS mechanism of Universal Health Coverage (UHC). It enables the redistribution of healthcare costs across different population groups. In China, this is exemplified by two major insurance schemes: the Urban Employee Basic Medical Insurance (UEBMI) and the Urban–Rural Resident Basic Medical Insurance (URRBMI). UEBMI is essential for formally employed urban workers and jointly financed by employers and employees, offering more generous benefits and higher reimbursement rates. In contrast, URRBMI is a voluntary, government-subsidized scheme covering informal workers, children, the elderly, and rural residents, with more limited benefit packages and lower reimbursement ceilings. Over the last two decades, the URRBMI premium has surged from RMB 10 (USD 1.4) in 2003 to RMB 380 (USD 53.1) in 2024, marking a 38-fold increase, which has in some cases encouraged disenrollment (Zhang et al., 2024).

UHC is beyond the self-financing and curative purposes. It also amplifies the importance of partnership and disease prevention. Transboundary diseases, climate change, and shared environmental risks require collective responses that transcend national borders. The Mekong Basin Disease Surveillance (MBDS) network comprises Cambodia, Laos, Myanmar, Thailand, Vietnam, and China (Yunnan province). MBDS was established to improve real-time sharing of disease surveillance data, coordinate outbreak responses, and build laboratory capacity (Phommasack et al., 2013). In East Asia, environmental health challenges have spurred innovative collaboration. The Trilateral Environmental Ministers Meeting (TEMM) involving China, Japan, and South Korea addresses transboundary air pollution, particularly the yellow dust originating from the Gobi Desert (Zhang, 2024). Another partnership was made by the Gulf Cooperation Council (GCC) countries. Recognizing the cross-border nature of food trade in the region, the GCC developed a coordinated regulatory framework through ministerial-level consensus and regional health summits. One significant outcome of this collaboration was the adoption of a unified nutrition labeling policy across all member states (Fadhil et al., 2022).

3.2.3 Challenges and the Future Ahead

Despite progress, several major challenges threaten the momentum of health financing and partnerships in Asia.

One of the foremost challenges in sustaining health programs in Asia is the transition from donor support, which can significantly disrupt program continuity. As countries experience economic growth and are reclassified as middle-income, they often "graduate" from eligibility for external assistance, such as that provided by Gavi, the Vaccine Alliance. However, this shift can create funding gaps, particularly in financing essential public health services like immunization. Countries such as Sri Lanka have transitioned in 2015 (Cernuschi et al., 2018; Kolesar et al., 2023). However, the impact of the economic and political crisis in 2022 may generate difficulties following donor transition, especially in procuring vaccines at affordable prices due to limited bargaining power and weaker domestic procurement systems. Other transitioned countries like Mongolia, Turkmenistan, Indonesia, and Vietnam could find similar challenges, which could exacerbate after the COVID-19 pandemic.

Second, geopolitical tensions and global uncertainties can indirectly affect health systems. The conflict between Iran and Israel, and the potential closure of the Strait of Hormuz, could disrupt oil flows and raise global energy prices. This would increase transportation and production costs for medical goods, many of which rely on petroleum-based raw materials or energy-intensive supply chains.

Third, there are concerns about the sustainability of external financing. The closure or downsizing of USAID programs in middle-income countries has left gaps in areas like HIV prevention, maternal health, and health systems strengthening. Without careful transition strategies, sudden exits can disrupt services and weaken institutional capacity.

Finally, medicine pricing and equitable access to essential drugs remain a significant challenge in many Asian countries, especially those with limited public health budgets. One key strategy to address this is compulsory licensing, a legal mechanism that allows governments to bypass patent protections and authorize the production or importation of generic versions of patented medicines in the interest of public health. This approach has been employed by countries such as India, Thailand, and Indonesia, particularly during public health emergencies or when medicine prices were prohibitively high. For instance, in the mid-2000s, Thailand issued compulsory licenses for several life-saving drugs, including antiretrovirals (ARVs) for HIV/AIDS, resulting in a sharp decrease in treatment costs and wider coverage (Kuanpoth, 2015). In recent years, voluntary licensing has emerged as a more collaborative alternative, where pharmaceutical patent holders grant licenses to generic manufacturers, often coordinated through mechanisms like the Medicines Patent Pool (MPP). This model, sometimes implemented on a royalty-free basis for low- and middle-income countries, played a critical role during the COVID-19 pandemic by enabling broader and quicker access to oral antivirals such as molnupiravir and nirmatrelvir/ritonavir (Paxlovid).

3.3 Global Health Partnerships and Their Impact on Health Outcomes

Zoonotic disease outbreaks have intensified across Asia, reflecting the growing entanglement of human, animal, and environmental health (Goldstein et al., 2022). However, integrated surveillance that spans these sectors remains limited, pointing to persistent challenges in translating One Health (OH) principles into practice. These limitations highlight broader issues in health governance and underscore the uneven, yet often essential, role that Global Health Partnerships (GHPs) play in shaping regional responses (Tegegne et al., 2024).

Global health partnerships are cooperative arrangements where various actors, including national governments, international agencies (like WHO), global funds, donor countries, private companies, and civil society organizations, coordinate efforts toward shared health goals. These partnerships gained prominence in the early twenty-first century with the advent of major global health initiatives targeting specific diseases or issues. Notably, the Global Fund (established in 2002) channels international financing to support country programs against HIV/AIDS, tuberculosis (TB), and malaria, while Gavi (founded in 2000) pools resources to expand vaccine access in low-income regions. WHO plays a complementary role by providing technical guidance, setting norms (e.g., treatment guidelines and vaccine prequalification), and coordinating health actions among partners. These collaborations align with broader agendas like the United Nations Sustainable Development Goals, especially SDG 3 ("Ensure healthy lives and promote well-being for all ages"), which explicitly recognizes the need for international cooperation (Cernuschi et al., 2018; Kolesar et al., 2023).

3.3.1 Typology of Global Health Partnerships in Asia's One Health Landscape

Public–private partnerships (PPPs) have become influential drivers of innovation and equity, particularly in zoonotic disease control. Initiatives like Gavi have expanded vaccine access through cofinancing mechanisms, strengthening national systems while promoting donor-prioritized diseases (WHO, 2022a). Similarly, platforms like the GHIT Fund channel investment into neglected diseases at the human–animal–environment interface, though their agendas often remain centered on biomedical innovation (GHIT, 2024). While these PPPs foster access and R&D, their transformative potential for OH is often constrained by vertical disease targeting and limited ecological integration.

Collaborations between multilateral institutions and bilateral donors have sought to institutionalize OH through policy harmonization and technical assistance. Recent investment efforts have combined immunization infrastructure with emerging surveillance functions, particularly in regions vulnerable to antimicrobial resistance (Sihombing et al., 2023). However, many such partnerships still reflect external policy agendas and asymmetrical governance structures, often excluding environmental actors from key decision-making processes (Abbas et al., 2022). Despite providing critical funding and expertise, their alignment with regional ownership and cross-sector equity remains limited.

Regional consortia facilitate coordinated responses to transboundary OH threats by promoting joint surveillance and governance frameworks. Networks in the Mekong region, for instance, have enabled more timely outbreak response and data sharing across countries (Phommasack et al., 2013). However, despite initial successes in outbreak containment, many face long-term sustainability challenges due to unpredictable financing and uneven institutional support (Hegde et al., 2024). These consortia highlight the promise of regional solidarity, while also revealing the fragility of initiatives reliant on short-term political or donor momentum.

University-led and research-based partnerships are key to strengthening OH capacity, particularly through workforce development and integrated surveillance systems. Training networks have made significant progress in some countries, yet regional disparities in workforce placement and intersectoral data sharing persist (SEAOHUN, 2023). Inconsistent adoption of integrated surveillance platforms is often linked to institutional silos and incompatible data infrastructures across ministries (Carter et al., 2024). A challenge remains in information integration, as most Southeast Asian health systems struggle with fragmented and non-interoperable data (de Smalen et al., 2021). These academic-led networks demonstrate the importance of knowledge generation and system building, while underscoring the operational and policy-level barriers that inhibit scalability. Philanthropic and experimental platforms contribute to agile, community-driven models for OH practice. Some have supported grassroots surveillance initiatives and technological innovation in diagnostics and data systems. However, these efforts often remain pilot-bound, lacking structural integration into public health systems. Without sustained government engagement and policy anchoring, their long-term impact and scalability remain uncertain. Such platforms not only offer valuable lessons in localization but also raise questions about fragmentation and replicability (Averhoff et al., 2022).

3.3.2 Case Studies and Challenges

Thailand's National Avian Influenza Surveillance System exemplifies institutionalized cross-sector coordination. Following the 2004 H5N1 outbreak, Thailand established the *Coordinating Unit for One Health* (CUOH), integrating surveillance efforts across the human (Ministry of Public Health), animal (Department of Livestock Development), and environmental (Department of National Parks) sectors. The system has enhanced surveillance responsiveness by implementing mobile reporting in live bird markets, establishing a unified laboratory network covering 43 provinces, and deploying joint field teams trained through the Field Epidemiology Training Program for Veterinarians (FETPV). The system introduced timeliness targets, including collecting samples within 24 h of abnormal events and obtaining laboratory results within 48 h, marking a significant step toward faster outbreak response (Innes et al., 2022). However, CUOH's sustainability remains challenged by its reliance on external funding. Despite its contributions to national health security, the program continues to depend heavily on donor support, which raises concerns about long-term resilience without greater integration into Thailand's domestic budget systems (Tangwangvivat et al., 2024).

MBDS is a pioneering regional health partnership involving six countries Cambodia, China (Yunnan province), Lao PDR, Myanmar, Thailand, and Vietnam established in the early 2000s to combat transboundary disease threats. It operates through formal memoranda of understanding among health ministries and fosters cross-border collaboration through joint outbreak investigations, real-time event-based surveillance, simulation exercises, and training of field epidemiologists (McPake et al., 2022). MBDS successfully facilitated early responses to avian influenza and dengue outbreaks, enhancing trust among member states. Its unique "trust-based" model has been cited as a regional prototype for collaborative health governance (Lawpoolsri et al., 2018). Nevertheless, differences in national capacities, uneven data-sharing mechanisms, and varying levels of institutional support remain key barriers to optimal effectiveness (Moore & Dausey, 2015).

One of the enduring challenges is the persistent fragmentation among ministries of health, agriculture, and environment, each operating within siloed mandates. While coordination mechanisms have been introduced in several countries, many remain ad hoc, under-resourced, or donor-driven (Sanga et al., 2024). In Indonesia, for instance, OH platforms are still largely project-based and have not yet been meaningfully embedded into national development planning or fiscal frameworks. This reflects a broader tendency to treat One Health as an auxiliary or optional initiative rather than a transformative framework for health governance (Adnyana et al., 2023). Environmental health, frequently described as the "third pillar" of OH, remains particularly marginalized, with environmental ministries often excluded from policymaking processes and intersectoral funding allocations (Dash & Rath, 2021).

Another critical issue is the misalignment between globally driven OH agendas and locally prioritized health needs (Cleaveland et al., 2017). Donor funding often favors high-profile concerns such as pandemic preparedness or antimicrobial resistance (AMR), while endemic but locally significant issues such as leptospirosis, food safety, or wildlife–human interface diseases receive less attention, particularly in countries like Laos or Indonesia. This asymmetry reinforces power imbalances in agenda-setting and weakens local ownership (Adnyana et al., 2023).

The overreliance on external funding sources continues to pose a barrier to sustainable OH implementation. Training networks like the Southeast Asia One Health University Network (SEAOHUN), while successful in workforce development, often struggle to secure domestic cofinancing or institutional mandates (SEAOHUN, 2023). Without long-term budget commitments, these programs remain vulnerable to donor fatigue, leading to workforce attrition and limited career pathways for OH professionals. This raises concerns about national health sovereignty and the capacity to build context-specific systems that are resilient beyond the life cycle of externally funded projects (Yopa et al., 2023).

While conceptual support for One Health is increasingly robust, its operationalization remains hindered by the lack of standardized frameworks for implementation and monitoring. Global guidelines such as the Quadripartite Joint Plan provide broad recommendations but often fall short on localized application tools (Milazzo et al., 2025). In most Asian contexts, indicators for cross-sector collaboration, ecological health integration, or joint response effectiveness are poorly defined or inconsistently applied (Sanga et al., 2024). As a result, OH risks remain an aspirational concept, with limited tools for performance evaluation or institutional accountability.

3.4 Global Health Diplomacy and Its Role in Addressing Global Health Challenges

Global Health Diplomacy (GHD) defines a multilevel, multi-actor negotiation and coordination approach that influences the global health policy environment by linking public health, international relations, and foreign policy goals. Kickbusch et al. define GHD as the strategic collaboration among a wide range of stakeholders, including nations, international organizations, civil society, and scientific experts, in advancing collective health goals through diplomatic instruments (Kickbusch, 2007). The World Health Organization (WHO) fosters GHD as a method for resolving transboundary health challenges, stating that international cooperation is required to promote health security, equity, and preparedness (Alwan, 2014).

In the Asian context, GHD is increasingly framed as both a soft power tool and a platform for collaboration, as evidenced by ASEAN's coordinated pandemic responses, regional antimicrobial resistance action plans, and collaborative frameworks such as the Asia-Pacific Strategy for Emerging Diseases (ASEAN, 2020;

WHO Western Pacific, 2017). Unlike general diplomacy, which is frequently focused on national interests, GHD in Asia is characterized by consensus-building norms and shared vulnerability, notably in dealing with new zoonotic risks, pandemic preparedness, and universal health coverage (UHC). Thus, GHD in Asia serves not just as an intermediary for policy negotiation but also as a regional devotion to health as a shared objective across political and cultural impediments. However, there is a need for more comprehensive efforts to address emerging health issues such as climate-related diseases, antimicrobial resistance, and noncommunicable diseases (Caballero-Anthony, 2018).

The COVID-19 pandemic provides valuable lessons learned about how efforts to deal with health problems require adequate global health diplomacy. With 60% of the world's population living in Asia, issues related to pandemic preparedness, zoonotic disease control, climate-induced health risks, and antimicrobial resistance require a GHD approach that is oriented toward regional interests. This will have a global impact if handled locally without such an approach. GHD promotes a One Health approach, integrating human, animal, and environmental health to combat zoonotic diseases, antimicrobial resistance (AMR), and climate-induced health risks (Dahal et al., 2017; Hernandez et al., 2025). GHD also supports the development of innovative, cost-effective solutions for resource-limited nations, such as universal health coverage and modified One Health approaches (Chen et al., 2019). By fostering coordination, communication, and collaboration across sectors and regions, GHD enhances pandemic preparedness and enables more effective responses to complex health challenges.

In practice, GHD is not only carried out by the government to government (G to G) as the actor but also involves regional organizations, non-state actors, and donors that have interest in health issues. In Asia, the key stakeholders in GHD include the World Health Organization's South-East Asia Regional Office (WHO SEARO) and Western Pacific Regional Office (WPRO), ASEAN, and individual health ministries. These actors support countries in addressing health risks related to climate change and are involved in multi-stakeholder diplomacy for noncommunicable diseases prevention and control. Moreover, China's Health Silk Road initiative, part of the Belt and Road Initiative (BRI), aims to enhance global health cooperation and combat infectious diseases across 69 countries (Chen et al., 2019). Regional civil society organizations (CSOs) play a role in implementing the One Health approach, which fosters collaboration between human, animal, and environmental health sectors in South Asian countries like Bangladesh, Bhutan, India, and Nepal (Goldstein et al., 2022). Table 3.1 presents the seven dimensions of global health diplomacy proposed by Kickbusch et al. (2007), the example of each dimension in Asia, and its relevance in one health context.

Kickbusch et al. proposed seven dimensions of global health diplomacy to better understand its contents (Kickbusch, 2007). Each has an essential function in addressing global health concerns. These include negotiating health objectives in the face of competing geopolitical interests, as experienced in the TRIPS waiver discussion, as well as building new governance models like ACPHEED and APSED III to improve regional preparedness. Diplomatic ties, such as ASEAN+3 FETN,

Table 3.1 Seven dimensions of global health diplomacy

Dimension	Description	Asian example	One Health relevance
Negotiating interests	Health vs. geopolitics	TRIPS waiver debate	Access to zoonotic disease countermeasures
New governance	Create/adapt institutions	ACPHEED, APSED III	Surveillance integration
Alliances	Political/ regional blocs	ASEAN+3 FETN	Coordinated outbreak response
Donor relations	Funding alignment	ADB & UHC in Philippines	Cross-sector donor mapping
Crisis response	Urgent coordination	COVID-19 ASEAN response fund	Early detection networks
Relationship building	Health as soft power	China's Health Silk Road	Trust-building in regional health
Peace and security	Health for ceasefires	Cross-border vaccination in Myanmar	Humanitarian access

help to coordinate epidemic responses, while donor relations, such as ADB's aid for universal health coverage in the Philippines, assure long-term cross-sector finance. Global health diplomacy is particularly important in disaster response, as evidenced by the COVID-19 ASEAN response fund, which facilitated early detection and joint regional action. Relationship building efforts, such as China's Health Silk Road, employ health as soft power to promote trust and strengthen regional ties. Finally, diplomacy promotes peace and security by facilitating humanitarian health initiatives, such as cross-border immunization efforts in conflict-affected places like Myanmar. Together, these components strengthen the One Health agenda by integrating human, animal, and environmental health concerns across national borders.

3.4.1 The ASEAN Leaders' Declaration on One Health Initiative

The ASEAN Leaders' Declaration on One Health Initiative was signed amid the 42nd ASEAN Summit in Labuan Bajo, Indonesia, upon May 10–11, 2023. The work was prompted by increasing awareness of the One Health plan for addressing health challenges in the region. This initiative consists of seven points of commitments that promotes the One Health action in region such as (ASEAN, 2023):

1. Strengthen ASEAN Member States' cross-sectoral collaboration in areas such as human, animal, plant, environmental, and food safety.
2. Encourage bilateral and multilateral cooperation to facilitate One Health implementation on a national and regional scale.
3. Collaborate with international and development partners to support One Health through sustainable and innovative financing.

4. Consolidate and link all One Health programs with relevant sectors, such as public health, agriculture, wildlife, the environment, and food systems.
5. Implement One Health in ASEAN sectoral bodies to promote collective prevention, detection, and response to future health hazards.
6. Increase regional and national capacity to improve the health of humans, animals, plants, and the environment.
7. Mandate ASEAN Health Ministers to work with other ASEAN sectoral ministers and stakeholders to coordinate, consult, and monitor One Health initiatives.

The declaration demonstrates how GHD enables countries to reconcile national interests with regional solidarity, enhance diplomatic ties across ministries, and encourage mutual responsibility for emerging health threats, all hallmarks of the One Health strategy. In this context, GHD provides both a mechanism and a platform for ASEAN states to align policies, pool resources, and rally political support for a common objective: safeguarding health at the human–animal–environment interface.

3.4.2 Belt and Road Initiative: China's Health Silk Road

China's Health Silk Road (HSR), a component of the Belt and Road Initiative, is an important example of bilateral global health diplomacy in Asia. The HSR, which aims to improve international healthcare collaboration and elevate the Global South's role in health governance, rose to prominence during the COVID-19 pandemic thanks to vaccine contributions, medical supplies, and infrastructure support. This health aid boosted China's diplomatic relations by portraying health as an instrument for mutual trust and preparation. While the program has been well received in countries such as the Middle East and North Africa, it has also prompted worries about transparency, product quality, and geopolitical impact, especially in light of strategic tensions with the United States. Despite these issues, the HSR helps shape global health governance and could potentially play an increasingly important role in future pandemic preparedness. However, insufficient awareness in some countries, such as Brazil, shows that further research is needed on the long-term impact and consequences for health sovereignty (Santiago & Rodrigues, 2023; Zeng et al., 2023; Zoubir & Tran, 2022).

3.4.3 World Health Assembly (WHA)

The World Health Assembly (WHA) is an iconic symbol of global health diplomacy, encouraging negotiations and collaboration among member countries to address major health concerns. This platform shows how health diplomacy may transcend traditional political boundaries, as evidenced by Taiwan's observer status, which was obtained after long talks that emphasized the connection between health and sovereignty concerns (Herington & Lee, 2014). The WHA has also played an important role in tackling global health crises, such as the current proposal to develop a pandemic treaty, which highlights the importance of international collaboration in health governance (Chattu et al., 2024).

3.5 Media and Health Communication in Asia

Health communication and mass media are essential resources for those with a professional or academic interest in health communication (Ahmed & Bates, 2016). Mass media plays a multifaceted role in global health (Jeyaraman et al., 2023; Pacheco, 2023). Mass media serves as communication tools to educate the public, disseminate health information, raise awareness of disease prevention, encourage public health initiatives, and promote positive health behaviors (Asemah, 2023; Ghahramani et al., 2022; Ouchene et al., 2024; Swarup Garg, 2023). Mass media serves as a crucial communication platform between health experts and the public, helping translate complex scientific information into understandable language (Reveilhac, 2022; Van Bekkum & Hilton, 2013). Mass media is also a means of holding the government and decision-makers accountable for health policies (Aghaei & Mowlaei, 2023; Mykkänen & Valentini, 2025; Renuka & Bhavsar, 2023).

Health communication in Asia is a growing and diverse field, characterized by not only rapid development and opportunities but also challenges (Paek et al., 2010; Pun et al., 2018). Mass media is crucial in facilitating the development of health communication in Asia. Asia is the world's largest and most populous continent, encompassing nearly a third of the world's land area and approximately 60% of the world's population, stretching from the Arctic Ocean in the north to the Indian Ocean in the south and from the Pacific Ocean in the east to Europe and the Mediterranean Ocean in the west (Antara, 2025). Not only is Asia the largest continent, but it is also a melting pot of cultures, religions, and histories. There are 48 countries with diverse forms of government, with authoritarian or semi-authoritarian forms of power (Hiariej, 1997; Rochayati, 2017; Zhupankhan et al., 2017). In terms of health communication, Asia attracts attention not only as the largest and most populous region in the world with high health disparities (Lee et al., 2015) but also as a region with a substantial high burden of disease (Kheng, 2022). A substantial burden of disease indicates a large disease burden and a high impact on individuals and society as a whole in terms of risk, morbidity, mortality, and significant socio-economic impacts due to a disease. With its vast territory, diversity of cultures, languages, and social norms, Asia presents a unique challenge for health communication in disseminating health information (Afifi et al., 2024).

Health communication in Asia is strengthened not only by mainstream media but also by advances in communication and information technology, including the advancement of revolutionary media in the way of digital or online materials. Asian countries are frequently at the cutting edge of embracing to technical breakthroughs and accelerating the diffusion of technology (Nageshwaran et al., 2021). Millions of individuals in Asia utilize social media platforms every day, including for health concerns (Willnat & Aw, 2014). Researchers have focused on digital media, particularly social media, in their studies on health communication and social media within the Asian context, including Mohsin et al. (2023), Duong et al. (2021), Wu et al. (2024), Nabi et al. (2023), Liu and Zou (2024), and Novera et al. (2024).

3.5.1 The Role of Mass Media in Health Communication in Asia

Mass media, often referred to as mass communication media, is a communication device or communication channel used to convey messages, information, and entertainment to a wide audience simultaneously (Anggarwal & Singh, 2022). The word "mass" in mass media indicates a very large number of people reached, while "media" means a channel or intermediary for messages or information to be conveyed. Mass media acts as an intermediary to reach a large public, overcoming the barriers of space and time. Mass media is generally grouped into several categories, namely (1) Print Media including newspapers, magazines, and tabloids that present information in the form of writing and images on paper, (2) Electronic Media including radio (audio) and television (audio-visual) that broadcast programs via electromagnetic waves or the Internet, (3) Digital Media: media that can be accessed via the Internet (online), such as news websites, blogs, podcasts, streaming services, and video platforms such as YouTube and social media, and (4) Out-of-Home (OOH) Media such as Billboards, posters, and transit ads (Lorimer, 2002; Rupesh Kadam, n.d.).

Mass media plays a crucial role in health development and health communication. It has the power to significantly impact large populations. The world faces numerous health challenges, and if these challenges are not communicated to the public, they can have devastating consequences for humanity (Saraf & Balamurugan, 2018). Mass media possesses countless important roles in society. For instance, it serves as a significant channel for conveying news, current events, and in-depth analysis to the general public, thereby impacting consciousness and public conversation. Second, it serves as a learning platform, providing educational resources such as documentaries, instructional programs, and digital courses. Third, mass media influences people's interactions with society by shaping norms, values, and behaviors. It also has a significant political impact by informing citizens, influencing election outcomes, and promoting accountability through investigative journalism. Furthermore, advertising in the media boosts consumer demand and economic activity. Finally, it promotes cultural contact by exchanging ideas, traditions, and values across borders, resulting in a deeper knowledge of global variety (Pacheco, 2023).

In the context of health communication in Asia, the role and function of mass media can be seen during the COVID-19 pandemic. The COVID-19 pandemic placed many countries around the world in a state of health emergency. The WHO declared COVID-19 a public health emergency of global concern (Nedelman, 2020). Each country adopted different policies in response to the COVID-19 pandemic (H. Chen et al., 2021). Each country also communicated differently in responding to and handling COVID-19. Several countries in Asia succeeded in responding and handling COVID-19 with clear health communication and appropriate mitigation measures. Taiwan responded quickly and moved swiftly to overcome COVID-19 by utilizing information based on big data integration, supported by a relatively high level of public discipline and cooperation. Similarly, Japan, Singapore, Vietnam, and Malaysia moved quickly with integrated communication and mitigation measures, thus successfully handling COVID-19. Furthermore, many Asian countries have been ambiguous in providing information about COVID-19, causing confusion among the public (Dugis, 2020; Nagler et al., 2020; Setyawan et al., 2021). In Indonesia, government health communications have not been able to build public trust in the handling of COVID-19. A content analysis of government communications in the mass media during the three phases of COVID-19 crisis management indicates that government health communications have not fully convinced the public about the guarantee of survival from COVID-19 (Prajarto, 2021). The Indonesian government's seemingly slow, inconsistent, and disjointed response in providing statements and information related to COVID-19 has contributed to Indonesia experiencing a significant impact from the COVID-19 pandemic. The WHO recorded that by the end of October 2020, more than 37 million people had been confirmed positive for COVID-19 in Indonesia (Basundoro & Karunia, 2021).

Mass media plays a significant role in changing circumstances, mindsets, and shaping public perspectives (Yuliza, 2020). Public trust in the COVID-19 virus is heavily influenced by information conveyed by the mass media. At the beginning of the COVID-19 virus's emergence and amidst the confusion surrounding its existence, most people were barely convinced of its existence. However, when the mass media presented accurate information about COVID-19, the public became convinced and trusted, and they were better prepared to take precautions. Similarly, when the government implemented a mandatory vaccination system to combat COVID-19, it initially met with varying speculation and even rejection from various segments of society. However, with the role played by the mass media in providing information and educating the public, public recognition of the vaccine has grown in a more positive direction. The examples presented demonstrate the significant role of the mass media during and in overcoming the COVID-19 pandemic (Rosyidi, 2021).

3.6 Conclusion

This chapter has argued that effective global health governance in Asia necessitates the integrated application of the One Health paradigm across all policy instruments. Our analysis reveals that while essential tools including the International Health Regulations (IHRs), innovative health financing, strategic partnerships, health diplomacy, and strategic health communication are available, they frequently operate in isolation. This siloed approach constitutes a critical vulnerability. The IHR lacks robust mandates for cross-sector coordination, health financing mechanisms remain unstable and inequitable, global partnerships often prioritize external agendas over local needs, and health communication strategies can be fragmented, impacting public trust and compliance. The COVID-19 pandemic starkly exposed these fractures, demonstrating that threats emerging from the human–animal–environment interface demand unified, synergistic responses that are effectively communicated to diverse publics. Therefore, the central implication is that Asia's future health security and its progress toward Universal Health Coverage (UHC) are fundamentally dependent on achieving systemic integration. The region must move beyond standalone solutions and instead forge synergistic systems in which reformed IHRs are operationalized through One Health, financed by sustainable and equitable domestic resources, supported by inclusive partnerships, strengthened by diplomatic cooperation, and underpinned by clear, evidence-based health communication that bridges the gap between policy and public action. By forging this integrated path, Asia can transform its significant challenges into an opportunity to lead the way in building a more resilient and equitable global health future.

Competing Interests The author(s) has no competing interests to declare that are relevant to the content of this manuscript.

References

Abbas, S. S., Shorten, T., & Rushton, J. (2022). Meanings and mechanisms of One Health partnerships: Insights from a critical review of literature on cross-government collaborations. *Health Policy and Planning, 37*(3), 385–399. https://doi.org/10.1093/heapol/czab134

Adnyana, I. M., Utomo, B., Eljatin, D. S., & Sudaryati, N. L. (2023). One Health approach and zoonotic diseases in Indonesia: Urgency of implementation and challenges. *Narra J, 3*(3). https://doi.org/10.52225/narra.v3i3.257

Afifi, S., Yaman, A., Bakti, I. G. M. Y., & Sumaedi, S. (2024). Health communication and social media: Asian perspective. In *Global knowledge, memory and communication*. https://doi.org/10.1108/GKMC-12-2023-0508

Aghaei, A., & Mowlaei, M. M. (2023). Government-controlled mass media as an obstacle to health policy making: The case of Iran. *International Journal of Social Determinants of Health and Health Services, 53*(2), 158–167. https://doi.org/10.1177/27551938221143640

Ahmed, R., & Bates, B. R. (Eds.). (2016). *Health communication and mass media*. Routledge. https://doi.org/10.4324/9781315586335

Ahsan, A., Wiyono, N. H., Amalia, N., Rusdjijati, R., Veruswati, M., Martini, S., Prabandari, Y. S., & Yuniar, A. M. (2024). Early assessment of tobacco excise sharing fund as policy for farmers' viable alternatives in Indonesia: Case study of four municipalities in Indonesia. *Humanities and Social Sciences Communications, 11*(1), 89. https://doi.org/10.1057/s41599-023-02585-y

Alwan, A. (2014). *Policy Brief: Health diplomacy*. https://applications.emro.who.int/docs/Policy_Brief_2014_EN_15340.pdf

Anggarwal, S., & Singh, S. P. (2022). Mass media and development communication. In *Home science and human ecology*. Board of Open Schooling and Skill Education.

Antara. (2025). *Mengenal batas wilayah Benua Asia dan keunikannya di peta dunia*. Antara. https://www.antaranews.com/berita/4796973/mengenal-batas-wilayah-benua-asia-dan-keunikannya-di-peta-dunia

ASEAN. (2020). *Asean strategic framework for public health emergencies*. https://asean.org/wp-content/uploads/2020/11/4-ASEAN-Strategic-Framework-on-PHE_Final.pdf

ASEAN. (2023). ASEAN Leaders' Declaration on One Health Initiative. In *ASEAN*. ASEAN.

Asemah, E. S. (Ed.). (2023). *Communication, media and society*. Jos University Press.

Averhoff, F., Berg, M., Rodgers, M., Osmanov, S., Luo, X., Anderson, M., Meyer, T., Landay, A., Gamkrelidze, A., Kallas, E. G., Ciuoderis, K., Hernandez, J. P., Henry, J. H., Osorio, J., Lindo, J., Deshommes, J., Anzinger, J., Manasa, J., Alkashvili, M., et al. (2022). The Abbott Pandemic Defense Coalition: A unique multisector approach adds to global pandemic preparedness efforts. *International Journal of Infectious Diseases, 117*, 356–360. https://doi.org/10.1016/j.ijid.2022.02.001

Barcellona, C., Khor, S. K., & Lim, J. (2023). Challenges and opportunities for regional collaboration for strategic purchasing in Southeast Asia. *The Lancet Regional Health - Southeast Asia, 15*, 100227. https://doi.org/10.1016/j.lansea.2023.100227

Bärnreuther, S. (2025). Financializing maternal and newborn care: Temporal tensions within a development impact bond in India. *Development and Change, 56*(1), 31–55. https://doi.org/10.1111/dech.12867

Basundoro, A. F., & Karunia, L. A. (2021). ANATOMI SEKURITISASI PANDEMI COVID-19: KOMPARASI ANTARA PAKISTAN DAN INDONESIA. *Jurnal Sentris, 2*(1), 1–20. https://doi.org/10.26593/sentris.v2i1.4609.1-20

Broberg, M. (2020). A critical appraisal of the World Health Organization's International Health Regulations (2005) in times of pandemic: It is time for revision. *European Journal of Risk Regulation, 11*(2), 202–209. https://doi.org/10.1017/err.2020.26

Burci, G. L., & Negri, S. (2022). The international health regulations as a WHO Constitutional Instrument: Internal governance and regime interactions. *International Organizations Law Review, 19*(1), 11–36. https://doi.org/10.1163/15723747-19010001

Buzgan, T., & Güner, Ö. (2020). *The effectiveness of the World Health Organization in pandemics and the future of the post-pandemic era* (pp. 95–113).

Caballero-Anthony, M. (2018). Health and human security challenges in Asia: New agendas for strengthening regional health governance. *Australian Journal of International Affairs, 72*(6), 602–616. https://doi.org/10.1080/10357718.2018.1537356

Carlson, C. J., & Phelan, A. L. (2022). International law reform for One Health notifications. *The Lancet, 400*(10350), 462–468. https://doi.org/10.1016/S0140-6736(22)00942-4

Carter, E. D., Stewart, D. E., Rees, E. E., Bezuidenhoudt, J. E., Ng, V., Lynes, S., Desenclos, J. C., Pyone, T., & Lee, A. C. K. (2024). Surveillance system integration: Reporting the results of a global multicountry survey. *Public Health, 231*, 31–38. https://doi.org/10.1016/j.puhe.2024.03.004

Cernuschi, T., Gaglione, S., & Bozzani, F. (2018). Challenges to sustainable immunization systems in Gavi transitioning countries. *Vaccine, 36*(45), 6858–6866. https://doi.org/10.1016/j.vaccine.2018.06.012

Chattu, V. K., Mol, R., Singh, B., Reddy, K. S., & Hatefi, A. (2024). Pandemic treaty as an instrument to strengthen global health security: Global health diplomacy at its crux. *Health Promotion Perspective, 14*(1), 9–18. https://doi.org/10.34172/hpp.42744

Chen, J., Bergquist, R., Zhou, X.-N., Xue, J.-B., & Qian, M.-B. (2019). Combating infectious disease epidemics through China's Belt and Road Initiative. *PLOS Neglected Tropical Diseases, 13*(4), e0007107. https://doi.org/10.1371/journal.pntd.0007107

Chen, H., Shi, L., Zhang, Y., Wang, X., Jiao, J., Yang, M., & Sun, G. (2021). Response to the COVID-19 pandemic: Comparison of strategies in six countries. *Frontiers in Public Health, 9*, 708496. https://doi.org/10.3389/fpubh.2021.708496

Cleaveland, S., Sharp, J., Abela-Ridder, B., Allan, K. J., Buza, J., Crump, J. A., Davis, A., Del Rio Vilas, V. J., De Glanville, W. A., Kazwala, R. R., Kibona, T., Lankester, F. J., Lugelo, A., Mmbaga, B. T., Rubach, M. P., Swai, E. S., Waldman, L., Haydon, D. T., Hampson, K., & Halliday, J. E. B. (2017). One Health contributions towards more effective and equitable approaches to health in low- and middle-income countries. *Philosophical Transactions of the Royal Society, B: Biological Sciences, 372*(1725), 20160168. https://doi.org/10.1098/rstb.2016.0168

Cook, A. D. (2021). Humanitarian diplomacy in ASEAN. *Asian Journal of Comparative Politics, 6*(3), 188–201. https://doi.org/10.1177/20578911211019247

Dahal, R., Upadhyay, A., & Ewald, B. (2017). One Health in South Asia and its challenges in implementation from stakeholder perspective. *Veterinary Record, 181*(23), 626–626. https://doi.org/10.1136/vr.104189

Dash, S., & Rath, A. P. (2021). Environmental health: The most neglected part of one health. *Environment Conservation Journal*, 133–136. https://doi.org/10.36953/ECJ.2021.22316

De La Rocque, S., Belot, G., Errecaborde, K. M. M., Sreedharan, R., Skrypnyk, A., Schmidt, T., Isla, N., Traore, T., Talisuna, A., Gongal, G., Samhouri, D., Caya, F., Carron, M., Kandel, N., Xing, J., & Chungong, S. (2021). Operationalisation of consensual One Health roadmaps in countries for improved IHR capacities and health security. *BMJ Global Health, 6*(7), e005275. https://doi.org/10.1136/bmjgh-2021-005275

de Smalen, A. W., Kitikiti, N., & Muthalagu, A. P. (2021). *Enabling digital health adoption in the Asia-Pacific*. Centre of regulatory excellence (CoRE). Duke-NUS Medical School.

DJSN. (2024). *Laporan Kinerja Program JKN Kuartal II Tahun 2024* [Quarterly]. DJSN.

Dugis, V. (2020). State response to the COVID-19 pandemic. *Jurnal Global & Strategis, 14*(2), 175. https://doi.org/10.20473/jgs.14.2.2020.175-188

Duong, H. T. et al. (2023). 'Preventing the COVID-19 Outbreak in Vietnam: Social Media Campaign Exposure and the Role of Interpersonal Communication'. *Health Communication, 38*(2), 394–401. https://doi.org/10.1080/10410236.2021.1953729.

Durrance-Bagale, A., Marzouk, M., Ananthakrishnan, A., Nagashima-Hayashi, M., Lam, S. T., Sittimart, M., & Howard, N. (2022). 'Science is only half of it': Expert perspectives on operationalising infectious disease control cooperation in the ASEAN region. *PLOS Global Public Health, 2*(5), e0000424. https://doi.org/10.1371/journal.pgph.0000424

Eccleston-Turner, M., Burci, G.-L., Liberman, J., & Sekalala, S. (2023). Implementation, compliance, and pandemic legal obligations. *Science, 380*(6647), 792–794. https://doi.org/10.1126/science.adh2080

Fadhil, I., Ali, R., Al-Raisi, S. S., Bin Belaila, B. A., Galadari, S., Javed, A., Sulaiman, K., Saeed, K., & Arifeen, S. (2022). Review of national healthcare systems in the Gulf Cooperation Council countries for noncommunicable diseases management. *Oman Medical Journal, 37*(3), e370. https://doi.org/10.5001/omj.2021.96

Fidler, D. P. (2005). From international sanitary conventions to global health security: The new international health regulations. *Chinese Journal of International Law, 4*(2), 325–392. https://doi.org/10.1093/chinesejil/jmi029

Fischer, J. E., & Katz, R. (2013). Moving forward to 2014: Global IHR (2005) implementation. *Biosecurity and Bioterrorism: Biodefense Strategy, Practice, and Science, 11*(2), 153–156. https://doi.org/10.1089/bsp.2013.0030

Ghahramani, A., De Courten, M., & Prokofieva, M. (2022). The potential of social media in health promotion beyond creating awareness: An integrative review. *BMC Public Health, 22*(1), 2402. https://doi.org/10.1186/s12889-022-14885-0

GHIT. (2024). *GHIT Fund Annual Report 2024*. https://www.ghitfund.org/assets/othermedia/annual_report_2024_eng.pdf

Goldstein, J. E., Budiman, I., Canny, A., & Dwipartidrisa, D. (2022). Pandemics and the human-wildlife interface in Asia: Land use change as a driver of zoonotic viral outbreaks. *Environmental Research Letters, 17*(6), 063009. https://doi.org/10.1088/1748-9326/ac74d4

Gostin, L. O., & Katz, R. (2016). The international health regulations: The governing framework for global health security. *The Milbank Quarterly, 94*(2), 264–313. https://doi.org/10.1111/1468-0009.12186

Guetiya Wadoum, R. E., Sevalie, S., Minutolo, A., Clarke, A., Russo, G., Colizzi, V., Mattei, M., & Montesano, C. (2021). The 2018–2020 Ebola outbreak in the Democratic Republic of Congo: A better response had been achieved through inter-state coordination in Africa. *Risk Management and Healthcare Policy, 14*, 4923–4930. https://doi.org/10.2147/RMHP.S327616

Hasan, M. Z., Ahmed, M. W., Mehdi, G. G., Khan, J. A. M., Islam, Z., Chowdhury, M. E., & Ahmed, S. (2022). Factors affecting the healthcare utilization from Shasthyo Suroksha Karmasuchi scheme among the below-poverty-line population in one subdistrict in Bangladesh: A cross sectional study. *BMC Health Services Research, 22*(1), 885. https://doi.org/10.1186/s12913-022-08254-1

Hegde, N. R., Talari, M., & Majumdar, S. S. (2024). One Health initiative in India: Genesis and hurdles in establishing the first consortium. *Veterinary World*, 2925–2931. https://doi.org/10.14202/vetworld.2024.2925-2931

Herington, J., & Lee, K. (2014). The limits of global health diplomacy: Taiwan's observer status at the world health assembly. *Globalization and Health, 10*(1), 71. https://doi.org/10.1186/s12992-014-0071-y

Hernandez, A., Lee, J., & Kang, H. (2025). Navigating the interconnected web of health: A comprehensive review of the One Health paradigm and its implications for disease management. *Yonsei Medical Journal, 66*(4), 203. https://doi.org/10.3349/ymj.2024.0108

Hiariej, E. (1997). (Tidak) Demokratis ala Asia: Review buku Clark D. Neher dan Ross Marlay, Democracy and Development in Southeast Asia; The llinds of Change, Westview Press, Inc., Colorado, 1995. *Jurnal Ilmu Sosial Dan Ilmu Politik, 1*(2), 57–64.

Innes, G. K., Lambrou, A. S., Thumrin, P., Thukngamdee, Y., Tangwangvivat, R., Doungngern, P., Noradechanon, K., Netrabukkana, P., Meidenbauer, K., Mehoke, T., Heaney, C. D., Hinjoy, S., & Elayadi, A. N. (2022). Enhancing global health security in Thailand: Strengths and challenges of initiating a One Health approach to avian influenza surveillance. *One Health, 14*, 100397. https://doi.org/10.1016/j.onehlt.2022.100397

International Monetary Fund. (2022). *Arsentyeva*. https://www.imf.org/en/Publications/WEO/Issues/2025/04/22/world-economic-outlook-april-2025

Jeyaraman, M., Ramasubramanian, S., Kumar, S., Jeyaraman, N., Selvaraj, P., Nallakumarasamy, A., Bondili, S. K., & Yadav, S. (2023). Multifaceted role of social media in healthcare: Opportunities, challenges, and the need for quality control. *Cureus*. https://doi.org/10.7759/cureus.39111

Katz, A. S., Brisbois, B., Zerger, S., & Hwang, S. W. (2018). Social impact bonds as a funding method for health and social programs: Potential areas of concern. *American Journal of Public Health, 108*(2), 210–215. https://doi.org/10.2105/AJPH.2017.304157

Kheng, K. S. (2022). The world needs more Asian leadership in global health. *Asiaglobal Papers, 6*, 1.

Kickbusch, I. (2007). Global health diplomacy: The need for new perspectives, strategic approaches and skills in global health. *Bulletin of the World Health Organization, 85*(3), 230–232. https://doi.org/10.2471/BLT.06.039222

Kickbusch, I., Novotny, T. E., Drager, N., Silberschmidt, G., & Alcazar, S. (2007). Global health diplomacy: Training across disciplines. *World Hospitals and Health Services the Official Journal of the International Hospital Federation, 43*(4), 20–22.

Kolesar, R. J., Spruk, R., & Tsheten, T. (2023). Evaluating country performance after transitioning from Gavi assistance: An applied synthetic control analysis. *Global Health: Science and Practice, 11*(4), e2200536. https://doi.org/10.9745/GHSP-D-22-00536

Kuanpoth, J. (2015). Compulsory licences: Law and practice in Thailand. In R. M. Hilty & K.-C. Liu (Eds.), *Compulsory licensing* (Vol. 22, pp. 61–77). Springer. https://doi.org/10.1007/978-3-642-54704-1_4

Lawpoolsri, S., Kaewkungwal, J., Khamsiriwatchara, A., Sovann, L., Sreng, B., Phommasack, B., Kitthiphong, V., Lwin Nyein, S., Win Myint, N., Dang Vung, N., Hung, P. S., Smolinski, M. W., Crawley, A., & Koo, M. (2018). Data quality and timeliness of outbreak reporting system among countries in Greater Mekong subregion: Challenges for international data sharing. *PLOS Neglected Tropical Diseases, 12*(4), e0006425. https://doi.org/10.1371/journal.pntd.0006425

Lee, A., Chua, H., Chan, M., Leung, P. W. L., Wong, J. W. S., & Chuh, A. A. T. (2015). Health disparity still exists in an economically well-developed society in Asia. *PLoS ONE, 10*(6), e0130424. https://doi.org/10.1371/journal.pone.0130424

Liu, Z. & Zou, W. (2024). 'Breaking Taboos in Women's Reproductive Health: The Communication Strategies Used by Top OB/GYN Influencers in Chinese Social Media', Health Communication, 39(4), 685–696. https://doi.org/10.1080/10410236.2023.2181677.

Lorimer, R. (2002). Mass communication: Some redefinitional notes. *Canadian Journal of Communication, 27*(1), 63–72. https://doi.org/10.22230/cjc.2002v27n1a1272

Mayank, V., & Saxena, N. (2024). Global governance of health and sovereignty: An agenda for reforms. *Kutafin Law Review, 11*(4), 657. https://doi.org/10.17803/2713-0533.2024.4.30.657-684

McPake, B., Gilbert, K., Vong, S., Ros, B., Has, P., Khuong, A. T., Phuc, P.-D., Hoang, Q. C., Nguyen, D. H., Siengsounthone, L., Luangphaxay, C., Annear, P., & McKinley, J. (2022). Role of regulatory capacity in the animal and human health systems in driving response to zoonotic disease outbreaks in the Mekong region. *One Health, 14*, 100369. https://doi.org/10.1016/j.onehlt.2022.100369

Milazzo, A., Liu, J., Multani, P., Steele, S., Hoon, E., & Chaber, A.-L. (2025). One Health implementation: A systematic scoping review using the Quadripartite One Health Joint Plan of Action. *One Health, 20*, 101008. https://doi.org/10.1016/j.onehlt.2025.101008

Mishra, A. K., & Dash, A. K. (2023). Development impact bonds in developing countries: An emerging innovation for achieving social outcomes. *Journal of Social and Economic Development, 25*(S1), 22–48. https://doi.org/10.1007/s40847-022-00213-0

Misnaniarti, Nugraheni, W. P., Laksono, A. D., Kusnali, A., Ardani, I., Latifah, L., Mubasyiroh, R., Yunitawati, D., & Warouw, T. S. (2025). National health insurance membership in Indonesia: Do socio-economic elements matter? *PLoS One, 20*(8), e0329781. https://doi.org/10.1371/journal.pone.0329781

Mohsin, F. M., Ali, S. H., Chong, S. K., Parikh, R. S., DiClemente, R. J., & Hu, L. (2023). Social media utilization within Asian American families and its role in healthy lifestyle behavioral influence: results from a nationwide survey. *Social Media+ Society, 9*(3), https://doi.org/10.1177/20563051231196544.

Moore, M., & Dausey, D. J. (2015). Local cross-border disease surveillance and control: Experiences from the Mekong Basin. *BMC Research Notes, 8*(1), 90. https://doi.org/10.1186/s13104-015-1047-6

Morris, R., & Wang, S. (2024). Building a pathway to One Health surveillance and response in Asian countries. *Science in One Health, 3*, 100067. https://doi.org/10.1016/j.soh.2024.100067

Mykkänen, M., & Valentini, C. (2025). Leveraging the power of news media: The media's role in publicizing Finnish Trade Associations' policy positions during a global health crisis. *International Journal of Strategic Communication*, 1–26. https://doi.org/10.1080/1553118X.2025.2493649

Nabi, M. N. U., Zohora, F. T., & Misbauddin, S. (2023). "Social media links with social capital to trust in healthcare facilities: empirical evidence from Bangladesh". Library Hi Tech, 41(1), 210–228, https://doi.org/10.1108/LHT-09-2022-0443.

Nageshwaran, G., Harris, R. C., & Guerche-Seblain, C. E. (2021). Review of the role of big data and digital technologies in controlling COVID-19 in Asia: Public health interest vs. privacy. *DIGITAL HEALTH, 7*, 20552076211002953. https://doi.org/10.1177/20552076211002953

Nagler, R. H., Vogel, R. I., Gollust, S. E., Rothman, A. J., Fowler, E. F., & Yzer, M. C. (2020). Public perceptions of conflicting information surrounding COVID-19: Results from a nationally representative survey of U.S. adults. *PLoS ONE, 15*(10), e0240776. https://doi.org/10.1371/journal.pone.0240776

Nedelman, M. (2020, January 30). *World Health Organization declares coronavirus a public health emergency of international concern*. CNN. https://www.cnn.com/2020/01/30/health/coronavirus-who-public-health-emergency-international-concern-declaration

Negri, S., & Eccleston-Turner, M. (2022). One Health and pathogen sharing: Filling the gap in the international health regulations to strengthen global pandemic preparedness and response. *International Organizations Law Review, 19*(1), 188–214. https://doi.org/10.1163/15723747-19010006

Novera, C. N., Connolly, R., Wanke, P., Rahman, M. A., & Azad, M. A. K. (2024). "Past, present and future impact of social media on health workers' mental health: a text mining approach". *Journal of Modelling in Management, 19*(1), 1–18. https://doi.org/10.1108/JM2-05-2022-0135.

Obermann, K., Jowett, M., & Kwon, S. (2018). The role of national health insurance for achieving UHC in the Philippines: A mixed methods analysis. *Global Health Action, 11*(1), 1483638. https://doi.org/10.1080/16549716.2018.1483638

Ouchene, D., Boussalah, H., & Ziane, K. (2024). The role of the media in health awareness. *International Journal of Health Sciences, 8*(S1), 477–482. https://doi.org/10.53730/ijhs.v8nS1.14808

Pacheco, T. (2023). The various aspects and challenges associated with mass media. *Social and Crimonology, 11*(3).

Paek, H.-J., Lee, A. L., Jeong, S.-H., Wang, J., & Dutta, M. J. (2010). The emerging landscape of health communication in Asia: Theoretical contributions, methodological questions, and applied collaborations. *Health Communication, 25*(6–7), 552–559. https://doi.org/10.1080/10410236.2010.496705

Pagotto, B. F., & Eccleston-Turner, M. (2024). The politics of public health emergencies of international concern. *Global Studies Quarterly, 4*(4), ksae083. https://doi.org/10.1093/isagsq/ksae083

Phommasack, B., Jiraphongsa, C., Ko Oo, M., Bond, K. C., Phaholyothin, N., Suphanchaimat, R., Ungchusak, K., & Macfarlane, S. B. (2013). Mekong Basin Disease Surveillance (MBDS): A trust-based network. *Emerging Health Threats Journal, 6*(1), 19944. https://doi.org/10.3402/ehtj.v6i0.19944

Prajarto, N. (2021). Content analysis on health communication of Covid-19 in online media from February to July 2021. *Jurnal Penelitian Komunikasi Dan Opini Publik, 25*(2), 132–148.

Pun, J. K. H., Chan, E. A., Wang, S., & Slade, D. (2018). Health professional-patient communication practices in East Asia: An integrative review of an emerging field of research and practice in Hong Kong, South Korea, Japan, Taiwan, and Mainland China. *Patient Education and Counseling, 101*(7), 1193–1206. https://doi.org/10.1016/j.pec.2018.01.018

Ratzan, S. C., Gostin, L. O., Meshkati, N., Rabin, K., & Parker, R. M. (2020). COVID-19: An urgent call for coordinated, trusted sources to tell everyone what they need to know and do. *Journal of Health Communication, 25*(10), 747–749. https://doi.org/10.1080/10810730.2020.1894015

Rencana Pembangunan Jangka Menengah Nasional Tahun 2020-2024, Pub. L. No. Nomor 18. (2020).

Renuka, M., & Bhavsar, K. (2023, July 28). *Mass media in public health—A catalyst for change*. https://www.icliniq.com/articles/diseases-and-disorders-common-medical-conditions/mass-media-in-public-health

Reveilhac, M. (2022). The deployment of social media by political authorities and health experts to enhance public information during the COVID-19 pandemic. *SSM - Population Health, 19*, 101165. https://doi.org/10.1016/j.ssmph.2022.101165

Rochayati, N. (2017). Dinamika Demokrasi Lokal di Asia Tenggara: Desentralisasi, Pilkada, dan Konflik Kekerasan di Indonesia dan Filipina. *Global: Jurnal Politik Internasional, 10*(2), 135. https://doi.org/10.7454/global.v10i2.277

Rosyidi, R. (2021). Peran Komunikasi Massa di Tengah Pandemi Covid-19. *Hudan Lin Naas: Jurnal Ilmu Sosial Dan Humaniora, 2*(1), 45–58.

Rupesh Kadam. (n.d.). *What is the difference between mass media and mass communication: A complete guide*. Retrieved September 2, 2025, from https://www.met.edu/blog/what_is_the_difference_between_mass_media_and_mass_communication

Sah, R., Reda, A., Lashin, B. I., Mohanty, A., Abdelaal, A., & Rodriguez-Morales, A. J. (2022). Public health emergencies of international concernin the 21st century. *Annals of Medicine and Surgery, 81*. https://doi.org/10.1016/j.amsu.2022.104417

Sakamoto, R. (2025). Aging in Southeast Asia and Japan: Challenges and opportunities. *Geriatrics & Gerontology International, 25*(7), 837–854. https://doi.org/10.1111/ggi.70062

Sanga, V. T., Karimuribo, E. D., & Hoza, A. S. (2024). One Health in practice: Benefits and challenges of multisectoral coordination and collaboration in managing public health risks: A meta-analysis. *International Journal of One Health*, 26–36. https://doi.org/10.14202/IJOH.2024.26-36

Santalucia, I., Sorrentino, M., Fiorilla, C., Tranquilli, S., Strazza, G., Montuori, P., Palladino, R., Fiore, M., Ferrante, M., & Triassi, M. (2025). Learning from COVID-19: A systematic review of the IHR-SPAR framework's role in the pandemic response. *International Journal of Environmental Research and Public Health, 22*(5), 695. https://doi.org/10.3390/ijerph22050695

Santiago, A. R., & Rodrigues, C. (2023). The impact of the Health Silk Road on Global South countries: Insights from Brazilian health agents. *Frontiers in Political Science, 5*, 1250017. https://doi.org/10.3389/fpos.2023.1250017

Saraf, R. A., & Balamurugan, J. (2018). The role of mass media in health care development: A review article. *Journal of Advanced Research in Journalism & Mass Communication, 5*(1), 39–43. https://doi.org/10.24321/2395.3810.201807

SEAOHUN. (2023). *Southeast Asia One Health University Network. SEAOHUN Annual Reports 2022–2023.* https://academy.seaohun.org/wp-content/uploads/2024/01/SEAOHUN-OHW-NG-Y4-SAR_Final_27Apr2023_single-page.pdf

Setyawan, D., Ra'is, D. U., & Rohman, A. (2021). Peran Komunikasi Publik dalam Menanggapi Gelombang Disinformasi Covid-19. *Publisia: Jurnal Ilmu Administrasi Publik, 6*(2), 165–175.

Sihombing, B., Bhatia, R., Srivastava, R., Aditama, T. Y., Laxminarayan, R., & Rijal, S. (2023). Response to antimicrobial resistance in South-East Asia Region. *The Lancet Regional Health - Southeast Asia, 18*, 100306. https://doi.org/10.1016/j.lansea.2023.100306

Sturtevant, J. L., Anema, A., & Brownstein, J. S. (2007). The new international health regulations: Considerations for global public health surveillance. *Disaster Medicine and Public Health Preparedness, 1*(2), 117–121. https://doi.org/10.1097/DMP.0b013e318159cbae

Swarup Garg, B. (Ed.). (2023). *Health promotion—Principles and approaches*. IntechOpen. https://doi.org/10.5772/intechopen.107637

Tangcharoensathien, V., Thammatach-aree, J., Witthayapipopsakul, W., Viriyathorn, S., Kulthanmanusorn, A., & Patcharanarumol, W. (2020). Political economy of Thailand's tax-financed universal coverage scheme. *Bulletin of the World Health Organization, 98*(2), 140–145. https://doi.org/10.2471/BLT.19.239343

Tangwangvivat, R., Rungsitiyakorn, R., Hoonaukit, C., Na Nan, S., Hooker, K. R., Bhunyakitikorn, W., Phiancharoen, C., Pinyopornpanish, P., Iamsirithaworn, S., & Wiratsudakul, A. (2024). Collective activities of the Thai Coordinating Unit for One Health (CUOH): Past activities and future directions. *One Health, 18*, 100728. https://doi.org/10.1016/j.onehlt.2024.100728

Tegegne, H. A., Freeth, F. T. A., Bogaardt, C., Taylor, E., Reinhardt, J., Collineau, L., Prada, J. M., & Hénaux, V. (2024). Implementation of One Health surveillance systems: Opportunities and challenges—Lessons learned from the OH-EpiCap application. *One Health, 18*, 100704. https://doi.org/10.1016/j.onehlt.2024.100704

The Economist. (2023). *Large parts of Asia are getting old before they get rich*. https://www.economist.com/leaders/2023/10/12/large-parts-of-asia-are-getting-old-before-they-get-rich

The Lancet Global Health. (2022). The future of the International Health Regulations. *The Lancet Global Health., 10*(7), e927. https://doi.org/10.1016/S2214-109X(22)00254-6

Van Bekkum, J. E., & Hilton, S. (2013). Primary care nurses' experiences of how the mass media influence frontline healthcare in the UK. *BMC Family Practice, 14*(1), 178. https://doi.org/10.1186/1471-2296-14-178

WHO. (2022a). *Applying a Primary Health Care approach to investments provided by Gavi, The Vaccine Alliance*. https://extranet.who.int/uhcpartnership/sites/default/files/media_documents/Gavi-Overview.pdf

WHO. (2022b). One health joint plan of action (2022–2026): Working together for the health of humans, animals, plants and the environment. https://www.who.int/publications/i/item/9789240059139

WHO Western Pacific. (2017). *Asia Pacific strategy for emerging diseases and public health emergencies: 2005. (APSED III: Advancing implementation of the International Health Regulations)Working together towards health security*. https://www.who.int/publications/i/item/9789290618171

Willnat, L., & Aw, A. (Eds.). (2014). *Social media, culture and politics in Asia*. Peter Lang US. https://doi.org/10.3726/978-1-4539-1241-6

World Bank. (2022). *The World Bank. Bangladesh—Global Health Expenditure database*. https://data.worldbank.org/indicator/SH.XPD.CHEX.GD.ZS?locations=BD

World Health Organization. (2023). *Trends in maternal mortality 2000 to 2020: Estimates by WHO, UNICEF, UNFPA, World Bank Group and UNDESA/Population Division* (1st ed.). World Health Organization.

World Health Organization. (2025). *Tracking every rupiah: Indonesia's bold step towards universal health coverage*. https://www.who.int/indonesia/news/detail/24-01-2025-tracking-every-rupiah%2D%2Dindonesia-s-bold-step-towards-universal-health-coverage

Wu, S., Zhang, J., & Du, L. (2024). '"I Do Not Trust Health Information Shared by My Parents": Credibility Judgement of Health (Mis)information on Social Media in China'. *Health Communication, 39*(1), 96–106. https://doi.org/10.1080/10410236.2022.2159143.

Yopa, D. S., Massom, D. M., Kiki, G. M., Sophie, R. W., Fasine, S., Thiam, O., Zinaba, L., & Ngangue, P. (2023). Barriers and enablers to the implementation of one health strategies in developing countries: A systematic review. *Frontiers in Public Health, 11*, 1252428. https://doi.org/10.3389/fpubh.2023.1252428

Yuliza. (2020). Peran Media Massa dalam Perubahan Sosial Budaya Masyarakat. *At-Tabayun-Journal Islamic Studies, 2*(2).

Zeng, W., Ding, M., & Liu, H. (2023). China's health Silk Road construction during the COVID-19 pandemic. *Global Public Health, 18*(1), 2185799. https://doi.org/10.1080/17441692.2023.2185799

Zhang, M. (2024). Deepening webs of functional trilateralism and challenges: A case of transboundary air pollution cooperation. In I. M. Zhang (Ed.), *China–Japan–South Korea trilateral cooperation* (pp. 33–49). Springer Nature. https://doi.org/10.1007/978-981-97-9148-4_3

Zhang, J., Zhao, D., & Zhang, X. (2024). China's universal medical insurance scheme: Progress and perspectives. *BMC Global and Public Health, 2*(1), 62. https://doi.org/10.1186/s44263-024-00096-9

Zhupankhan, A., Tussupova, K., & Berndtsson, R. (2017). Could changing power relationships lead to better water sharing in Central Asia? *Water, 9*(2), 139. https://doi.org/10.3390/w9020139

Zoubir, Y. H., & Tran, E. (2022). China's Health Silk Road in the Middle East and North Africa amidst COVID-19 and a contested world order. *Journal of Contemporary China, 31*(135), 335–350. https://doi.org/10.1080/10670564.2021.1966894

Chapter 4
Epidemiology in One Health

Denada Jihan Dampi, Danindra Ario Wiryawan, Vivi Rosalin Rajagukguk, Bayu Satria Wiratama, and Khrisdiana Putri

Abbreviations

AIDS	Acquired Immunodeficiency Syndrome
ASEAN	Association of Southeast Asian Nations
BBPK	*Balai Besar Pelatihan Kesehatan* (National Health Training Center)
COHFE	Competency Framework for One Health Epidemiology
COVID-19	Coronavirus Disease 2019
DHIS2	District Health Information Software 2
EMPRES-i+	Emergency Prevention System for Transboundary Animal and Plant Pests and Diseases
EWARS	Early Warning and Response System
FAO	Food and Agriculture Organization of the United Nations
FETP	Field Epidemiology Training Program
HPAI	Highly Pathogenic Avian Influenza

D. J. Dampi (✉) · D. A. Wiryawan · V. R. Rajagukguk
Master of Public Health Program, Faculty of Medicine, Public Health, and Nursing, Universitas Gadjah Mada, Sleman, Indonesia
e-mail: denadajihandampi@mail.ugm.ac.id; danindra.ario.wiryawan@mail.ugm.ac.id; vivirosalinrajagukguk@mail.ugm.ac.id

B. S. Wiratama
Department of Biostatistics, Epidemiology, and Population Health, Faculty of Medicine, Public Health, and Nursing, Universitas Gadjah Mada, Sleman, Indonesia
e-mail: bayu.satria@ugm.ac.id

K. Putri
Department of Public Health, Faculty of Veterinary Medicine, Universitas Gadjah Mada, Yogyakarta, Indonesia

One Health Centre of Excellence, Universitas Gadjah Mada, Yogyakarta, Indonesia
e-mail: khrisdiana@ugm.ac.id

© The Author(s), under exclusive license to Springer Nature Singapore Pte Ltd. 2026

A. U. Rauf, T. Wibawa (eds.), *The One Health Concept in Asian Contexts*, https://doi.org/10.1007/978-981-95-9880-9_4

HIV	Human Immunodeficiency Virus
NoV	Norovirus
PDSR	Participatory Disease Surveillance and Response
PODD	Participatory One Health Digital Disease Detection
RNA	Ribonucleic Acid
RBF	Rat-Bite Fever
SARS	Severe Acute Respiratory Syndrome
SARS-CoV-2	Severe Acute Respiratory Syndrome Coronavirus 2
SEAOHUN	Southeast Asia One Health University Network
SMS	Short Message Service
VPPs	Veterinary Paraprofessionals
WHO	World Health Organization
WOAH	World Organization for Animal Health (formerly OIE)

4.1 One Health Approach and Its Implications for Epidemiology

The One Health approach provides a transformative framework for advancing epidemiology to address the multifaceted health challenges of the twenty-first century. As a concept, One Health is defined as the collaborative efforts of multiple disciplines to attain optimal health for people, animals, plants, and the environment (Centers for Disease Control and Prevention, 2023). This approach acknowledges that many health threats originate at the interfaces among humans, animals, and ecosystems. Approximately 60% of known human pathogens are zoonotic, and more than 75% of emerging infectious diseases in humans originate from animal reservoirs (World Organization for Animal Health, 2025). These statistics underscore the necessity for epidemiology to adopt a systems-based perspective that transcends traditional disciplinary and institutional boundaries, particularly in Asia, where dense populations, high biodiversity, and intense human–animal interactions amplify the risk of zoonotic spillovers.

Asia's vulnerability to emerging zoonoses is evidenced by the region's experience with outbreaks such as severe acute respiratory syndrome (SARS), avian influenza, and Nipah virus. The 2003 SARS outbreak, which was traced to wildlife markets in China, and repeated H5N1 epizootics in Southeast Asia demonstrated the insufficiency of siloed, sector-specific responses. Similarly, the emergence of Nipah virus in Malaysia in 1998, which was initially misdiagnosed, highlighted the need for cross-sectoral epidemiologic investigations to accurately identify and control zoonotic threats (Centers for Disease Control and Prevention, 1999). These events catalyzed regional and global endorsement of the One Health paradigm, beginning with the 2007 ministerial declaration in New Delhi and reinforced by the international response to the COVID-19 pandemic (Centers for Disease Control and Prevention, 2025; Government of India, 2007).

Within this context, One Health reframes epidemiology not merely as a reactive science, but as a proactive discipline focused on prevention through systemic interventions. A conventional response to rabies, for instance, might rely primarily on human post-exposure prophylaxis. In contrast, a One Health approach emphasizes mass dog vaccination, community education, and ecological management to eliminate the source of transmission and prevent exposure entirely. This strategy has been proven both effective and feasible across settings, including resource-constrained regions. Research demonstrates that large-scale dog vaccination can significantly reduce and potentially eliminate rabies reservoirs, thereby interrupting zoonotic transmission to humans (Vos et al., 2021). This paradigm aligns with the broader ethos of One Health, which centers on prevention, equity, and the protection of vulnerable populations through integrated and anticipatory public health strategies.

From a methodological standpoint, the implementation of One Health requires integrated surveillance systems that synthesize data from human, animal, and environmental health sectors. Yet in most countries, these surveillance streams remain fragmented, with limited interoperability and weak coordination mechanisms. An innovative solution to this challenge is the four-way linking model, which integrates epidemiological, laboratory, human, and animal health data into a single coordinated platform. This model enables joint risk assessments, facilitates early detection of zoonotic threats, and supports synchronized responses across sectors. Its institutionalization has been observed in countries such as Egypt, where the four-way linking model has laid the groundwork for a formalized One Health surveillance system (Allal et al., 2019). That integration demonstrates the potential of multisectoral coordination to enhance surveillance capacity and strengthen early warning systems.

In parallel with institutional innovation, technological advancements have played a pivotal role in operationalizing One Health. Molecular and genomic tools have enabled the detection of pathogens across species and from environmental reservoirs such as water and soil. For example, metagenomic surveys of wildlife are increasingly used to identify viruses with zoonotic potential before they spill over into human populations (Cui et al., 2023; Mishra et al., 2019; Wani et al., 2024). Digital health platforms such as District Health Information Software-2 (DHIS2) have expanded to include veterinary modules, allowing for the creation of unified dashboards and cross-sectoral alert systems that enhance situational awareness (DHIS, 2023). Moreover, artificial intelligence and machine learning are being piloted to analyze large volumes of heterogeneous data, enabling the detection of early warning signals that may elude traditional surveillance methods (Guo et al., 2023; Villanueva-Miranda et al., 2025).

The role of Field Epidemiology Training Programs (FETPs) has also evolved in response to the complexities of One Health. Initially designed to build capacity in human health surveillance, FETPs are increasingly incorporating veterinarians and veterinary paraprofessionals (VPPs) into their cohorts. This expansion supports multisectoral outbreak investigations and reflects the interdisciplinary realities of zoonotic disease transmission (Seffren et al., 2022). In support of this shift, the FAO, WHO, and WOAH jointly developed the Competency Framework for One Health Epidemiology (COHFE), which outlines technical and functional competencies across 14 domains. This framework provides guidance for curriculum development to ensure that field epidemiologists can work effectively within One Health systems (World Organization for Animal Health, 2025). However, challenges remain, with fewer than half of FETPs reporting sufficient coverage of veterinary-relevant competencies. Nonetheless, these efforts mark a crucial step toward institutionalizing a multisectoral epidemiology workforce capable of addressing zoonotic and environmental health threats (Al Nsour et al., 2018, 2021).

The FETPs in Asia play a crucial role in strengthening epidemiological capacity and improving public health responses to outbreaks, particularly zoonotic diseases. By adopting the One Health approach, which links human, animal, and environmental health, countries like Thailand have developed sustainable models that integrate veterinary and human health surveillance, enhancing control of diseases such as avian influenza (Iamsirithaworn et al., 2014). Japan and South Korea also emphasize interdisciplinary training and rapid response, with FETP graduates and trainers actively participating in outbreak investigations and risk communication across the region (Lee et al., 2017; Sunagawa, 2025; TEPHINET, 2025). In Indonesia, the FETP managed by the Ministry of Health is implemented through BBPK Ciloto for Frontline and Intermediate training and through universities including Universitas Indonesia, Universitas Gadjah Mada, Universitas Airlangga, Universitas Udayana, Universitas Hasanuddin, Universitas Diponegoro, and Universitas Andalas for Advanced training (Field Epidemiology Training Program (FETP) Indonesia, 2018). The program strengthens epidemiological capacity across all levels of the health system and equips public health professionals with skills in disease surveillance, outbreak investigation, and rapid response, focusing on diseases connected to One Health, such as avian influenza, leptospirosis, and rabies.

Avian influenza serves as a key example of One Health challenges. FETPs in Thailand and Vietnam have established robust surveillance systems to monitor poultry populations, enabling early detection of potential human infections (Dwyer & Kirkland, 2011; Gongal et al., 2020; Iamsirithaworn et al., 2014; Qiu et al., 2021). Graduates are trained to conduct field investigations, implement control measures, and coordinate with multiple sectors, highlighting the importance of collaboration among human health, veterinary, and environmental professionals. Regional networks further facilitate data sharing and joint outbreak responses, addressing cross-border health threats effectively.

Despite these successes, challenges remain, including securing sustainable funding, strengthening laboratory capacity, and increasing public awareness in rural poultry farming areas. Continued investment in FETPs, combined with One Health principles, ensures that epidemiologists are equipped to manage emerging zoonotic diseases. Across Asia, these programs have proven vital in enhancing surveillance, training public health personnel, and fostering rapid, coordinated responses to outbreaks such as avian influenza, ultimately reinforcing regional and global health security (Field Epidemiology Training Program (FETP) Indonesia, 2018; TEPHINET, 2025).

In addition, the emergence of COVID-19 renewed global recognition of the importance of One Health. Although the term itself was not explicitly used in early pandemic documents, the methodology of the WHO-convened Global Study of Origins of SARS-CoV-2 was informed by One Health principles. Investigations included genomic comparisons of SARS-CoV-2 with related coronaviruses in bats and pangolins, environmental sampling in live animal markets, and assessments of biosafety practices in laboratories handling zoonotic pathogens (World Health Organization, 2021). These investigations illustrate the integration of human, animal, and environmental health perspectives in tracing the origins of the pandemic. They also provide a real-world example of how the One Health framework can guide collaborative scientific inquiry during global health emergencies. Despite these advances, the implementation of One Health remains uneven and challenged by structural and operational barriers. Although global initiatives such as the *Quadripartite One Health Joint Plan of Action* have garnered political support, their practical execution often lacks full sectoral integration. A recent systematic review found that while many One Health programs included components of policy engagement and capacity building, fewer than half involved all three sectors, and environmental health remained the most underrepresented (Milazzo et al., 2025).

Similar challenges are evident in Southeast Asia, where national One Health platforms exist but are often hampered by fragmented financing mechanisms, limited infrastructure for cross-sectoral coordination, and donor-driven agendas with weak national ownership. Platforms such as the Southeast Asia One Health University Network (SEAOHUN) and ASEAN centers have provided valuable support for training and dialogue, yet more robust and formalized structures are needed to enable joint surveillance, data sharing, and coordinated outbreak response (Lâm et al., 2025).

The One Health approach is reshaping the landscape of epidemiology, both in Asia and globally. By broadening the discipline's focus to include the interconnected domains of human, animal, and environmental health, One Health strengthens the preventive orientation of epidemiological practice and enhances methodological integration across sectors. Although the path to full implementation remains complex, the demonstrated benefits in areas such as pandemic preparedness, zoonotic disease control, and surveillance innovation provide compelling justification for its continued advancement. Achieving the full potential of One Health requires long-term investment in surveillance infrastructure, workforce training, institutional coordination, and inclusive governance.

4.2 Zoonotic Diseases and Their Epidemiological Characteristics

Zoonoses refer to diseases and infections that can be naturally transmitted between vertebrate animals and humans, representing a major public health concern due to the shared pathogens and established epidemiological connections between species (Rahman et al., 2020; World Health Organization, 2021). These diseases are prevalent worldwide and significantly impact public health, quality of life, and economic growth (Di Bari et al., 2023; Welburn et al., 2015). It is estimated that over 60% of newly emerging infectious diseases globally originate from zoonotic sources (Institute of Medicine (US) Committee on Emerging Microbial Threats to Health et al., 1992).

Zoonotic diseases show distinct epidemiological characteristics in Southeast Asia, with systematic evidence from 2011 to 2022 highlighting frequent associations with poultry, pigs, ruminants, companion animals, and wildlife (Nguyen et al., 2024). The region is marked by a significant burden of zoonoses, where evolving disease patterns and gaps in surveillance reflect the dynamic nature of their epidemiology (Bordier & Roger, 2013). Live animal markets, where humans, domestic animals, and wildlife interact, further shape the epidemiological risk landscape, making them critical hotspots for emerging infectious diseases and highlighting the importance of stricter regulatory interventions (Naguib et al., 2021).

Environmental and ecological determinants also influence the epidemiology of zoonotic diseases in Asia. Disruption of natural habitats, coupled with exposure to contaminated food, water, and soil, contributes to transmission dynamics involving wildlife reservoirs (Nguyen et al., 2025). In addition, biodiversity loss, urban expansion, and agricultural intensification in southern China and Southeast Asia have historically driven spillover events and remain central epidemiological factors that increase the likelihood of future pandemics (Goldstein et al., 2022). These elements, combined with Asia's dense populations, rapid socioeconomic change, and favorable climatic conditions, create an environment where novel pathogens can emerge and spread more easily (Horby et al., 2014; Yumba et al., 2024).

Epidemiological challenges are further compounded by weak public health systems and sociocultural practices that increase exposure to zoonotic pathogens in many Asian countries (Binot et al., 2015). Addressing these vulnerabilities requires a stronger cross-sectoral One Health approach to effectively monitor, prevent, and respond to zoonotic risks (Bhatia & Narain, 2010). The continuing emergence of zoonotic diseases poses a serious epidemiological threat to global health, with Southeast Asia remaining a hotspot due to biodiversity, population density, and frequent human–animal interactions (Hossain et al., 2025). Vietnam exemplifies these risks, as more than half of its population lives in rural areas with daily contact with animals, emphasizing the urgent need for context-specific epidemiological strategies to mitigate future outbreaks (Chu et al., 2019).

Several Southeast Asian countries continue to face a high burden of leptospirosis, with Malaysia and Thailand implementing national surveillance systems to monitor annual incidence and mortality (Ganasen, 2025). The region is also regarded as a major hotspot for emerging zoonotic diseases, where wildlife trade in open markets contributes to the risk of viral spillover, including avian influenza, severe acute respiratory syndrome (SARS), and Nipah virus infections (Bhatia & Narain, 2010). Rodent-associated zoonoses, such as hantavirus pulmonary syndrome, leptospirosis, and rickettsiosis, further exacerbate public health challenges in Southeast Asia (Pimentel & Taylor, 2014), while zoonotic pathogens overall account for nearly 60% of newly emerging human diseases worldwide (Hossain et al., 2025). These diseases carry the potential to trigger large-scale health crises and economic disruption, making prevention strategies critical. Such measures must consider the epidemiological profile of each pathogen and its prevalence in different animal hosts (Chaudhuri et al., 2024). In response, the World Health Organization underscores the need for stronger awareness, multisectoral and multidisciplinary collaboration, as well as the implementation of scheduled control programs, reduced exposure to animals, and protective measures in endemic regions to minimize outbreaks and their severity (Bhatia & Narain, 2010).

To date, a total of 217 rodent species have been identified as vectors or reservoirs of various infectious diseases. These include 31 helminth-related diseases, 28 viral infections, 26 bacterial infections, 14 protozoan diseases, 8 rickettsial infections, and 4 fungal diseases (Ristiyanto, 2016). The diversity of pathogens carried by rodents highlights their significant potential to pose public health risks, particularly in areas with high levels of human–rodent contact, such as densely populated settlements, agricultural regions, and areas with poor sanitation. This underscores the importance of rodent population control and breaking the transmission chain as key strategies in preventing zoonotic diseases. In detail, bacteria, viruses, parasites, and fungi can be described as follows.

4.2.1 Bacteria

Bacteria are one of the main groups of pathogens responsible for zoonotic diseases. These microorganisms are capable of surviving and multiplying within animal hosts, and can be transmitted to humans through various routes, including direct contact, consumption of contaminated food, vector bites, or environmental exposure (Glaser et al., 1994). Direct transmission can occur through bites or scratches from animals, such as in rat-bite fever (RBF), which is caused by *Streptobacillus moniliformis*, a facultative anaerobic gram-negative bacillus commonly found in the nasopharynx of rodents, particularly rats (Elliott, 2007).

Transmission can also occur through the consumption of contaminated animal products resulting from improper handling or processing. Examples include yersiniosis caused by *Yersinia enterocolitica* and listeriosis caused by *Listeria monocytogenes*. *Y. enterocolitica* is widespread in the environment and among animals, with pigs serving as the primary reservoir of pathogenic strains for humans (Huovinen et al., 2010). Outbreaks are frequently associated with untreated water, unpasteurized milk, or contaminated poultry products, particularly affecting individuals with compromised immune systems (Sabina et al., 2011).

In addition, zoonotic bacteria can be transmitted via vectors, such as *Rickettsia felis*, which is spread by fleas. These insects act as both vectors and reservoirs for the pathogen, and human infections have been linked to the presence of *R. felis* (Edouard et al., 2014; Parola et al., 2003). Environmental transmission is also possible, as in the case of leptospirosis caused by the spirochete *Leptospira*, the etiological agent of Weil's disease in Japan. This disease remains an endemic public health issue across the Asia-Pacific region, particularly in areas where people are exposed to contaminated water and poor sanitation conditions.

4.2.2 *Viruses*

Zoonotic viruses are a group of pathogens capable of crossing the species barrier from animals to humans through various transmission routes, including bites, droplets, or consumption of wild animal meat. Such transmission can cause serious illnesses and, in some cases, trigger global pandemics. A classic example is rabies, or hydrophobia, which can be transmitted through animal bites, non-bite exposures, and, on rare occasions, human-to-human transmission, although bites from rabid animals remain the most common route (Altantogtokh et al., 2023). Animals frequently associated with rabies include dogs, raccoons, skunks, bats, and foxes. The rabies virus, classified under the genus *Lyssavirus* within the family *Rhabdoviridae*, possesses a lipid envelope and a negative-sense single-stranded RNA genome (Drew, 2004). As no effective treatment for rabies currently exists, preventive measures and cross-sectoral collaboration remain the cornerstone of control efforts.

Beyond rabies, Coronavirus Disease 2019 (COVID-19), caused by Severe Acute Respiratory Syndrome Coronavirus 2 (SARS-CoV-2), is another zoonosis with far-reaching impacts. SARS-CoV-2 is transmitted through direct contact, droplets, airborne particles, and via fomites, objects, or surfaces contaminated with secretions from infected individuals (Burke et al., 2020; Chan et al., 2020; Ghinai et al., 2020; Hamner et al., 2020; Huang et al., 2020; Liu et al., 2020; Luo et al., 2020; Pung et al., 2020; WHO, 2020). This diverse range of transmission mechanisms makes COVID-19 highly capable of spreading within communities.

Foodborne transmission is also possible for certain zoonotic viruses. Norovirus (NoV) is the leading cause of nonbacterial gastroenteritis and is highly contagious, spreading through direct contact, fomites, and contaminated food (Lopman et al., 2003; Mead et al., 1999). Since the genus *Norovirus* includes strains infecting humans, pigs, cattle, and mice, the potential for zoonotic transmission remains (U.S. Department of Health and Human Services, 2001). NoV can infect individuals of all age groups and has been responsible for large outbreaks in closed environments, as exemplified by rapid spread aboard cruise ships (Cramer et al., 2006).

4.2.3 *Parasites*

Zoonotic parasites are classified into four main categories based on their distinct modes of transmission. Direct zoonotic parasites infect humans directly from animals without requiring an intermediate host, examples of which include *Entamoeba histolytica*, *Cryptosporidium parvum*, *Toxoplasma gondii*, *Hymenolepis nana*, *Trichinella spiralis*, and *Sarcoptes scabiei*. Metazoonoses require an invertebrate intermediate host, such as insects or arthropods, before infecting humans, as seen in *Babesia bovis*, *Clonorchis sinensis*, and *Dirofilaria immitis*. Cyclozoonoses involve a vertebrate intermediate host, including *Taenia solium* and *Echinococcus granulosus*. Meanwhile, saprozoonoses are transmitted through contaminated soil or water, exemplified by *Ancylostoma caninum* and *Strongyloides stercoralis* (Youn, 2009).

Additionally, carnivorous parasites found in dogs and cats have the potential to infect humans, while anthroponotic parasites may be transmitted from humans to animals. Wild rodents play a significant role in the spread of zoonotic parasites, particularly intestinal helminths belonging to nematodes, trematodes, and cestodes. Zoonotic intestinal protozoa, such as *Cryptosporidium* spp. and *Giardia* spp., are also frequently detected in wild rodents, with reported prevalence rates ranging from 15% to 50% (Tijjani et al., 2020). *Cryptosporidium* infection in rodents has been reported at rates of 5–39% and poses a risk of transmission to humans, potentially causing acute diarrhea. Therefore, rodent population control represents a key preventive strategy within the framework of the One Health approach (Lv et al., 2009).

4.2.4 Fungi

Approximately 300 of the 1.5 million known fungal species are recognized to have a causal relationship with human disease. Fungal infections in animals can be classified into several categories. First, infections that are not transmissible to humans, such as aspergillosis, mucormycosis, candidiasis, and infections caused by melanizing fungi. Second, endemic infections in which transmission occurs indirectly through the environment, including coccidioidomycosis, histoplasmosis, paracoccidioidomycosis, and blastomycosis. Third, zoophilic fungal pathogens whose transmission is almost direct, such as chytridiomycosis and white-nose syndrome in bats. Fourth, fungi that can be transmitted directly from animals to humans, including zoophilic dermatophytes, microsporidia, and dimorphic fungi (Seyedmousavi et al., 2018). A notable example is *Histoplasma capsulatum*, the etiological agent of histoplasmosis, which is commonly found in soil contaminated with bat or bird droppings. This infection is often asymptomatic in immunocompetent individuals but can be potentially fatal in immunocompromised patients, such as those with HIV/AIDS or individuals receiving immunosuppressive therapy.

4.3 Environmental Factors Influencing Disease Transmission

The One Health paradigm recognizes that human, animal, and ecosystem health are intimately connected. Environmental changes—both gradual (e.g., climate change, biodiversity loss) and abrupt (e.g., deforestation, extreme weather)—alter the ecological and social interfaces where pathogens, animal hosts, vectors, and people interact. These alterations influence pathogen survival, host abundance, contact rates, and human vulnerability, thereby shaping disease emergence, re-emergence, and transmission dynamics across local to global scales. Understanding how environmental drivers act singly and in combination is essential.

4.3.1 *Climate Change and Weather Extremes*

Climate variables such as temperature, humidity, and precipitation are key drivers of disease transmission. Climate change can alter the geographic distribution, seasonality, and intensity of infectious diseases (Button, 2023). Climate change significantly alters the habitats and behaviors of disease vectors—mosquitoes, ticks, and flies—acting as a public health emergency. For example, vector-borne diseases like malaria and dengue fever depend heavily on temperature and stagnant water bodies for mosquito breeding; thus, warming climates and altered rainfall patterns facilitate their spread. Rising temperatures accelerate pathogen and vector reproduction rates, increasing the risk of transmission to human and animal populations (WHO, 2022).

Similarly, increased rainfall and flooding can create breeding grounds for mosquitoes, thereby contributing to the spread of diseases like dengue fever and Zika virus (Watts et al., 2018). On the other hand, drought conditions may force wildlife into closer contact with human settlements in search of food and water, increasing the likelihood of spillover events. For instance, Asia has seen a 9.5% increase in dengue vector abundance over the past 110 years. Even a 1 °C increase in temperature nearly doubles the population at risk for dengue in Taiwan. Weather extremes like heatwaves, droughts, heavy rainfall, and cyclones further modulate transmission, creating breeding environments or disrupting vector habitats in complex, nonlinear ways (Zain et al., 2024).

4.3.2 *Land Use and Urbanization*

Changes in land use, such as deforestation, agricultural expansion, and urban sprawl, can disrupt ecosystems and increase contact among wildlife, livestock, and human populations. These interactions create opportunities for pathogens to jump species barriers, a process known as spillover (Plowright et al., 2017). Deforestation in tropical regions, for instance, has been linked to outbreaks of diseases such as Ebola, Nipah virus, and Malaria. When natural habitats are fragmented, reservoir hosts like bats and rodents are displaced and may seek shelter in peri-urban areas, elevating the risk of zoonotic transmission (Gibb et al., 2020). Urbanization can also affect vector habitats. Poorly planned urban infrastructure often leads to stagnant water accumulation and waste buildup, which are conducive to the proliferation of *Aedes* mosquitoes, the primary vectors for Dengue, Chikungunya, and Zika viruses.

4.3.3 Pollution, Chemical Exposure, Environmental Persistence, and Foodborne Pathogen Transmission

Environmental media such as air, soil, and water enable pathogen persistence and dispersal. Climate-related events—floods, storms, dust—facilitate the spread of foodborne pathogens like *Salmonella, Escherichia coli, Listeria*, and antibiotic-resistant bacteria via water contamination, aerosols, or dust storms (Balta et al., 2024). Air pollution is linked to respiratory illnesses and may exacerbate airborne disease transmission dynamics (Button, 2023).

Furthermore, bioaccumulation of toxic substances like heavy metals and persistent organic pollutants in food chains poses health risks and can induce immune suppression (Humboldt-Dachroeden & Mantovani, 2021). Pollution also encourages antimicrobial resistance by facilitating gene exchange and mutations among microbes in the environment (WHO, 2022). Persistent pathogens in soil, water, and built environments can sustain transmission even outside outbreak periods, complicating control efforts. Climate events exacerbate these pathways by redistributing pathogens across environments and hosts, reinforcing the need for integrated One Health strategies that address environmental reservoirs.

4.3.4 Socioecological and Behavioral Factors

Environmental risk factors intersect with human behaviors and socioecological conditions, including population density, occupational exposure, and leisure activities, thereby affecting individual and community susceptibility to infections (Yeh et al., 2018). These complex interactions necessitate comprehensive epidemiological models that integrate environmental, social, and biological data for effective disease prediction and control.

Socioecological factors, defined as the social and environmental conditions influencing health, include socioeconomic status, gender, and migrant status, which affect outcomes through material, structural, and behavioral mechanisms (Myer et al., 2008; Spallek et al., 2012; Zha, 2019). In Southeast Asia, the region's diverse social, economic, and political contexts have led to disparities in health status and fragmented health systems, posing significant challenges for national public health responses (Chongsuvivatwong et al., 2011). Similarly, behavioral factors such as smoking, alcohol consumption, poor nutrition, physical inactivity, and obesity are major contributors to noncommunicable diseases, including cardiovascular illnesses, and are shaped by genetic, environmental, and cultural influences in the Asia-Pacific (Galeone et al., 2021; Vasan, 2025). Both socioecological and behavioral determinants strongly influence morbidity and premature mortality, particularly from noncommunicable diseases (Galeone et al., 2021), while rapid yet unequal socioeconomic development and differing demographic and epidemiological transitions have deepened health disparities across the region (Chongsuvivatwong et al., 2011). Added to this are challenges such as urban poverty, low government spending on health, and the dual burden of communicable and noncommunicable diseases, which continue to shape the epidemiological landscape and public health priorities in South and Southeast Asia (Vasan, 2025).

4.3.5 Surveillance, Modeling, and One Health Governance

To manage environmentally driven disease risks, integrated surveillance and modeling tools are essential. Harmonizing climatic, ecological, vector, and health data enables predictive systems like early warning models and nowcasting platforms to guide timely interventions (Charnley et al., 2025). Governance must be multisectoral and multilevel. The One Health approach requires cross-disciplinary collaboration—public health, veterinary, environmental sectors—to co-develop policy, surveillance, and response systems that are adaptive, inclusive, and climate-smart (Robbiati et al., 2024). Environmental factors, such as climate change, pollution, and socioecological and behavioral shifts, are interconnected drivers of disease transmission in One Health, necessitating multidisciplinary approaches for prevention. By addressing these elements, public health efforts can reduce the global burden of emerging diseases (Humboldt-Dachroeden & Mantovani, 2021).

To better understand how the One Health approach has been operationalized across countries, various models of governance and coordination have been established in Asia. Figure 4.1 compares One Health models in Bangladesh, Singapore, Thailand, and Hong Kong. Despite differences in implementation details, all operate at the ministerial level and share common features. They can be classified into three types: coordinating committee, working group, and blended models (Beltramo et al., 2024).

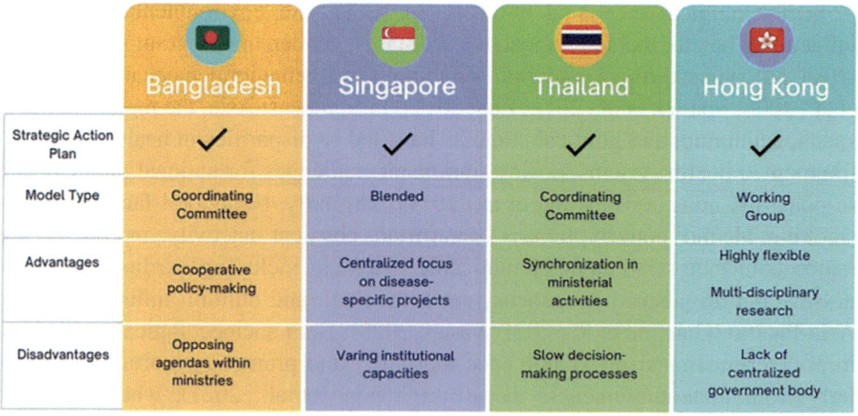

Fig. 4.1 Comparison of One Health models in Bangladesh, Singapore, Thailand, and Hong Kong, including their strengths and limitations. (From Beltramo et al., 2024, licensed under CC-BY 4.0)

4.4 One Health Surveillance Systems

One Health surveillance integrates the monitoring of human, animal, and environmental health to support the early detection of zoonotic threats and to enable more accurate risk assessments. This approach accelerates response processes and provides a foundation for evidence-based disease prevention and control policies. The prevention and control of emerging pathogens heavily rely on local-level surveillance, which serves to detect health events affecting humans, animals, plants, and the environment at an early stage. Although in the context of human disease outbreaks, One Health is often perceived merely as a link between human and animal health, its scope extends far beyond this. One Health represents an integrated and comprehensive framework aimed at balancing and optimizing the health of humans, animals, and ecosystems in a sustainable manner (Adisasmito et al., 2023).

One Health data collection that integrates various sources of clinical data is a critical component in disease and outbreak surveillance and control efforts. One approach that can be applied is *participatory surveillance*, a two-way communication process for receiving and transmitting data as follow-up, while also expanding engagement to broader segments of the community (Smolinski, 2016). This process is not merely about gathering data from the community for monitoring purposes, but also about ensuring that such data actively contribute to ongoing disease surveillance and provide feedback to the monitored population. Through the implementation of an integrated data collection system of this kind, disease or outbreak control, particularly for zoonotic diseases, can be more effectively monitored and addressed by stakeholders and actors involved in the response.

Advancements in technology have significantly transformed One Health surveillance by enhancing the integration of data from human, animal, and environmental health sectors. These innovations enable faster detection and more coordinated responses to emerging threats, particularly in Asia where zoonotic spillover risks are high. Modern surveillance systems increasingly combine real-time reporting, cross-sectoral data sharing, and predictive analytics, creating opportunities for earlier intervention and improved disease control.

At the regional level, platforms such as the Food and Agriculture Organization's EMPRES-i+ provide countries with tools to visualize outbreak patterns, monitor transboundary animal disease events, and access early warnings from both official and unofficial sources (FAO, 2025). The system integrates epidemiological, laboratory, and geospatial datasets, with analytical features that allow users to model disease spread and identify potential hotspots. This predictive capacity supports preemptive measures across borders, aligning with the One Health principle of addressing threats at their source.

Complementing these regional initiatives, community-based surveillance models have proven essential for early detection in rural and high-risk areas where formal health infrastructure may be limited. Thailand's Participatory One Health Digital Disease Detection (PODD) system enables trained community volunteers to report unusual events in animals, humans, or the environment through a smartphone application, which automatically categorizes the risk level and triggers rapid investigation (Yano et al., 2018). In Indonesia, the Participatory Disease Surveillance and Response (PDSR) program was established to control highly pathogenic avian influenza (HPAI), deploying trained village-level officers who worked directly with poultry owners to detect and respond to outbreaks. Between 2006 and 2008, PDSR teams investigated more than 7000 HPAI events, confirming outbreaks through rapid field diagnostics and implementing control measures such as culling and disinfection (Azhar et al., 2010). The Indonesian Integrated Animal Health Information System (iSIKHNAS) employs mobile phone–based SMS reporting from field officers and simplified office worksheets to collect data quickly and directly from the source. The system is designed to make information readily available, easily visualized, and accessible for analysis, ensuring that stakeholders can use it effectively whenever needed (https://isikhnas.pertanian.go.id). Similarly, in Vietnam, participatory surveillance has been embedded within national zoonotic disease control programs for avian influenza and rabies, improving coordination between veterinary and public health services and strengthening targeted interventions at the animal–human interface (Bordier et al., 2021).

Building upon these community and regional surveillance frameworks, emerging technologies have further advanced predictive analytics within One Health surveillance. By integrating epidemiological, environmental, and climatic datasets, predictive systems can forecast disease risks before case numbers peak. For example, the WHO-developed Early Warning and Response System (EWARS) incorporates meteorological indicators and time-series epidemiological data to predict outbreaks of vector-borne diseases such as dengue and chikungunya. Field trials in Brazil, Malaysia, and Mexico demonstrated that EWARS could forecast outbreaks several weeks in advance, enabling targeted vector control measures ahead of peak transmission periods (Hussain-Alkhateeb et al., 2018). Similar analytical approaches are now being piloted in Asian contexts to anticipate livestock disease spread using climate and movement data, as well as to model zoonotic spillover risks from wildlife populations, thereby strengthening proactive prevention measures across the One Health spectrum.

One Health is a health paradigm emphasizing that human, animal, plant, and environmental health are interconnected and mutually influential. This approach is inherently collaborative, involving various stakeholders from the human health, animal health, agriculture, environmental, academic, and civil society sectors. It is also multisectoral, integrating the roles and perspectives of government agencies, international organizations, the private sector, and local communities. Globally, the multisectoral One Health approach has been exemplified through formal collaboration initiated by the Tripartite organizations, namely, the Food and Agriculture Organization of the United Nations (FAO), the World Organization for Animal Health (OIE), and the World Health Organization (WHO), which jointly build interagency collaboration in accordance with their respective mandates (WHO, 2020). Such global collaboration has proven capable of controlling outbreaks caused by zoonotic diseases, enabling more regulated and targeted control efforts that focus on the interrelated aspects of the three main components: people, animals, and the environment, which interact to determine the occurrence of disease.

The rapid expansion of technology access worldwide has created significant opportunities for health surveillance systems to move beyond formal reporting mechanisms by directly engaging communities and stakeholders in rapid local-level data collection. Through the use of mobile devices, online applications, and various digital communication channels, the reporting of symptoms, disease incidents, and risk factors can now be conducted in real time, thereby accelerating early detection and timely responses to potential outbreak threats. This direct engagement approach has been applied across a range of diseases, from endemic infectious diseases to emerging pathogens with pandemic potential and has been proven effective in extending the reach and improving the sensitivity of surveillance systems (Smolinski, 2016). With active cross-sectoral stakeholder support within the One Health framework, such integration not only strengthens early detection capabilities but also serves as a critical component in the control and mitigation of outbreaks, particularly zoonotic diseases, through collaborative efforts that involve the human, animal, and environmental health sectors. The ultimate goal is to achieve optimal health for all living beings, recognizing that challenges such as zoonoses, antimicrobial resistance, climate change, and food safety cannot be addressed by a single sector alone, but require cross-border and interdisciplinary collaboration.

4.5 Conclusion

The One Health approach is increasingly essential for advancing epidemiology in Asia, where close interactions among humans, animals, and the environment drive the emergence and reemergence of zoonotic diseases such as SARS, avian influenza, Nipah virus, and COVID-19. This chapter highlights how environmental change, urbanization, biodiversity loss, and sociocultural practices significantly influence disease dynamics, increasing the risk of spillover events and shaping the region's epidemiological landscape. Advances in genomic technologies, integrated surveillance, digital platforms, artificial intelligence, and participatory reporting systems have strengthened early detection and cross-sectoral coordination. Field Epidemiology Training Programs (FETPs) further enhance workforce capacity by integrating human, animal, and environmental health professionals, enabling more effective outbreak investigations and response. However, persistent barriers including fragmented governance structures, limited environmental health expertise, insufficient laboratory capacity, and funding gaps continue to hinder full One Health implementation. While regional networks such as SEAOHUN and various national One Health platforms have supported collaboration, many programs still lack comprehensive multisectoral integration, with environmental sectors being the least represented. Overall, realizing the full potential of One Health in Asia requires sustained investment in surveillance infrastructure, capacity building, interoperable data systems, and inclusive, cross-sectoral governance mechanisms. By strengthening collaboration among human health, veterinary, and environmental sectors, Asian countries will be better equipped to prevent, detect, and respond to zoonotic threats, enhance pandemic preparedness, and safeguard regional and global health security in the face of increasingly complex epidemiological challenges.

Competing Interests The authors have no competing interests to declare that are relevant to the content of this manuscript.

References

Adisasmito, W. B., Almuhairi, S., Barton Behravesh, C., Bilivogui, P., Bukachi, S. A., Casas, N., Becerra, N. C., Charron, D. F., Chaudhary, A., Ciacci Zanella, J. R., Cunningham, A. A., Dar, O., Debnath, N., Dungu, B., Farag, E., Gao, G. F., Hayman, D. T. S., Khaitsa, M., Koopmans, M. P. G., et al. (2023). One Health action for health security and equity. *The Lancet, 401*(10376), 530–533. https://doi.org/10.1016/S0140-6736(23)00086-7

Al Nsour, M., Iblan, I., & Tarawneh, M. R. (2018). Jordan field epidemiology training program: Critical role in national and regional capacity building. *JMIR Medical Education, 4*(1), e12. https://doi.org/10.2196/mededu.9516

Al Nsour, M., Khader, Y., Bashier, H., & Alsoukhni, M. (2021). Evaluation of advanced field epidemiology training programs in the Eastern Mediterranean region: A multi-country study. *Frontiers in Public Health, 9*, 684174. https://doi.org/10.3389/fpubh.2021.684174

Allal, L., Mahrous, H., Saad, A., Refaei, S., Attia, M., Mahrous, I., Fahim, M., Elfadaly, S., & Abdelnabi, A. (2019). From Four-Way Linking to a One Health Platform in Egypt: Institutionalisation of a multidisciplinary and multisectoral One Health system: -EN- -FR- Du maillage quadri-directionnel à la Plateforme Une seule santé en Égypte : institutionnalisation d'un système multidisciplinaire et multisectoriel Une seule santé -ES- El paso de la conexión cuatridimensional al dispositivo de Una sola salud, o la institucionalización de un sistema pluridisciplinar y multisectorial de Una sola salud en Egipto. *Revue Scientifique et Technique de l'OIE, 38*(1), 261–270. https://doi.org/10.20506/rst.38.1.2958

Altantogtokh, D., Boldbaatar, B., Matulis, G., Lilak, A. A., Tsogbadrakh, N., Chimedtseren, B., Ariunbold, K., & Von Fricken, M. E. (2023). Rabies exposure from infected horse bite in an urban setting: A case study from Mongolia. *Zoonotic Diseases, 4*(1), 1–7. https://doi.org/10.3390/zoonoticdis4010001

Azhar, M., Lubis, A. S., Siregar, E. S., Alders, R. G., Brum, E., McGrane, J., Morgan, I., & Roeder, P. (2010). Participatory disease surveillance and response in Indonesia: Strengthening veterinary services and empowering communities to prevent and control highly pathogenic avian influenza. *Avian Diseases, 54*(s1), 749–753. https://doi.org/10.1637/8713-031809-Reg.1

Balta, I., Lemon, J., Murnane, C., Pet, I., Vintila, T., McCleery, D., Callaway, T., Douglas, A., Stef, L., & Corcionivoschi, N. (2024). The One Health aspect of climate events with impact on foodborne pathogens transmission. *One Health, 19*, 100926. https://doi.org/10.1016/j.onehlt.2024.100926

Beltramo, B., Kolluru, S., Slager, L., Wall, L., Ostwald, K., & Rasali, D. (2024). Comparative analysis of One Health policies in Asia for exploring opportunities for British Columbia in Canada. *International Journal of Environmental Research and Public Health, 22*(1), 34. https://doi.org/10.3390/ijerph22010034

Bhatia, R., & Narain, J. P. (2010). Review paper: The challenge of emerging zoonoses in Asia Pacific. *Asia-Pacific Journal of Public Health, 22*(4), 388–394. https://doi.org/10.1177/1010539510370908

Binot, A., Duboz, R., Promburom, P., Phimpraphai, W., Cappelle, J., Lajaunie, C., Goutard, F. L., Pinyopummintr, T., Figuié, M., & Roger, F. L. (2015). A framework to promote collective action within the One Health community of practice: Using participatory modelling to enable interdisciplinary, cross-sectoral and multi-level integration. *One Health, 1*, 44–48. https://doi.org/10.1016/j.onehlt.2015.09.001

Bordier, M., & Roger, F. (2013). Zoonoses in South-East Asia: A regional burden, a global threat. *Animal Health Research Reviews, 14*(1), 40–67. https://doi.org/10.1017/S1466252313000017

Bordier, M., Goutard, F. L., Antoine-Moussiaux, N., Pham-Duc, P., Lailler, R., & Binot, A. (2021). Engaging stakeholders in the design of One Health surveillance systems: A participatory approach. *Frontiers in Veterinary Science, 8*, 646458. https://doi.org/10.3389/fvets.2021.646458

Burke, R. M., Midgley, C. M., Dratch, A., Fenstersheib, M., Haupt, T., Holshue, M., Ghinai, I., Jarashow, M. C., Lo, J., McPherson, T. D., Rudman, S., Scott, S., Hall, A. J., Fry, A. M., & Rolfes, M. A. (2020). Active monitoring of persons exposed to patients with confirmed COVID-19—United States, January–February 2020. *MMWR. Morbidity and Mortality Weekly Report, 69*(9), 245–246. https://doi.org/10.15585/mmwr.mm6909e1

Button, D. (2023). The influence of environmental factors on disease development and spread. *Journal of Primary Care and General Practice, 8*(1). https://doi.org/10.35841/aapcgp.8.1.189

Centers for Disease Control and Prevention. (1999). *Outbreak of Hendra-Like Virus—Malaysia and Singapore, 1998–1999*. CDC. https://www.cdc.gov/mmwr/preview/mmwrhtml/00056866.htm

Centers for Disease Control and Prevention. (2023). *One Health*. https://www.cdc.gov/one-health/index.html

Centers for Disease Control and Prevention. (2025). *One Health history*. https://www.cdc.gov/one-health/about/one-health-history.html

Chan, J. F.-W., Yuan, S., Kok, K.-H., To, K. K.-W., Chu, H., Yang, J., Xing, F., Liu, J., Yip, C. C.-Y., Poon, R. W.-S., Tsoi, H.-W., Lo, S. K.-F., Chan, K.-H., Poon, V. K.-M., Chan, W.-M., Ip, J. D., Cai, J.-P., Cheng, V. C.-C., Chen, H., et al. (2020). A familial cluster of pneumonia associated with the 2019 novel coronavirus indicating person-to-person transmission: A study of a family cluster. *The Lancet, 395*(10223), 514–523. https://doi.org/10.1016/S0140-6736(20)30154-9

Charnley, G. E. C., Alcayna, T., Almuedo-Riera, A., Antoniou, C., Badolo, A., Bartumeus, F., Boodram, L.-L., Bueno-Marí, R., Codeço, C., Codeço Coelho, F., Costa, F., Cox, H., Haddad, N., Hamid, N. A., Kittayapong, P., Korukluoğlu, G., Michaelakis, A., Maciel-de-Freitas, R., Montalvo, T., et al. (2025). Strengthening resilience to emerging vector-borne diseases in Europe: Lessons learnt from countries facing endemic transmission. *The Lancet Regional Health - Europe, 53*, 101271. https://doi.org/10.1016/j.lanepe.2025.101271

Chaudhuri, S., Biswas, S., & Rana, T. (2024). Introduction. In T. Rana (Ed.), *The handbook of zoonotic diseases of goats* (pp. 1–17). CABI. https://doi.org/10.1079/9781800622852.0001

Chongsuvivatwong, V., Phua, K. H., Yap, M. T., Pocock, N. S., Hashim, J. H., Chhem, R., Wilopo, S. A., & Lopez, A. D. (2011). Health and health-care systems in Southeast Asia: Diversity and transitions. *The Lancet, 377*(9763), 429–437. https://doi.org/10.1016/S0140-6736(10)61507-3

Chu, D.-T., Ngoc, T. U., Chu-Dinh, T., Ngoc, V. T. N., Van Nhon, B., Pham, V.-H., Nghia, L. L., Anh, L. Q., Van Pham, T. H., & Truong, N. D. (2019). The possible zoonotic diseases transferring from pig to human in Vietnam. *European Journal of Clinical Microbiology & Infectious Diseases, 38*(6), 1003–1014. https://doi.org/10.1007/s10096-018-03466-y

Cramer, E., Blanton, C., Blanton, L., Vaughanjr, G., Bopp, C., & Forney, D. (2006). Epidemiology of gastroenteritis on cruise ships, 2001–2004. *American Journal of Preventive Medicine, 30*(3), 252–257. https://doi.org/10.1016/j.amepre.2005.10.027

Cui, X., Fan, K., Liang, X., Gong, W., Chen, W., He, B., Chen, X., Wang, H., Wang, X., Zhang, P., Lu, X., Chen, R., Lin, K., Liu, J., Zhai, J., Liu, D. X., Shan, F., Li, Y., Chen, R. A., et al. (2023). Virus diversity, wildlife-domestic animal circulation and potential zoonotic viruses of small mammals, pangolins and zoo animals. *Nature Communications, 14*(1), 2488. https://doi.org/10.1038/s41467-023-38202-4

DHIS. (2023). *DHIS2 for One Health*. https://dhis2.org/one-health/

Di Bari, C., Venkateswaran, N., Fastl, C., Gabriël, S., Grace, D., Havelaar, A. H., Huntington, B., Patterson, G. T., Rushton, J., Speybroeck, N., Torgerson, P., Pigott, D. M., & Devleesschauwer, B. (2023). The global burden of neglected zoonotic diseases: Current state of evidence. *One Health, 17*, 100595. https://doi.org/10.1016/j.onehlt.2023.100595

Drew, W. L. (2004). *Rabies* (Vol. 4). McGraw Hill.

Dwyer, D. E., & Kirkland, P. D. (2011). Influenza: One Health in action. *New South Wales Public Health Bulletin, 22*(6), 123. https://doi.org/10.1071/NB11005

Edouard, S., Bhengsri, S., Dowell, S. F., Watt, G., Parola, P., & Raoult, D. (2014). Two human cases of *Rickettsia felis* infection, Thailand. *Emerging Infectious Diseases, 20*(10), 1780–1781. https://doi.org/10.3201/eid2010.140905

Elliott, S. P. (2007). Rat bite fever and *Streptobacillus moniliformis*. *Clinical Microbiology Reviews, 20*(1), 13–22. https://doi.org/10.1128/CMR.00016-06

FAO. (2025). *Food and Agriculture Organization of the United Nations One Health: A collaborative approach to preventing the next pandemic*. https://www.fao.org/one-health/highlights/preventing-the-next-pandemic/en#:~:text=The%20power%20of%20collaboration,response%20when%20an%20outbreak%20occurs

Field Epidemiology Training Program (FETP) Indonesia. (2018). *FETP di Indonesia*. https://fetpindonesia.or.id/page/content/1/about-fetp-indonesia

Galeone, C., Bonzi, R., Turati, F., Pelucchi, C., Rota, M., & La Vecchia, C. (2021). Social epidemiology: The challenges and opportunities of worldwide data consortia. In P. Mariani & M. Zenga (Eds.), *Data science and social research II* (pp. 175–185). Springer. https://doi.org/10.1007/978-3-030-51222-4_14

Ganasen, T. (2025). Rodent-borne zoonotic diseases in Southeast Asia: A narrative review. *Tropical Biomedicine, 42*(2), 100–122. https://doi.org/10.47665/tb.42.2.003

Ghinai, I., McPherson, T. D., Hunter, J. C., Kirking, H. L., Christiansen, D., Joshi, K., Rubin, R., Morales-Estrada, S., Black, S. R., Pacilli, M., Fricchione, M. J., Chugh, R. K., Walblay, K. A., Ahmed, N. S., Stoecker, W. C., Hasan, N. F., Burdsall, D. P., Reese, H. E., Wallace, M., et al. (2020). First known person-to-person transmission of severe acute respiratory syndrome coronavirus 2 (SARS-CoV-2) in the USA. *The Lancet, 395*(10230), 1137–1144. https://doi.org/10.1016/S0140-6736(20)30607-3

Gibb, R., Redding, D. W., Chin, K. Q., Donnelly, C. A., Blackburn, T. M., Newbold, T., & Jones, K. E. (2020). Zoonotic host diversity increases in human-dominated ecosystems. *Nature, 584*(7821), 398–402. https://doi.org/10.1038/s41586-020-2562-8

Glaser, C. A., Angulo, F. J., & Rooney, J. A. (1994). Animal-associated opportunistic infections among persons infected with the human immunodeficiency virus. *Clinical Infectious Diseases, 18*(1), 14–24. https://doi.org/10.1093/clinids/18.1.14

Goldstein, J. E., Budiman, I., Canny, A., & Dwipartidrisa, D. (2022). Pandemics and the human-wildlife interface in Asia: Land use change as a driver of zoonotic viral outbreaks. *Environmental Research Letters, 17*(6), 063009. https://doi.org/10.1088/1748-9326/ac74d4

Gongal, G., Ofrin, R., De Balogh, K., Oh, Y., Kugita, H., & Dukpa, K. (2020). Operationalization of One Health and tripartite collaboration in the Asia-Pacific region. *WHO South-East Asia Journal of Public Health, 9*(1), 21. https://doi.org/10.4103/2224-3151.282991

Government of India. (2007). *Vision and road map released at the conclusion of the three-day international ministerial conference on avian and pandemic influenza*. https://www.woah.org/app/uploads/2021/03/newdelhi-roadmapfinal.pdf

Guo, W., Lv, C., Guo, M., Zhao, Q., Yin, X., & Zhang, L. (2023). Innovative applications of artificial intelligence in zoonotic disease management. *Science in One Health, 2*, 100045. https://doi.org/10.1016/j.soh.2023.100045

Hamner, L., Dubbel, P., Capron, I., Ross, A., Jordan, A., Lee, J., Lynn, J., Ball, A., Narwal, S., Russell, S., Patrick, D., & Leibrand, H. (2020). High SARS-CoV-2 attack rate following exposure at a choir practice—Skagit County, Washington, March 2020. *MMWR. Morbidity and Mortality Weekly Report, 69*(19), 606–610. https://doi.org/10.15585/mmwr.mm6919e6

Horby, P. W., Hoa, N. T., Pfeiffer, D. U., & Wertheim, H. F. L. (2014). Drivers of emerging zoonotic infectious diseases. In A. Yamada, L. H. Kahn, B. Kaplan, T. P. Monath, J. Woodall, & L. Conti (Eds.), *Confronting emerging zoonoses* (pp. 13–26). Springer. https://doi.org/10.1007/978-4-431-55120-1_2

Hossain, H., Chowdhury, M. S. R., Khan, S. S., Ahmad, T., Brishty, K. A., Rahman, M., Rahman, M. N., & Akter, S. (2025). Emerging zoonotic diseases: Epidemiology, public health impact, and the urgent need for a unified "One Health" approach. *The Pakistan Veterinary Journal*. https://doi.org/10.29261/pakvetj/2025.115

Huang, C., Wang, Y., Li, X., Ren, L., Zhao, J., Hu, Y., Zhang, L., Fan, G., Xu, J., Gu, X., Cheng, Z., Yu, T., Xia, J., Wei, Y., Wu, W., Xie, X., Yin, W., Li, H., Liu, M., et al. (2020). Clinical features of patients infected with 2019 novel coronavirus in Wuhan, China. *The Lancet, 395*(10223), 497–506. https://doi.org/10.1016/S0140-6736(20)30183-5

Humboldt-Dachroeden, S., & Mantovani, A. (2021). Assessing environmental factors within the One Health approach. *Medicina, 57*(3), 240. https://doi.org/10.3390/medicina57030240

Huovinen, E., Sihvonen, L. M., Virtanen, M. J., Haukka, K., Siitonen, A., & Kuusi, M. (2010). Symptoms and sources of Yersinia enterocolitica-infection: A case-control study. *BMC Infectious Diseases, 10*(1), 122. https://doi.org/10.1186/1471-2334-10-122

Hussain-Alkhateeb, L., Kroeger, A., Olliaro, P., Rocklöv, J., Sewe, M. O., Tejeda, G., Benitez, D., Gill, B., Hakim, S. L., Gomes Carvalho, R., Bowman, L., & Petzold, M. (2018). Early warning and response system (EWARS) for dengue outbreaks: Recent advancements towards widespread applications in critical settings. *PLoS ONE, 13*(5), e0196811. https://doi.org/10.1371/journal.pone.0196811

Iamsirithaworn, S., Chanachai, K., & Castellan, D. (2014). Field epidemiology and One Health: Thailand's experience. In A. Yamada, L. H. Kahn, B. Kaplan, T. P. Monath, J. Woodall, & L. Conti (Eds.), *Confronting emerging zoonoses* (pp. 191–212). Springer. https://doi.org/10.1007/978-4-431-55120-1_9

Institute of Medicine (US) Committee on Emerging Microbial Threats to Health, Lederberg, J., Shope, R. E., & Oaks, S. C., Jr. (1992). *Emerging infections: Microbial threats to health in the United States* (p. 2008). National Academies Press. https://doi.org/10.17226/2008

Lâm, S., Dang-Xuan, S., Unger, F., Meeyam, T., Pham-Duc, P., Wacharapluesadee, S., & Nguyen-Viet, H. (2025). Operationalizing regional One Health initiatives in Southeast Asia: Ways forward. *One Health, 20*, 101034. https://doi.org/10.1016/j.onehlt.2025.101034

Lee, M.-S., Kim, E.-Y., & Lee, S.-W. (2017). Experience of 16 years and its associated challenges in the Field Epidemiology Training Program in Korea. *Epidemiology and Health, 39*, e2017058. https://doi.org/10.4178/epih.e2017058

Liu, J., Liao, X., Qian, S., Yuan, J., Wang, F., Liu, Y., Wang, Z., Wang, F.-S., Liu, L., & Zhang, Z. (2020). Community transmission of severe acute respiratory syndrome Coronavirus 2, Shenzhen, China, 2020. *Emerging Infectious Diseases, 26*(6). https://doi.org/10.3201/eid2606.200239

Lopman, B. A., Adak, G. K., Reacher, M., & Brown, D. W. G. (2003). Two epidemiologic patterns of *Norovirus* outbreaks: Surveillance in England and Wales, 1992–2000. *Emerging Infectious Diseases, 9*(1), 71–77. https://doi.org/10.3201/eid0901.020175

Luo, L., Liu, D., Liao, X., Wu, X., Jing, Q., Zheng, J., Liu, F., Yang, S., Bi, B., Li, Z., Liu, J., Song, W., Zhu, W., Wang, Z., Zhang, X., Chen, P., Liu, H., Cheng, X., Cai, M., et al. (2020). *Modes of contact and risk of transmission in COVID-19 among close contacts*. https://doi.org/10.1101/2020.03.24.20042606

Lv, C., Zhang, L., Wang, R., Jian, F., Zhang, S., Ning, C., Wang, H., Feng, C., Wang, X., Ren, X., Qi, M., & Xiao, L. (2009). *Cryptosporidium* spp. in wild, laboratory, and pet rodents in China: Prevalence and molecular characterization. *Applied and Environmental Microbiology, 75*(24), 7692–7699. https://doi.org/10.1128/AEM.01386-09

Mead, P. S., Slutsker, L., Dietz, V., McCaig, L. F., Bresee, J. S., Shapiro, C., Griffin, P. M., & Tauxe, R. V. (1999). Food-related illness and death in the United States. *Emerging Infectious Diseases, 5*(5), 607–625. https://doi.org/10.3201/eid0505.990502

Milazzo, A., Liu, J., Multani, P., Steele, S., Hoon, E., & Chaber, A.-L. (2025). One Health implementation: A systematic scoping review using the Quadripartite One Health Joint Plan of Action. *One Health, 20*, 101008. https://doi.org/10.1016/j.onehlt.2025.101008

Mishra, N., Fagbo, S. F., Alagaili, A. N., Nitido, A., Williams, S. H., Ng, J., Lee, B., Durosinlorun, A., Garcia, J. A., Jain, K., Kapoor, V., Epstein, J. H., Briese, T., Memish, Z. A., Olival, K. J., & Lipkin, W. I. (2019). A viral metagenomic survey identifies known and novel mammalian viruses in bats from Saudi Arabia. *PLoS ONE, 14*(4), e0214227. https://doi.org/10.1371/journal.pone.0214227

Myer, L., Susser, E., Link, B., & Morroni, C. (2008). Social epidemiology. In *International encyclopedia of public health* (pp. 74–87). Elsevier. https://doi.org/10.1016/B978-012373960-5.00196-9

Naguib, M. M., Li, R., Ling, J., Grace, D., Nguyen-Viet, H., & Lindahl, J. F. (2021). Live and wet markets: Food access versus the risk of disease emergence. *Trends in Microbiology, 29*(7), 573–581. https://doi.org/10.1016/j.tim.2021.02.007

Nguyen, T. T., Mai, T. N., Dang-Xuan, S., Nguyen-Viet, H., Unger, F., & Lee, H. S. (2024). Emerging zoonotic diseases in Southeast Asia in the period 2011–2022: A systematic literature review. *Veterinary Quarterly, 44*(1), 1–15. https://doi.org/10.1080/01652176.2023.2300965

Nguyen, H. T. T., Lindahl, J. F., Bett, B., Nguyen-Viet, H., Lâm, S., Nguyen-Tien, T., Unger, F., Dang-Xuan, S., Bui, T. X., Le, H. T., Lundkvist, Å., Ling, J., & Lee, H. S. (2025). Understanding zoonotic pathogens and risk factors from wildlife in Southeast Asia: A systematic literature review. *Veterinary Quarterly, 45*(1), 1–17. https://doi.org/10.1080/01652176.2025.2475990

Parola, P., Sanogo, O. Y., Lerdthusnee, K., Zeaiter, Z., Chauvancy, G., Gonzalez, J. P., Miller, R. S., Telford, S. R., Wongsrichanalai, C., & Raoult, D. (2003). Identification of *Rickettsia* spp. and *Bartonella* spp. in fleas from the Thai-Myanmar border. *Annals of the New York Academy of Sciences, 990*(1), 173–181. https://doi.org/10.1111/j.1749-6632.2003.tb07359.x

Pimentel, L. C., & Taylor, E. V. (2014). Surveillance for zoonotic diseases. In N. M. M'ikanatha & J. K. Iskander (Eds.), *Concepts and methods in infectious disease surveillance* (1st ed., pp. 92–106). Wiley. https://doi.org/10.1002/9781118928646.ch10

Plowright, R. K., Parrish, C. R., McCallum, H., Hudson, P. J., Ko, A. I., Graham, A. L., & Lloyd-Smith, J. O. (2017). Pathways to zoonotic spillover. *Nature Reviews Microbiology, 15*(8), 502–510. https://doi.org/10.1038/nrmicro.2017.45

Pung, R., Chiew, C. J., Young, B. E., Chin, S., Chen, M. I.-C., Clapham, H. E., Cook, A. R., Maurer-Stroh, S., Toh, M. P. H. S., Poh, C., Low, M., Lum, J., Koh, V. T. J., Mak, T. M., Cui, L., Lin, R. V. T. P., Heng, D., Leo, Y.-S., Lye, D. C., et al. (2020). Investigation of three clusters of COVID-19 in Singapore: Implications for surveillance and response measures. *The Lancet, 395*(10229), 1039–1046. https://doi.org/10.1016/S0140-6736(20)30528-6

Qiu, C., Yang, G., & Lu, P. (2021). Outline of human avian influenza. In C. Qiu, Y. Shi, & P. Lu (Eds.), *Avian influenza in human* (pp. 1–6). Springer. https://doi.org/10.1007/978-981-16-1429-3_1

Rahman, M. T., Sobur, M. A., Islam, M. S., Ievy, S., Hossain, M. J., El Zowalaty, M. E., Rahman, A. T., & Ashour, H. M. (2020). Zoonotic diseases: Etiology, impact, and control. *Microorganisms, 8*(9), 1405. https://doi.org/10.3390/microorganisms8091405

Ristiyanto, R. (2016). *Penyakit Tular Rodensia* (1st ed.). UGM Press.

Robbiati, C., Milano, A., Declich, S., & Dente, M. G. (2024). One Health prevention and preparedness to vector-borne diseases: How should we deal with a multisectoral, multilevel and multigroup governance? *One Health Outlook, 6*(1), 21. https://doi.org/10.1186/s42522-024-00114-8

Sabina, Y., Rahman, A., Ray, R. C., & Montet, D. (2011). *Yersinia enterocolitica*: Mode of transmission, molecular insights of virulence, and pathogenesis of infection. *Journal of Pathogens, 2011*, 1–10. https://doi.org/10.4061/2011/429069

Seffren, V., Lowther, S., Guerra, M., Kinzer, M. H., Turcios-Ruiz, R., Henderson, A., Shadomy, S., Baggett, H. C., Harris, J. R., Njoh, E., & Salyer, S. J. (2022). Strengthening the global one health workforce: Veterinarians in CDC-supported field epidemiology training programs. *One Health, 14*, 100382. https://doi.org/10.1016/j.onehlt.2022.100382

Seyedmousavi, S., Bosco, S. D. M. G., De Hoog, S., Ebel, F., Elad, D., Gomes, R. R., Jacobsen, I. D., Jensen, H. E., Martel, A., Mignon, B., Pasmans, F., Piecková, E., Rodrigues, A. M.,

Singh, K., Vicente, V. A., Wibbelt, G., Wiederhold, N. P., & Guillot, J. (2018). Fungal infections in animals: A patchwork of different situations. *Medical Mycology, 56*(suppl_1), S165–S187. https://doi.org/10.1093/mmy/myx104

Smolinski, M. (2016). Innovations in participatory disease surveillance. *International Journal of Infectious Diseases, 53*, 10. https://doi.org/10.1016/j.ijid.2016.11.030

Spallek, J., Kuntz, B., & Schott, T. (2012). Sozialepidemiologie. *Public Health Forum, 20*(3), 4–8. https://doi.org/10.1016/j.phf.2012.06.015

Sunagawa, T. (2025). A perspective on field epidemiology in Japan: Insights from human resource development in the Field Epidemiology Training Program. *Global Health & Medicine, 7*(2), 172–174. https://doi.org/10.35772/ghm.2025.01023

TEPHINET. (2025). *Japan Field Epidemiology Training Program*. https://www.tephinet.org/training-programs/japan-field-epidemiology-training-program

Tijjani, M., Majid, R. A., Abdullahi, S. A., & Unyah, N. Z. (2020). Detection of rodent-borne parasitic pathogens of wild rats in Serdang, Selangor, Malaysia: A potential threat to human health. *International Journal for Parasitology: Parasites and Wildlife, 11*, 174–182. https://doi.org/10.1016/j.ijppaw.2020.01.008

U.S. Department of Health and Human Services. (2001). *"Norwalk-Like Viruses" Public health consequences and outbreak management*. https://www.cdc.gov/mmwr/PDF/rr/rr5009.pdf

Vasan, S. S. (2025). Mens health: Unique health challenges in Southeast Asia and the far East. In F. L. H. Rajiwate & P. H. C. Lim (Eds.), *Men's health* (pp. 265–270). Springer Nature. https://doi.org/10.1007/978-3-031-76898-9_19

Villanueva-Miranda, I., Xiao, G., & Xie, Y. (2025). Artificial intelligence in early warning systems for infectious disease surveillance: A systematic review. *Frontiers in Public Health, 13*, 1609615. https://doi.org/10.3389/fpubh.2025.1609615

Vos, A., Nokireki, T., Isomursu, M., et al. (2021). Oral vaccination of foxes and raccoon dogs against rabies with the 3rd generation oral rabies virus vaccine, SPBN GASGAS, in Finland. *Acta Veterinaria Scandinavica, 63*, 40. https://doi.org/10.1186/s13028-021-00605-y

Wani, A. K., Chopra, C., Dhanjal, D. S., Akhtar, N., Singh, H., Bhau, P., Singh, A., Sharma, V., Pinheiro, R. S. B., Américo-Pinheiro, J. H. P., & Singh, R. (2024). Metagenomics in the fight against zoonotic viral infections: A focus on SARS-CoV-2 analogues. *Journal of Virological Methods, 323*, 114837. https://doi.org/10.1016/j.jviromet.2023.114837

Watts, N., Amann, M., Ayeb-Karlsson, S., Belesova, K., Bouley, T., Boykoff, M., Byass, P., Cai, W., Campbell-Lendrum, D., Chambers, J., Cox, P. M., Daly, M., Dasandi, N., Davies, M., Depledge, M., Depoux, A., Dominguez-Salas, P., Drummond, P., Ekins, P., et al. (2018). The Lancet Countdown on health and climate change: From 25 years of inaction to a global transformation for public health. *The Lancet, 391*(10120), 581–630. https://doi.org/10.1016/S0140-6736(17)32464-9

Welburn, S. C., Beange, I., Ducrotoy, M. J., & Okello, A. L. (2015). The neglected zoonoses—The case for integrated control and advocacy. *Clinical Microbiology and Infection, 21*(5), 433–443. https://doi.org/10.1016/j.cmi.2015.04.011

WHO. (2020). *Shortage of personal protective equipment endangering health workers worldwide*. https://www.who.int/newsroom/detail/03-03-2020-shortage-of-personalprotective-equipment-endangeringhealthworkers-worldwide

WHO. (2022). *New report highlights the impact of changes in environment on One Health*. https://www.who.int/europe/news/item/01-07-2022-new-report-highlights-the-impact-of-changes-in-environment-on-one-health

World Health Organization. (2021). *WHO-convened Global Study of Origins of SARS-CoV-2: China Part—Joint WHO-China Study (14 January–10 February 2021)*. https://www.who.int/publications/i/item/who-convened-global-study-of-origins-of-sars-cov-2-china-part

World Organization for Animal Health. (2025). *One Health*. https://www.woah.org/en/what-we-do/global-initiatives/one-health/

Yano, T., Phornwisetsirikun, S., Susumpow, P., Visrutaratna, S., Chanachai, K., Phetra, P., Chaisowwong, W., Trakarnsirinont, P., Hemwan, P., Kaewpinta, B., Singhapreecha, C.,

Kreausukon, K., Charoenpanyanet, A., Robert, C. S., Robert, L., Rodtian, P., Mahasing, S., Laiya, E., Pattamakaew, S., et al. (2018). A participatory system for preventing pandemics of animal origins: Pilot study of the Participatory One Health Disease Detection (PODD) System. *JMIR Public Health and Surveillance, 4*(1), e25. https://doi.org/10.2196/publichealth.7375

Yeh, H.-Y., Chen, K.-H., & Chen, K.-T. (2018). Environmental determinants of infectious disease transmission: A focus on One Health concept. *International Journal of Environmental Research and Public Health, 15*(6), 1183. https://doi.org/10.3390/ijerph15061183

Youn, H. (2009). Review of zoonotic parasites in medical and veterinary fields in the Republic of Korea. *The Korean Journal of Parasitology, 47*(Suppl), S133. https://doi.org/10.3347/kjp.2009.47.S.S133

Yumba, E. E. K., Kuzin, A. A., & Zobov, A. E. (2024). Features of the epidemiological surveillance system of rabies and monkeypox in the Republic of Cameroon. *Bulletin of the Russian Military Medical Academy, 25*(4), 681–690. https://doi.org/10.17816/brmma492246

Zain, A., Sadarangani, S. P., Shek, L. P.-C., & Vasoo, S. (2024). Climate change and its impact on infectious diseases in Asia. *Singapore Medical Journal, 65*(4), 211–219. https://doi.org/10.4103/singaporemedj.SMJ-2023-180

Zha, P. (2019). Social epidemiology. In D. F. Pacquiao & M. M. Douglas (Eds.), *Social pathways to health vulnerability* (pp. 159–180). Springer. https://doi.org/10.1007/978-3-319-93326-9_7

Chapter 5
Antimicrobial Resistance

Nilna Sa'adatar Rohmah, Ridwan Balatif, Muhamad Imam Utama, Rizki Andini Nawawi, Farida Nur Oktoviani, Mustofa, Tri Wibawa, and Abdul Rahman Siregar

Abbreviations

AMR	Antimicrobial resistance
ARGs	Antimicrobial resistance genes
ASEAN	Association of Southeast Asian Nations
CRAB	Carbapenem-resistant *Acinetobacter baumannii*
DHFR	Dihydrofolate reductase
DHPS	Dihydropteroate synthase
DNA	Deoxyribonucleic acid
ECM	Extracellular matrix

N. S. Rohmah (✉) · M. I. Utama
Department of Biostatistics, Epidemiology and Population Health, Faculty of Medicine, Public Health, and Nursing, Universitas Gadjah Mada, Yogyakarta, Indonesia
e-mail: nilnasaadatarrohmahskm@mail.ugm.ac.id; muhamadimamutama@mail.ugm.ac.id

R. Balatif · F. N. Oktoviani · T. Wibawa
Department of Microbiology, Faculty of Medicine, Public Health, and Nursing, Universitas Gadjah Mada, Sleman, Yogyakarta, Indonesia
e-mail: ridwanbalatif@mail.ugm.ac.id; farida.nur.o@ugm.ac.id; twibawa@ugm.ac.id

R. A. Nawawi
Department of Clinical Microbiology, Faculty of Medicine, Universitas Sriwijaya, Palembang, Indonesia
e-mail: rizkiandininawawi@fk.unsri.ac.id

Mustofa
Department of Pharmacology and Therapy, Faculty of Medicine, Public Health and Nursing, Universitas Gadjah Mada, Yogyakarta, Indonesia
e-mail: mustofafk@ugm.ac.id

A. R. Siregar
Faculty of Biology, Universitas Gadjah Mada, Yogyakarta, Indonesia
e-mail: ar.siregar@ugm.ac.id

© The Author(s), under exclusive license to Springer Nature Singapore Pte Ltd. 2026

A. U. Rauf, T. Wibawa (eds.), *The One Health Concept in Asian Contexts*,
https://doi.org/10.1007/978-981-95-9880-9_5

ESKAPE	*Enterococcus faecium*, *Staphylococcus aureus*, *Klebsiella pneumoniae*, *Acinetobacter baumannii*, *Pseudomonas aeruginosa*, and *Enterobacter* species
GAP	Global Action Plan
GLASS	Global Antimicrobial Resistance and Use Surveillance System
HGT	Horizontal gene transfer
IPC	Infection prevention and control
LMICs	Low- and middle-income countries
MDR	Multidrug resistance
MDROs	Multidrug-resistant organisms
MDR-TB	Multidrug-resistant tuberculosis
MGE	Mobile genetic elements
MRSA	Methicillin-resistant *Staphylococcus aureus*
NAPs	National action plans
PBP	Penicillin-binding protein
QRDR	Quinolone-resistance-determining region
ROS	Reactive oxygen species
TB	Tuberculosis
TMP-SMX	Trimethoprim-sulfamethoxazole
WWTPs	Wastewater treatment plants
XDR-TB	Extensively drug-resistant tuberculosis

5.1 Introduction to AMR

Antimicrobial resistance (AMR) has become one of the most critical global health challenges of the twenty-first century. AMR occurs when microorganisms such as bacteria, viruses, fungi, and parasites develop mechanisms that protect them from the effects of these drugs. This phenomenon is primarily driven by the overuse and misuse of antibiotics in human healthcare, agriculture, and veterinary practices, as well as environmental contamination from pharmaceutical residues. The rise of AMR compromises the treatment of common infections, making diseases like multidrug-resistant tuberculosis (MDR-TB), methicillin-resistant *Staphylococcus aureus* (MRSA), and resistant malaria increasingly difficult to treat. The impact of AMR extends beyond healthcare, escalating costs, prolonging hospital stays, and leading to higher morbidity and mortality, especially among vulnerable populations such as the elderly, children, and those with weakened (Alomari et al., 2024; Ifedinezi et al., 2024; Warrier et al., 2023).

To address AMR effectively, it is essential to adopt the One Health approach, which integrates human, animal, and environmental health. This approach recognizes that resistance is not confined to humans but spreads through animals and environmental factors like wastewater, agricultural runoff, and environmental contamination. By understanding the interconnectedness between these sectors,

One Health provides a comprehensive framework for combating AMR, acknowledging that pathogens causing resistance can spread not only among humans but also from animals and through environmental factors (La Rosa et al., 2025; Msemakweli et al., 2024).

Understanding the scale of AMR, both globally and locally, is essential for framing its significance as a public health problem. From a statistical perspective, it is estimated that globally AMR caused 1.27 million deaths directly and 4.95 million deaths indirectly in 2019. In Indonesia, AMR surveillance is currently conducted in 20 selected hospitals across various regions, with data analyzed under the Global Antimicrobial Resistance and Use Surveillance System (GLASS). The 2019 GLASS report for Indonesia showed an increase in antimicrobial resistance for certain bacteria such as *Escherichia coli* and *Klebsiella pneumoniae*, including resistance to carbapenems, fluoroquinolones, and third-generation cephalosporins (Limato et al., 2022; Murray et al., 2025; Siahaan et al., 2022).

5.2 Mechanisms of AMR

AMR remains one of the largest global problems due to increasing infections by resistant microorganisms and difficulties in developing new antimicrobials to overcome it. Humanity's war against AMR has been going on since the twentieth century. With the introduction of penicillin to the markets in 1941, various strains of penicillin-resistant *Staphylococcus aureus* started to emerge in the following year. Similarly, when methicillin was discovered and introduced in 1960 to treat penicillin-resistant *S. aureus,* methicillin-resistant *S. aureus* emerged again in the same year (Uddin et al., 2021).

In 2021, approximately 4.71 million deaths were associated with AMR and 1.14 million deaths were attributable to AMR. In Southeast Asia and Oceania, AMR-related deaths are estimated to rise from 52.7 deaths per 100,000 (2021) to 92 per 100,000 (2050). Globally, three pathogens cause the highest AMR-related mortality, namely methicillin-resistant *S. aureus* (130 thousand), carbapenem-resistant *Acinetobacter baumannii* (CRAB) (78.1 thousand), and carbapenem-resistant *Streptococcus pneumoniae* (71.6 thousand). A similar pattern of etiologies is also observed in Southeast Asia and Oceania (Naghavi et al., 2024). In Indonesia, AMR organism infections are estimated to cause 34–133 thousand deaths in 2019 (Gach et al., 2024). Infections caused by resistant microorganisms would decrease treatment success of common infections like typhoid fever, influenza, and candidiasis. This will in turn increase complication and mortality risks. In addition, AMR infections would also increase treatment costs owing to the need for alternative antimicrobes that might cost more (Abushaheen et al., 2020). Without effective preventive measures, AMR is projected to be the leading cause of death worldwide by 2050 (Tang et al., 2023).

(a) Antimicrobial Resistance

Various literature sources use the terms "antimicrobial resistance" and "antibiotic resistance" interchangeably. The term "antimicrobial" refers to drugs used to treat infectious diseases caused by microbes, such as viruses, bacteria, fungi, and parasites. Antimicrobials work by inhibiting or eradicating these microbes through mechanisms such as inhibition of cell wall synthesis, disruption of cellular energy generation, damages in nucleic acid or protein synthesis, and modulation of metabolic pathways (Eshboev et al., 2024). AMR occurs when microbes can survive in the presence of antimicrobials, in other words rendering antimicrobials ineffective. Antibiotic resistance specifically refers to resistance occurring in bacteria (Karvanen & Cars, 2024). This section will focus on the underlying mechanisms of antibiotic resistance.

Antibiotic use may trigger resistance in bacteria by inducing mutations. Spontaneous mutation rates in bacteria are generally kept low by cellular mechanisms, such as DNA repair. However, when disruptions to cellular functions due to environmental factors occur, such as by antibiotic exposure, mutation rates increase to overcome bacterial cell mortality. Both lethal and sublethal doses of antibiotics may induce mutagenesis. Antibiotics directly damaging DNA, such as quinolones, may directly increase mutation rate. However, other antibiotics not acting on DNA, such as β-lactams and aminoglycosides, are thought to also affect mutation rates by disrupting bacterial metabolic functions, thereby triggering cellular stress by formation of reactive oxygen species (ROS). Generated ROS will damage DNA and induce mutagenesis (Blázquez et al., 2018). Selective pressure also drives multiplication of resistant bacteria. In a population of bacterial cells, a small number of bacteria typically carry resistant genes. When the population is exposed to antibiotics, susceptible bacteria will be eradicated, while resistant bacteria will survive. This situation advantages resistant bacteria and drives their growth, eventually taking over the population (Hasan et al., 2022).

Antibiotic resistance may occur through three mechanisms: preventing intracellular antibiotic accumulation, modifying the target molecules of antibiotics, and enzymatic inactivation of antibiotics (Halawa et al., 2024). These mechanisms may occur as intrinsic, adaptive, and acquired resistance. Intrinsic resistance refers to the innate resistance capabilities of the bacteria, such as outer membrane components in Gram-negative bacteria or the absence of cell walls in *Mycoplasma* bacteria which causes resistance to β-lactam agents. Adaptive resistance occurs when bacteria receive environmental pressure, triggering cellular stress responses. This would speed up bacterial cellular modifications to overcome the action of antibiotics, such as biofilm formation, decreasing cell membrane permeability, and production of antibiotic-degrading enzymes. Acquired resistance involves the transfer of resistant traits across bacterial species (horizontal gene transfer, HGT) or genetic mutations (Elshobary et al., 2025; Ho et al., 2024). Resistance mechanisms to antibiotics are illustrated in Fig. 5.1 and elaborated in the following section.

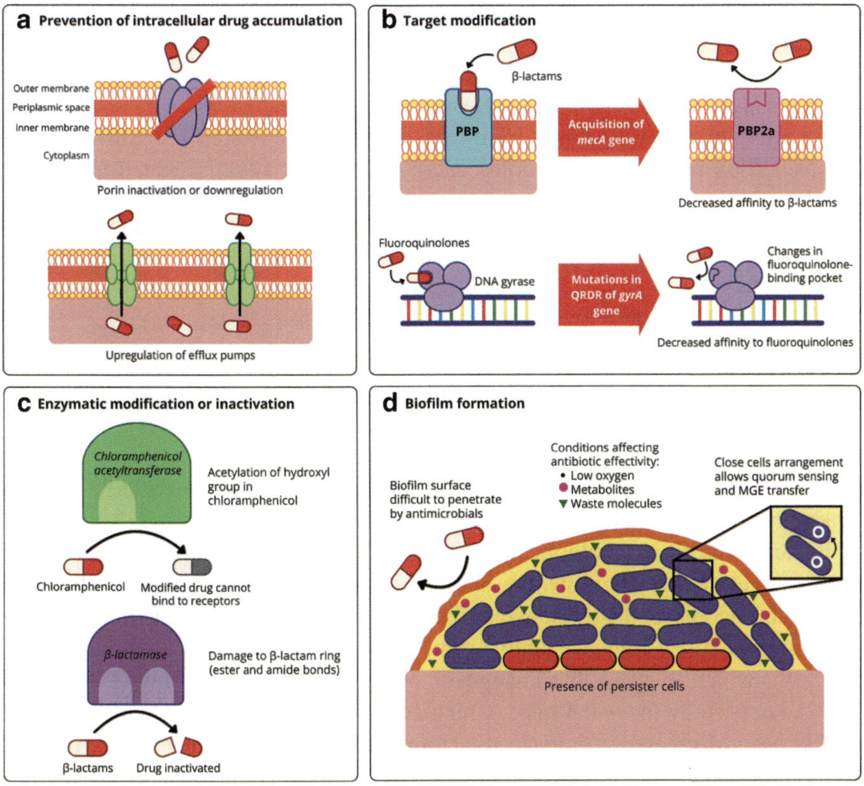

Fig. 5.1 Some main mechanisms of resistance to antibiotics. Mechanisms A to C are specific to certain antibiotics, and other mechanisms may vary by antibiotic or organism. (**a**) Prevention of antibiotic accumulation by downregulating expression of porin channels, porin inactivation, and increasing efflux pumps, (**b**) modification of antibiotic targets, where mutations may cause changes in the target sites such as PBP for penicillin and QRDR for fluoroquinolones, preventing these antibiotics from binding to targets and rendering them ineffective, (**c**) modification of drugs by enzymes, modifying or damaging the antibiotic structure and causing inactivation, and (**d**) biofilm formation confers resistance through a difficult-to-penetrate surface, conditions affecting antimicrobial effectivity within the matrix (low oxygen presence of metabolites and waste molecules), transfer of mobile genetic elements and cell communication by quorum sensing, and presence of persister cells. *PBP* penicillin-binding protein, *QRDR* quinolone-resistance-determining region, *MGE* mobile genetic elements. (Authors' original work)

1. Preventing intracellular accumulation of antibiotics

Gram-negative bacteria possess porin canals, which act as entry points of several antibiotic classes, such as β-lactams and quinolones. Decreasing the number of porin canals may inhibit antibiotic entry into the bacterial cells, thereby causing resistance to the antibiotic (Halawa et al., 2024). Mutations triggering porin protein inactivation or downregulation, such as OprD, cause decreased bacterial permeability to several antibiotic classes, such as aminoglycosides, carbapenem, and fluoroquinolones (Belay et al., 2024; Lee & Ko, 2012). Other mechanisms may be present in particular bacteria, such as membrane permeability reduction resulted from alteration of the porin channels and outer membrane structure of *Escherichia coli* and *Klebsiella pneumoniae* involving mutation in OmpK35, OmpK36, OmpF, and OmpC (García-Sureda et al., 2011; Hassen & Jouini, 2025).

An alternative mechanism is by increasing antibiotic excretion by using efflux pumps. Efflux pumps are a complex energy-dependent system located in the cell membrane. These pumps act in excretion of toxic molecules, including antibiotics, therefore decreasing intracellular antibiotic concentration and decreasing antibiotic effectivity (Belay et al., 2024).

2. Modification of antibiotic targets

Modification of antibiotic target sites will reduce the antibiotic's ability to bind to its target, therefore reducing its effectiveness. These changes often occur because of spontaneous mutations in protein-coding genes. For example, mutations affecting quinolone-resistance-determining region (QRDR) in DNA gyrase (topoisomerase II) and topoisomerase IV would trigger fluoroquinolone resistance in both Gram-positive and Gram-negative bacteria (Belay et al., 2024).

Bacteria can resist antibiotics through complete substitution or bypass of the drug's target site. Bacteria evolve alternative targets that perform the same biochemical functions as the original ones but are no longer susceptible to inhibition by the antibiotic. A key clinical example is methicillin-resistant *Staphylococcus aureus* (MRSA), which involves the change of penicillin-binding proteins (PBPs) into PBP2a encoded by the *mecA* gene, which confers β-lactam resistance to *S. aureus*. PBP2a has a decreased affinity to β-lactam antibiotics, decreasing their effectiveness (Fergestad et al., 2020). Another example is vancomycin-resistant enterococci (VRE), where resistance arises from structural changes in the peptidoglycan, directed by the *van* gene clusters. Enterococci develop resistance to vancomycin by replacing the C-terminal d-alanine in their peptidoglycan with d-lactate or D-serine, creating a d-Ala-d-Lac or d-Ala-d-Ser structure, respectively (Almeida-Santos et al., 2025).

An alternative strategy to evade antimicrobial effects involves bypassing the inhibited metabolic pathway by overproducing the antibiotic's target. A notable example of this is resistance to trimethoprim-sulfamethoxazole (TMP-SMX). An additional mechanism of TMP-SMX resistance involves increased expression of the drug targets, dihydrofolate reductase (DHFR) or dihydropteroate synthase (DHPS) (Ahmad et al., 2025).

3. Enzymatic inactivation of antibiotics

Some enzymes, such as β-lactamase, can damage and inactivate antibiotics. The enzyme β-lactamase is able to damage the ester and amide bonds in β-lactam antibiotics. Another example is chloramphenicol-acetyltransferase, which changes the structure of chloramphenicol by acetylation of hydroxyl groups. This causes chloramphenicol to not bind to the target ribosomes, rendering it ineffective (Halawa et al., 2024).

4. Biofilm formation

Biofilm is an organized structure of microbes encapsulated by an extracellular matrix (ECM) and attached to biotic or abiotic surfaces. Biofilm formation confers benefits to its constituent microbes by forming collective recalcitrance. Recalcitrance signifies the survival capability of biofilms at the presence of high concentrations of antibiotics. Biofilm-forming microbes may even be 10–1000 times less susceptible to various antimicrobials compared to their planktonic forms (Uruén et al., 2020). The biofilm matrix mostly consists of water (97%), followed by an extracellular polymeric matrix made of polysaccharides, protein, nucleic acids, lipid, mineral ions, and cell detritus (Al-Madboly et al., 2024).

Biofilm formation exerts several mechanisms in decreasing effectiveness of antimicrobials. First, the complex, sticky biofilm surface makes it difficult for antimicrobials to penetrate the matrix and reach the target microbes underneath. Second, the environment inside a biofilm contains metabolites, waste molecules, and low oxygen levels, which may also affect the pH. Some antibiotics, such as tobramycin and ciprofloxacin, showed decreased bactericidal activities in low-oxygen environments. Changes in pH also decrease aminoglycoside effectivity. Third, the microbes in a biofilm are arranged close to each other, supporting communication by quorum sensing, as well as transfer of mobile genetic elements. Finally, a small subpopulation of microbes in a biofilm is in a spore-like state, conferring resistance to extreme conditions. This small subpopulation is also known as persister cells (Prinzi & Rohde, 2023).

(b) Spread of Resistance Genes

Antibiotic use in livestock farming constitutes approximately 50% of total global antibiotic consumption. As a result, the gastrointestinal tracts and fecal matter of livestock and poultry represent major reservoirs of drug-resistant bacterial strains and antibiotic resistance genes, thereby playing a pivotal role in the dissemination of antimicrobial resistance. The transmission of resistance genes occurs via horizontal gene transfer (HGT), which encompasses conjugation (the transfer of genetic material between bacteria through sex pili), transformation (the uptake and incorporation of free DNA fragments into the bacterial genome), and transduction (the bacteriophage-mediated transfer of genetic material) (Jian et al., 2021; Murray et al., 2025).

5.3 Consequences of AMR on Public Health

(a) Health impacts

Antimicrobials, such as antibiotics, are important for saving human lives from infectious diseases. Since the first discovery of penicillin by Alexander Fleming, there have been several other antimicrobial substances discovered. However, following the discovery of antimicrobial substances, microorganisms also quickly develop resistance. The discovery of new antimicrobial agents could not keep pace with the emergence of resistant microorganisms. The period from 1940 to 1960 was known as the "Golden Era of Antibiotics," during which several types of antimicrobials were discovered, but since then, the emergence of antimicrobial resistance has grown rapidly (Salam et al., 2023; Tang et al., 2023).

Common infectious diseases that were once effectively treated with available antimicrobials are now becoming more severe due to reduced treatment effectiveness. This ineffectiveness has led to greater reliance on second-line antimicrobials, which are more expensive, have more severe side effects, and require longer treatment durations. Prolonged illness not only worsens patient health outcomes but also places a significant resource burden on healthcare facilities due to extended care needs. Beyond the direct impact of the disease itself, it is estimated that by 2050, there will be 10 million deaths attributed to AMR annually (Ahmed et al., 2024; O'Neil, 2016).

Several microorganisms of particular concern in the context of AMR are grouped under the acronym ESKAPE, referring to *Enterococcus faecium*, *Staphylococcus aureus*, *Klebsiella pneumoniae*, *Acinetobacter baumannii*, *Pseudomonas aeruginosa*, and *Enterobacter* species. These bacteria are considered a global priority in AMR control, because they have been identified as resistant not only to one antibiotic but also to multiple antibiotics from different classes. Resistance to three or more antibiotic classes is referred to as multidrug resistance (MDR). ESKAPE pathogens have demonstrated resistance to oxazolidinones, lipopeptides, macrolides, fluoroquinolones, tetracyclines, β-lactams, β-lactam-β-lactamase inhibitor combinations, and even last-line antibiotics such as carbapenems, glycopeptides, and clinically unfavorable polymyxins. This extensive resistance makes the treatment and management of infections caused by these bacteria significantly more complex and resource-intensive. Besides, ESKAPE pathogens are also known to be the leading causes of hospital-acquired infection (Ahmed et al., 2024; De Oliveira et al., 2020; Miller & Arias, 2024).

Mycobacterium tuberculosis, the cause of tuberculosis (TB), harbors another well-documented example of multidrug resistance. Standard TB treatment, which relies on a combination of antibiotics, has increasingly become ineffective in some cases. *M. tuberculosis* resistance to rifampicin and isoniazid is referred to as multidrug-resistant tuberculosis (MDR-TB). When MDR-TB becomes resistant to fluoroquinolone antibiotics or other second-line antibiotics (capreomycin, kanamycin, or amikacin), it is referred to as extensively drug-resistant TB (XDR-TB). MDR-TB and XDR-TB pose serious treatment challenges and public health threats, as these drug-resistant strains can be transmitted to others, perpetuating the spread of resistance. Patients with these conditions are known to have higher mortality rates or more adverse side effects of the drug both during and after completing the treatment (Ausi et al., 2021; Liebenberg et al., 2022; Prestinaci et al., 2015).

The growing prevalence of multidrug-resistant and extensive drug-resistant infections, such as those caused by ESKAPE pathogens and *Mycobacterium tuberculosis*, underscores the profound health burden of AMR. These infections not only increase morbidity and mortality but also prolong hospital stays, complicate treatment regimens, and require the use of more costly and toxic drugs. Such challenges inevitably translate into substantial economic consequences for both healthcare systems and society, making the economic impact of AMR an equally pressing concern.

(b) Economic burden

The consequences of AMR extend far beyond patient outcomes, imposing a substantial economic burden that includes not only direct healthcare costs but also productivity losses, agricultural impacts, and wider societal effects. The cost of AMR can be described in three different levels: patients, healthcare system, and economic level. At the patient level, infections caused by drug-resistant pathogens have a higher mortality rate than those caused by nonresistant variants. Antimicrobial resistance also hinders the progression of elimination of priority infectious diseases such as tuberculosis, HIV, and malaria. Healthcare systems are challenged on multiple fronts, such as reduced effectiveness of prophylaxis and chemotherapy, increased healthcare expenditure, and extended durations of hospitalization. The estimated global cost attributable to AMR is projected to range from USD 300 billion to over USD 1 trillion annually by 2050. Additionally, procedures requiring use of antibiotics will be more susceptible to unfavorable outcomes. From a wider economic perspective, AMR affects the health and productivity of the workforce. Billions of dollars can be lost from AMR, which stems from loss of productivity, higher treatment cost, or even abandonment of procedures that will be deemed too dangerous (Dadgostar, 2019; O'Neil, 2016; Roope et al., 2019; Tahmasebi et al., 2025).

Human populations are not the only victims of AMR. Animals, especially livestock, have higher exposure to antibiotics. In this setting, antibiotics are often administered via feed or water. This blanket treatment approach is driven by the economic impracticality of treating individual animals. The World Bank estimates that by 2050, AMR could wipe away 3.8% of global gross domestic products each year and push 28 million people into poverty. Losses resulting from the impact of drug resistance on livestock could cost global GDP up to $950 billion, while the spread of resistant pathogens from livestock to humans could cost up to $5.2 trillion. Loss of livestock is not the only effect of AMR on animals. The use of structurally similar antibiotics in livestock to the one used in humans also creates a public health concern. Livestock excrement can contain antimicrobial resistance genes (ARGs). The excrements can disseminate in the environment and cause contamination, facilitating ARGs spread to other livestock and farm workers. Foodborne pathogens with ARGs have already been identified, further confirming the risk of animal products contaminated by resistant microorganisms. An endemic of AMR pathogens can wipe out the entire farm or even other farms, thus threatening food security (Allcock et al., 2017; EcoAMR series, 2024; Samreen et al., 2021; The World Bank, 2024; World Health Organization, 2023).

In the ongoing tug-of-war between the development of new antimicrobial agents and emerging resistance, humanity risks losing within just a few years. This underscores the urgent need to invest in research and development of new antimicrobial agents, alongside funding to generate evidence that can inform policymakers, support innovation, and raise public awareness about the dangers of AMR. The estimated cost needed to provide 15 new drugs and diagnostics over a 10-year period is around US$16 billion. However, the development of antimicrobial agents remains unattractive to industry, as low returns on investment, high development costs, short product lifespans, and greater profitability in other therapeutic areas discourage innovation. Addressing this challenge requires a paradigm shift toward a collaborative model for drug development, bringing together academia, pharmaceutical companies, and governments to share the risks and costs for the benefit of public health (Allcock et al., 2017; O'Neil, 2016; Sugden et al., 2016).

(c) Vulnerable populations

Antimicrobial resistance cases are reported worldwide, disregarding international and socioeconomic boundaries. Identifying vulnerable populations is crucial for guiding effective treatment decisions and targeted interventions. People with disabilities, elderly and pediatric populations, immunocompromised people, chronic disease patients, and marginalized people are known to be vulnerable to AMR. Geographic disparities may also render some regions more vulnerable to AMR (Adebisi, 2024; Shamas et al., 2024).

People with disabilities often require frequent healthcare visits, increasing their exposure to environments where antibiotics are heavily used and resistant bacteria can thrive. Many also have chronic conditions or weakened immune systems, such as those with Down syndrome. Reliance on medical devices—common among individuals with spinal cord injuries or severe cerebral palsy—further heightens the risk, as these can provide entry points for pathogens and foster difficult-to-treat, biofilm-associated infections. The elderly also face heightened vulnerability due to a combination of immunosenescence, frailty, multimorbidity, and frequent healthcare encounters. These aging-related changes increase infection risk and reduce the body's ability to clear resistant pathogens. Chronic diseases further elevate susceptibility, with conditions such as diabetes increasing the likelihood of developing infections that are difficult to treat due to resistance (Adebisi, 2024; Theodorakis et al., 2024).

Children, particularly neonates and infants, are vulnerable to AMR due to immature immune systems, frequent medical care, and higher exposure to hospital environments. Those who are immunocompromised—whether from cancer treatment, organ transplantation, or other causes—face even greater risks. Frequent antibiotic use, invasive procedures, and reduced infection-fighting capacity make resistant infections both more likely and more difficult to treat in these populations (Hocking et al., 2021; McNeil, 2014; Okeke et al., 2024; Tillotson & Zinner, 2017).

Marginalized communities face a disproportionate burden of AMR due to socioeconomic, ethnic, and geographic barriers that restrict access to timely and adequate healthcare. These disparities can delay diagnosis, limit treatment options, and increase the risk of poor outcomes. Geographic remoteness further compounds the problem by reducing access to health and social services, as seen in higher prevalence rates of resistant pathogens in rural and remote areas. In both rural and urban settings, factors such as household crowding, high population density, and widespread community antibiotic use facilitate the transmission of resistant bacteria (Alomari et al., 2024; Blakiston & Freeman, 2020, 2020; Mohanty et al., 2024; Wozniak et al., 2022).

5.4 Factors Contributing to AMR

(a) Human factors

One of the primary drivers of AMR is the overuse and misuse of antibiotics in clinical settings. Antibiotic misuse occurs when antibiotics are prescribed for infections that do not require them, such as viral infections (e.g., the common cold or flu). This misapplication of antibiotics places selective pressure on bacteria, encouraging them to evolve resistance. Studies indicate that approximately 50% of antibiotic prescriptions are unnecessary, contributing significantly to the global AMR crisis (Kardos, 2017; Padma, 2022). Additionally, inadequate infection control practices in healthcare settings amplify AMR. In overcrowded hospitals with poor hygiene and sanitation, the spread of resistant bacteria is accelerated. For instance, improper sterilization of medical equipment and insufficient hand hygiene can foster transmission of multidrug resistant organisms (MDROs) (Wen & Lei, 2024).

The lack of awareness among both healthcare providers and patients is another contributing factor. Many healthcare providers prescribe antibiotics prematurely, influenced by patient demand or insufficient diagnostic tools. Inadequate education regarding the risks of AMR perpetuates misconceptions among patients, such as the belief that antibiotics can treat viral infections. Public health campaigns and antimicrobial stewardship programs are critical to mitigate such practices (Battula & Kumar, 2024). Moreover, in low- and middle-income countries (LMICs), the unrestricted sale of antibiotics, and the practice of self-medication significantly exacerbate AMR. Antibiotics are often available over the counter, which increases the likelihood of inappropriate use and accelerates the development of resistant strains. Addressing this issue requires stricter regulations, enhanced education for healthcare professionals, and greater public awareness, alongside coordinated global efforts to tackle AMR (Battula & Kumar, 2024; Msemakweli et al., 2024). Despite regulations, antibiotics remain widely available without prescription in Indonesia. Evidence from Wulandari et al. (2021) confirmed that inappropriate dispensing practices persist in both licensed and unlicensed outlets, underscoring weak enforcement and the urgent need to integrate drug outlet practices into AMR strategies. This misalignment between policy and practice represents a critical gap within Indonesia's AMR National Action Plan, particularly from One Health perspective, where misuse at the community level may amplify resistance across human, animal, and environmental interfaces.

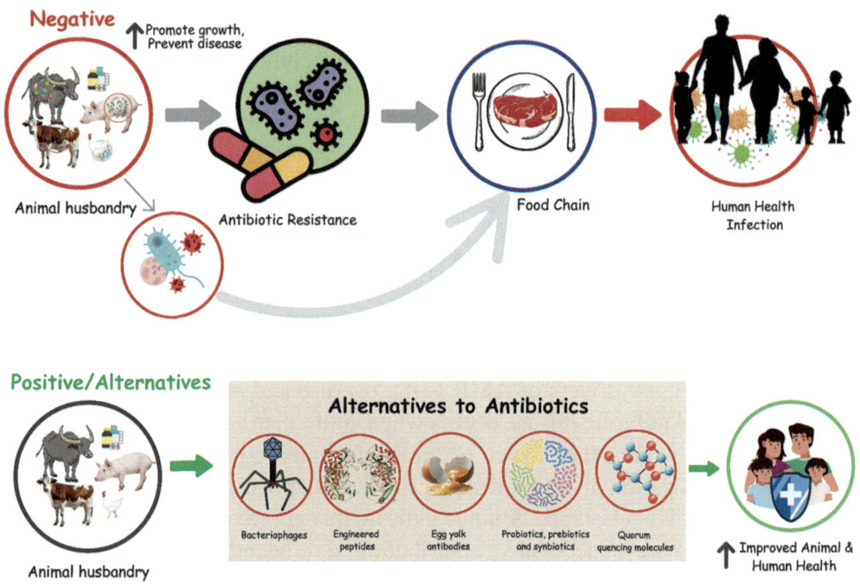

Fig. 5.2 The pathway of antibiotic resistance from animal husbandry to humans and alternatives for promoting growth and preventing disease in animals. The negative pathway (top) illustrates how the use of antibiotics in livestock farming can lead to resistance spreading through the food chain and impacting human health. The positive/alternative pathway (bottom) outlines innovative solutions to improve both animal and human health. (Authors' original work)

(b) Animal health and agriculture

The use of antibiotics in agriculture, particularly in livestock farming, is a major factor contributing to the rise of AMR. In many regions, antibiotics are used not only to treat infections in animals but also as preventive measures and growth promoters. The routine inclusion of antibiotics in animal feed or water is common practice to improve growth rates and prevent diseases, especially in overcrowded and unsanitary conditions (Low et al., 2021). However, this widespread and non-therapeutic use of antibiotics in animal husbandry creates a selective pressure, encouraging the development of resistant bacteria that can spread to humans through direct contact, consumption of contaminated animal products, and environmental exposure (Skandalis et al., 2021) (Fig. 5.2).

In addition to the public health risks, the use of antibiotics in livestock farming also exacerbates environmental contamination. Animal manure exposed to antibiotics contains both the drugs and resistant bacteria, which can contaminate soil and water, further spreading AMR within ecosystems. Therefore, reducing dependency on antibiotics through better vaccination practices and biosecurity in farming operations should be considered as a solution to mitigate environmental impact and enhance resilience against AMR (Wang, 2025).

(c) Environmental factors

One of the significant environmental contributors to the spread of AMR is wastewater contamination from various sectors, including healthcare, pharmaceutical, manufacturing, and agriculture. Wastewater from these sources contains high concentrations of antibiotics and resistant bacteria, which are often discharged into water bodies without proper treatment. This creates selective pressure on microorganisms, enabling resistant strains to survive and proliferate (La Rosa et al., 2025).

While wastewater treatment plants (WWTPs) can reduce some contaminants, many still fail to remove all antibiotics and resistant bacteria before the treated water is released back into the environment. Advancing technologies, such as membrane filtration and biological treatment processes, show promise in reducing antibiotic concentrations. However, these methods are still not entirely effective at removing resistant bacteria, highlighting the need for further technological advancements (Mardalisa et al., 2023) (Fig. 5.3).

In addition to agriculture runoff, pharmaceutical residues from healthcare and pharmaceutical manufacturing significantly contribute to environmental contamination. These residues often enter sewage systems and water sources due to inadequate

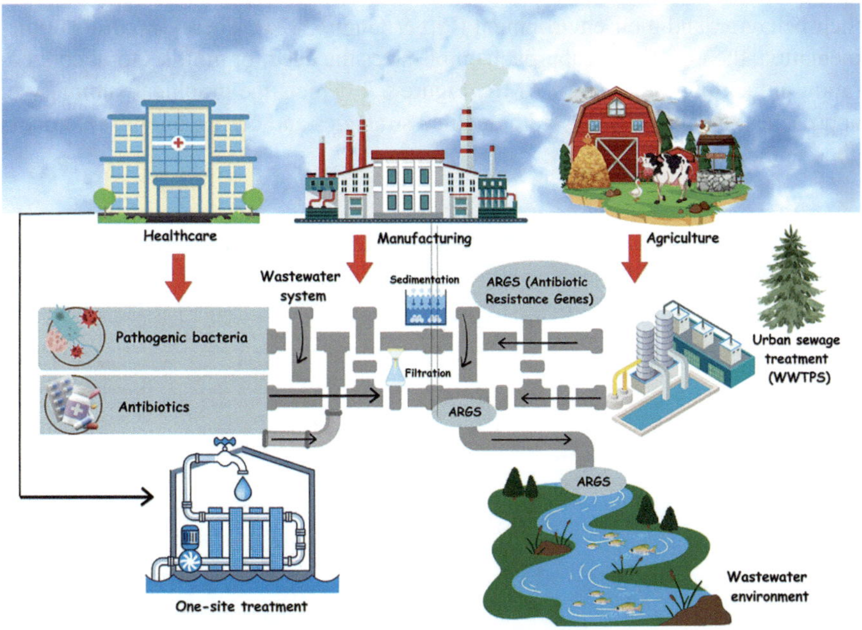

Fig. 5.3 The flow of ARGs into the environment from various factors. Wastewater from healthcares, pharmaceutical manufacturing, and farms serves as a major pathway for the spread of antibiotics, pathogenic bacteria, and ARGs. While wastewater treatment plants (WWTPs) attempt to reduce these contaminants, ARGs can persist and enter the surrounding water environment, contributing to global antimicrobial resistance (AMR). (Authors' original work)

disposal practices and insufficient wastewater treatment capabilities. The persistence of these pollutants in the environment exacerbates AMR by providing a continuous source of resistance for microbial populations. This highlights the need for more robust wastewater treatment systems capable of effectively removing pharmaceutical contaminants (Nguyen et al., 2024).

Furthermore, agricultural runoff, which includes antibiotic residues from livestock farming, remains a key contributor to the environmental spread of AMR. Animal manure containing antibiotics and resistant bacteria often contaminate soil and water, which in turn affects agricultural produce and surrounding ecosystems. To reduce the environmental impact of AMR, a more sustainable approach to farming is necessary, including reducing antibiotic use in livestock, improving waste management systems, and strengthening regulatory frameworks to limit antibiotic residues in the environment (Robles-Jimenez et al., 2025).

5.5 Strategies to Combat AMR

One Health acknowledges the interlinkage between the health of humans, animals, their behavior, and their environment (Pitt & Gunn, 2024). Therefore, in its implementation, the One Health approach emphasizes the need for multisectoral collaboration in tackling the issue of AMR. Figure 5.4 depicts the graphical summary of approaches to combat AMR, with detailed strategies and corresponding references cited in the following sections.

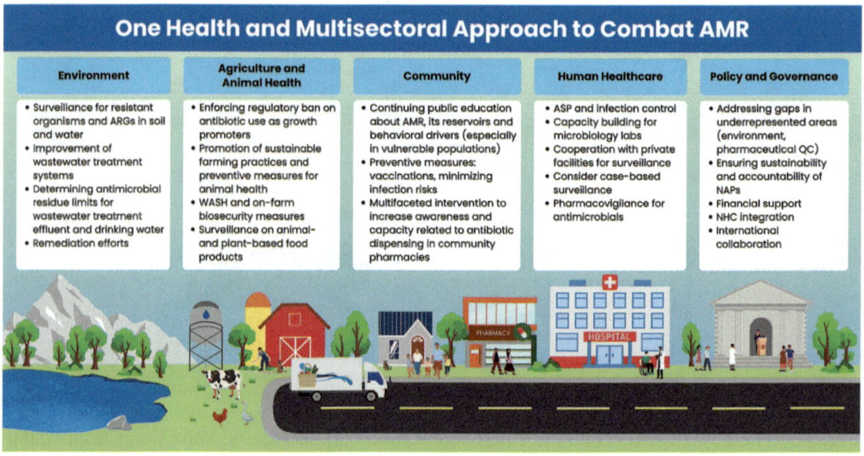

Fig. 5.4 Graphical synthesis of the multisectoral approach to combat the spread and emergence of AMR involving interlinking sectors. *AMR* antimicrobial resistance, *ARGs* antimicrobial resistance genes, *ASPs* antimicrobial stewardship programs, *NAPs* national action plans, *NHC* national healthcare coverage, *QC* quality control, *WASH* water, sanitation, and hygiene. (Authors' original work)

(a) Antimicrobial Stewardship Programs

Antibiotic stewardship programs are considered instrumental in preventing and limiting AMR in clinical settings. Stewardship programs comprise various interventions from education, antibiotic use guidelines, new diagnostic tests, and restricting use of certain antibiotics (Harun et al., 2024). Implementation of such programs are still facing complex challenges attributable to limited program funding, longer turnaround time, lack of competent microbiologists and laboratory personnel, and low capacity of microbiology laboratories related to infrastructure and costs. These challenges are especially pronounced in LMICs (Gandra et al., 2020; Lim et al., 2021).

Promoting infection prevention and control (IPC) programs is essential to support antimicrobial stewardship programs. Incentivizing healthcare facilities to meet antimicrobial stewardship and IPC standards has shown a positive impact in implementing IPC strategies in hospitals. For example, the Ministry of Health, Labor and Welfare in Japan has facilitated financial incentive provision for healthcare facilities meeting IPC standards since 1996 (Nomoto et al., 2022). This was later expanded starting in 2018, where comprehensive implementation of antimicrobial stewardship programs was also financially incentivized (Maeda et al., 2021). However, financial incentivization alone does not suffice to bolster IPC and stewardship program implementation, and a multimodal approach is necessary considering the complexity of factors and stakeholders involved in IPC programs.

(b) Regulatory and Policy Measures

In accordance with the One Health Joint Action Plan and the WHO's Global Action Plan (GAP) on AMR, countries develop their own national action plans (NAPs) for their own implementation. However, several gaps in the policies and implementation of NAPs remain. For instance, some NAPs, like those of Association of Southeast Asian Nations (ASEAN) members, are yet to determine research and surveillance priorities in the environmental sector. In addition, sustained engagement and accountability, especially with regard to funding and program monitoring and evaluation, may be inadequate (Chua et al., 2021). The lack of monitoring and evaluation also highlights gaps in how the national policies are implemented at healthcare facilities (Zay Ya et al., 2024).

Strengthening the governance aspects of combatting AMR requires constant support from policymakers and continuous analysis to address existing issues, effectively monitor implementation, and ensure sustainability of national AMR programs. A relatively successful story is how Thailand's NAP on AMR, first endorsed in 2016, established two key strategic foundations for its implementation. First, a national policy committee on AMR was established to supervise and guide implementation of strategies outlined in the NAP. This committee involves various stakeholders including civil society organizations, professional organizations, private sector, and academia alongside government agencies. Second, a comprehensive scientific platform utilizing pooled funding and strategic partners for data collection was developed as the scientific arm of the committee, which generates evidence to guide the development, implementation, and monitoring of AMR-related policies. This has led to major progress in establishing governance mechanisms, monitoring of how the NAP has been implemented, as well as exceeding targets on some indicators, such as dropping antimicrobial consumption in animals by nearly half by 2021 (Sumpradit et al., 2021).

Government financial support for antimicrobial stewardship and AMR surveillance programs, while necessary for program sustainability in the long run, is not without its own set of challenges. Many antimicrobial stewardship programs are underfunded in public healthcare facilities, and this may be especially pronounced in public hospitals and facilities managed under regional governments (such as city, regency, or province). Additional cost-related issues may arise from insurance or national health system coverage. Under some national healthcare coverage systems like Indonesia's *Jaminan Kesehatan Nasional* (JKN) program, cost analysis, especially related to diagnostic stewardship, remains difficult due to minimal funding. Antibiotic reviews may be of limited use as well, considering limited choices of antimicrobials in the covered list of medications under the national plan (Limato et al., 2022). Considering how AMR significantly increases healthcare costs, national healthcare systems will benefit from incorporating antimicrobial stewardship and infection control measures in their planning and policies.

In LMICs, the costs for a national surveillance system may take up more than 5% of the general government health expenditures, which may not be sustainable for these countries (Painter et al., 2025). Many antimicrobial stewardship and surveillance programs receive assistance from external financial support such as the WHO, United States Centre for Disease Control and Prevention (US CDC), or Fleming Fund, but these financial assistances may only provide partial support and "filling up gaps" in surveillance by reaching a limited number of sites (Gandra et al., 2020; Painter et al., 2025). A global funding initiative may be beneficial in hastening surveillance, bolstering supply chains, and sustained access to effective antimicrobials, especially considering the number of deaths attributable to AMR keeps rising (Painter et al., 2025).

Widespread access to antibiotics without prescription remains a concern in Asian countries. Drug stores are the main points where people easily access antibiotics (Sulis & Gandra, 2021). A study involving Asian and African countries in 2021 reported that 91% of surveyed households in Bangladesh and 72.5% in Vietnam reported obtaining antibiotics for mild illnesses in drug stores, contrasting the situation in Mozambique and South Africa where most households predominantly seek care in public healthcare facilities (Do et al., 2021). Similar practices had also been reported in China, where 86.8% of surveyed community pharmacies dispense antibiotics without prescription. This practice tended to be more common in prefectural-level cities or counties than in provincial capitals (Gong et al., 2020). Indonesia also faces this problem, as antibiotic dispensing without prescription occurred in 69% of pharmacies. This occurred more frequently in pharmacies attached to clinics and standalone pharmacies than drug stores. Additionally, widespread antibiotic dispensing without prescription happens in both urban and rural pharmacies (Ferdiana et al., 2021; Wulandari et al., 2021). While regulatory frameworks exist, such as making unrestricted sale and purchase of antibiotics without prescription a criminal offense, these practices continue anyway, in part due to perceptions of easier access to drugstores than to visit healthcare facilities (Adhikari et al., 2021; Nguyen et al., 2022). While most antibiotics sold without prescription were from Access group (such as cefalexin or amoxicillin), there has been a concerning rise in the sales of antibiotics from the Watch group in Bangladesh and Vietnam (Nguyen et al., 2022; Sulis & Gandra, 2021).

Antibiotics are often used to stimulate growth and productivity of farmed animals, despite existing regulatory bans on these practices (Pitt & Gunn, 2024). Additional concern about regulatory compliance may arise for countries and regions where most of the animal farming sector is held by small enterprises with backyard systems (Sundram et al., 2024). Reducing the need for antibiotics through vaccinations and development of sustainable alternatives for disease prevention and health maintenance of farm animals, such as through organic farming, would be necessary to prevent further spread of AMR. Water, sanitation, and hygiene (WASH) systems in farming communities can also be leveraged integratively with biosecurity measures to prevent spread of resistant organisms (Jimenez et al., 2023).

(c) Surveillance

Surveillance systems are still showing heterogeneity between countries, especially in low- and middle-income countries (LMICs), as no standard sets of surveillance activities are clearly defined. Most laboratories in AMR surveillance programs, such as the WHO's GLASS, use clinical isolates in their reporting. One example of a consistent surveillance system is implemented in Taiwan through the Taiwan Surveillance of Antimicrobial Resistance (TSAR) program, which is an ongoing biennial multicenter study on pathogens from both inpatient and outpatient settings in Taiwan hospitals. The program has been ongoing since 1998, allowing for a long-term observation of changes in pathogens and resistance patterns (Huang et al., 2024). However, data in existing AMR surveillance programs may be underrepresented, as most surveillance systems do not distinguish data from healthcare-associated and community-acquired infections (Gandra et al., 2020; Lim et al., 2021). Case-based surveillance systems, such as "A Clinically Oriented Antimicrobial Resistance Surveillance Network" (ACORN), which has undergone pilot implementation in Laos, Cambodia, and Vietnam, may be considered to aid existing national surveillance systems, as it takes into account clinical data otherwise overlooked in laboratory sample-based surveillance (van Doorn et al., 2022). However, implementation of case-based surveillance in LMICs may be hampered by the varying degrees of electronic medical record implementation across countries, lack of supporting facilities, and the need to localize surveillance items for personnel training and reporting systems (Lim et al., 2021).

While water and soil environments are known to harbor resistant organisms and ARGs, there is a gap in environmental surveillance and remediation efforts compared to human and animal surveillance stewardship strategies. While evidence had shown the potential of antibiotic residues, resistant organisms, or ARG exposure through drinking water, no standard currently exists for antibiotic residues in drinking water, posing a threat of AMR development through chronic exposure of antibiotics at subtherapeutic levels (Hanna et al., 2023; Nava et al., 2022). In addition, environmental surveillance data for AMR in many countries are still scarce (Hanna et al., 2023).

Substandard or counterfeit antibiotics are often found in places with low compliance to antibiotic consumption and prescribing (Zabala et al., 2022). Various factors might also influence antibiotics quality, such as pharmaceutical outlet conditions with improper storage conditions (Islam et al., 2017). The role of antimicrobial quality control in most national action plans to tackle AMR remains undefined. In theory, administration of antibiotic preparations containing less than indicated, or even excessive, active ingredient content should be associated with the estimated AMR prevalence. This may also be true for mortality attributed to AMR (Maffioli et al., 2024, 2025). Due to scarce data on the prevalence of substandard and counterfeit antibiotics in many regions, it is necessary to strengthen postmarketing surveillance and pharmaceutical quality control measures.

(d) Public Education

Public involvement in most NAPs for AMR uses the top-down approach. However, this approach may have overlooked some high-risk populations, such as those with a lower socioeconomic and education level (Chua et al., 2021). Building the right knowledge, attitude, and practices related to AMR in the general public needs to consider the needs of these high-risk populations. University-based community service activities and bottom-up efforts from communities and grassroots movements may help in reaching and educating the prevention of AMR.

High rates of antibiotic procurement without prescription as self-medication might have been attributable to the public perception of easier access to drugstores compared to actually seeking treatment at healthcare facilities. In addition, many buyers obtaining antibiotics without prescription do not know the correct dosing and usage duration of antibiotics (Nguyen et al., 2022; Sulis & Gandra, 2021). Several drivers for this behavior exist from both the consumer and pharmacy. People tend to attempt self-medication for mild illnesses with antibiotics because of the perceived need for more money and/or time for consultations at primary health centers and private practices. Without prescription, people could obtain antibiotics using used packages from prior antibiotic use or occasionally through pharmacist recommendations. Misconceptions about antibiotics further drive inappropriate antibiotic dispensing, especially perceptions of antibiotics as a "powerful" medication for any condition, including those not attributable to bacterial infections. From the perspective of pharmacists and pharmacy owners, denying to dispense antibiotics without prescription was perceived to decrease income, and pharmacists suffer from a power imbalance with the pharmacy owner influencing dispensing practices (Ferdiana et al., 2021).

Measures have been employed to increase public awareness and prevent antibiotic sales without prescription. India is an Asian country facing the problem of extensive over-the-counter sales of antibiotics. The Indian government introduced the "Red Line campaign" initiative in 2016, labeling antibiotics and several other prescription-only drugs regulated under Schedule H1 with a bold red line on the blister pack. While it was hoped to increase public awareness about antibiotic use and deter antibiotic purchases without prescription, the program lacks sustained public campaigns and public awareness might have faded after the initial introduction (Mathew et al., 2022). Indonesia has also introduced a community-based program promoting responsible self-medication since 2015. The Ministry of Health program, called *Gerakan Masyarakat Cerdas Menggunakan Obat* (GeMa CerMat, "Community Smart Use of Medication Movement"), involved training pharmacists to provide information about medicines to their communities. However, slow implementation has led to a relatively unchanged self-medication behavior, including antibiotic use (Ferdiana et al., 2021). Considering how these practices continue to happen despite bans and regulations, public outreach efforts need to address this knowledge gap and emphasize the importance of precautionary measures, such as vaccination. Furthermore, comprehensive strategies aimed at community pharmacies can significantly decrease the distribution of antibiotics without prescription. A multifaceted approach involving online educational sessions, awareness campaigns, peer supervision, and rewards in the form of branding and certification for community pharmacists participating in the program significantly decreased the likelihood of antibiotic dispensing without prescription (Ferdiana et al., 2024).

There is also a lack of awareness in the general public about antibiotic use in farm and companion animals (Bhatt et al., 2023; Rhys-Davies & Ogden, 2020). Raising public awareness on the role of animals in AMR spread is necessary to support AMR preventive measures. Promotion of sustainable farming practices, such as organic farming, may also be used to reach small farming enterprises and further prevent AMR in animals.

5.6 Conclusion

(a) Summary of key insights

Antibiotic resistance is a global problem estimated to be the main cause of death worldwide in the future. Antibiotics can cause mutagenesis in DNA that triggers resistance through direct damaging effects on DNA and indirectly through compounds formed as a result of metabolic disorders (e.g., ROS). Antibiotic resistance may be intrinsic, adaptive, or acquired. Mechanisms underlying antibiotic resistance consist of prevention of intracellular accumulation of antibiotics, antibiotic target modification, enzymatic inactivation of antibiotics, and biofilm formation. Antibiotic resistance genes can spread from one bacterium to another through transformation, conjugation, and transduction.

The threat of AMR has consequences that reach far and wide, ranging from direct patient outcomes to economic losses and agricultural and environmental impacts. These impacts are disproportionately affecting vulnerable populations, such as those with medical conditions, certain age groups like children, and marginalized communities with barriers to education and healthcare. Multidrug and extensive drug resistance microorganisms are on a concerning rise, which further complicates management of infectious diseases with available antimicrobials.

Antibiotic overuse and misuse had been widely recognized as AMR drivers by exerting selection pressure and inducing mutagenesis or HGT. Furthermore, inadequate infection control measures and lack of surveillance in some crucial areas such as animal health and environmental factors cannot be overlooked as equally important contributors to the emergence and spread of AMR. In Asian countries, the main issue is the purchase of antibiotics without a doctor's prescription. Most of these antibiotics are purchased through drugstores, and this phenomenon occurs in both urban and rural areas. Additionally, the general public lacks awareness regarding antimicrobial use in farm and companion animals. While regulatory frameworks and action plans on global and national levels are available, the implementation of these programs and integration across sectors might have remained suboptimal, especially in LMICs.

(b) Call to action

The One Health Joint Action Plan on AMR and the WHO's GAP on AMR outline the importance of multisectoral collaborative approach in mitigating AMR. However, several challenges and limitations remain to be addressed, which are especially pronounced for LMICs and vulnerable populations. Some Asian countries like Japan, Thailand, and Taiwan have shown success with continuous active surveillance, multisectoral involvement, incentivization of IPC improvement, and good public awareness on AMR. Yet, many LMICs in Asia still struggle with weak regulatory enforcement, as well as logistical and financial limitations. In addition to robust political will, financial and infrastructure support across sectors from individual countries, international cooperation is paramount in the surveillance and mitigation of AMR, as well as addressing the gaps and inequalities between high-income countries and LMICs.

Globalization has enabled the movement of goods and people across borders faster than ever before. While a global joint action plan on AMR exists as a guideline for adaptation implementation in individual countries, the possible transfer of resistant microorganisms and ARGs through international trade and travel has mostly remained unaddressed by individual countries and regional associations. This calls for an international consensus to fill in this gap and prevent cross-border spread of AMR.

Various campaign programs to raise public awareness on antibiotic use, such as the "Red Line campaign" in India or GeMa CerMat in Indonesia, have been carried out. So far, this approach has not provided satisfactory results in part due to low sustainability. Public involvement in preventing and mitigating AMR needs to start by continuing education and raising awareness to hopefully drive behavioral changes. However, this effort needs to also consider the needs and circumstances of vulnerable populations. The top-down model ascribed by many NAPs may need to change and accommodate the role of public movements, such as those of communities and educational institutions. Additionally, continued public education and engagement is necessary to create a collective consciousness about AMR.

Competing Interests The author(s) has no competing interests to declare that are relevant to the content of this manuscript.

References

Abushaheen, M. A., Muzaheed, Fatani, A. J., Alosaimi, M., Mansy, W., George, M., Acharya, S., Rathod, S., Divakar, D. D., Jhugroo, C., Vellappally, S., Khan, A. A., Shaik, J., & Jhugroo, P. (2020). Antimicrobial resistance, mechanisms and its clinical significance. *Disease-a-Month, 66*(6), 100971. https://doi.org/10.1016/j.disamonth.2020.100971

Adebisi, Y. A. (2024). Antimicrobial resistance and people living with disabilities. *The Lancet, 403*(10441), 2289. https://doi.org/10.1016/S0140-6736(24)00429-X

Adhikari, B., Pokharel, S., Raut, S., Adhikari, J., Thapa, S., Paudel, K., Neupane, S., Neupane, S. R., Yadav, R., Shrestha, S., Rijal, K. R., Marahatta, S. B., Cheah, P. Y., & Pell, C. (2021). Why do people purchase antibiotics over-the-counter? A qualitative study with patients, clinicians and dispensers in central, eastern and western Nepal. *BMJ Global Health, 6*(5), e005829. https://doi.org/10.1136/bmjgh-2021-005829

Ahmad, M., Aduru, S. V., Smith, R. P., Zhao, Z., & Lopatkin, A. J. (2025). The role of bacterial metabolism in antimicrobial resistance. *Nature Reviews Microbiology, 23*(7), 439–454. https://doi.org/10.1038/s41579-025-01155-0

Ahmed, S. K., Hussein, S., Qurbani, K., Ibrahim, R. H., Fareeq, A., Mahmood, K. A., & Mohamed, M. G. (2024). Antimicrobial resistance: Impacts, challenges, and future prospects. *Journal of Medicine, Surgery, and Public Health, 2*, 100081. https://doi.org/10.1016/j.glmedi.2024.100081

Allcock, S., Young, E. H., Holmes, M., Gurdasani, D., Dougan, G., Sandhu, M. S., Solomon, L., & Török, M. E. (2017). Antimicrobial resistance in human populations: Challenges and opportunities. *Global Health, Epidemiology and Genomics, 2*, e4. https://doi.org/10.1017/gheg.2017.4

Al-Madboly, L. A., Aboulmagd, A., El-Salam, M. A., Kushkevych, I., & El-Morsi, R. M. (2024). Microbial enzymes as powerful natural anti-biofilm candidates. *Microbial Cell Factories, 23*(1), 1–16. https://doi.org/10.1186/s12934-024-02610-y

Almeida-Santos, A. C., Novais, C., Peixe, L., & Freitas, A. R. (2025). Vancomycin-resistant Enterococcus faecium: A current perspective on resilience, adaptation, and the urgent need for novel strategies. *Journal of Global Antimicrobial Resistance, 41*, 233–252. https://doi.org/10.1016/j.jgar.2025.01.016

Alomari, R., Abdel-Razeq, A., & Shamiah, H. (2024). Comprehensive assessment of the global burden of antimicrobial resistance: Trends and insights from 2000 to 2023. *American Journal of BioMedicine, 12*(4), 151–168. https://doi.org/10.18081/2333-5106/2024.12/151

Ausi, Y., Santoso, P., Sunjaya, D., & Barliana, M. I. (2021). Between curing and torturing: Burden of adverse reaction in drug-resistant tuberculosis therapy. *Patient Preference and Adherence, 15*, 2597–2607. https://doi.org/10.2147/PPA.S333111

Battula, P., & Kumar, B. (2024). Assessment of antimicrobial resistance risks due to physician and patient practices: An observational study. *Tropical Journal of Pharmaceutical Research, 23*(10), 1761–1767. https://doi.org/10.4314/tjpr.v23i10.22

Belay, W. Y., Getachew, M., Tegegne, B. A., Teffera, Z. H., Dagne, A., Zeleke, T. K., Abebe, R. B., Gedif, A. A., Fenta, A., Yirdaw, G., Tilahun, A., & Aschale, Y. (2024). Mechanism of antibacterial resistance, strategies and next-generation antimicrobials to contain antimicrobial resistance: A review. *Frontiers in Pharmacology, 15*, 1444781. https://doi.org/10.3389/fphar.2024.1444781

Bhatt, V., Ponnampalavanar, S. S. L. S., Chong, C. W., Tang, L. Y., Krishnasamy, K., Goh, S. S. L., & Teh, C. S. J. (2023). Socio-demographic factors and public knowledge of antibiotic resistance. *Healthcare, 11*(16), Article 16. https://doi.org/10.3390/healthcare11162284

Blakiston, M. R., & Freeman, J. T. (2020). Population-level exposures associated with MRSA and ESBL-E. coli infection across district health boards in Aotearoa New Zealand: An ecological study. *133*(1510).

Blázquez, J., Rodríguez-Beltrán, J., & Matic, I. (2018). Antibiotic-induced genetic variation: how it arises and how it can be prevented. *Annual Review of Microbiology*, *72*(2018), 209–230. https://doi.org/10.1146/annurev-micro-090817-062139

Chua, A. Q., Verma, M., Hsu, L. Y., & Legido-Quigley, H. (2021). An analysis of national action plans on antimicrobial resistance in Southeast Asia using a governance framework approach. *The Lancet Regional Health—Western Pacific, 7*, 100084. https://doi.org/10.1016/j.lanwpc.2020.100084

Dadgostar, P. (2019). Antimicrobial resistance: Implications and costs. *Infection and Drug Resistance, 12*, 3903–3910. https://doi.org/10.2147/IDR.S234610

De Oliveira, D. M. P., Forde, B. M., Kidd, T. J., Harris, P. N. A., Schembri, M. A., Beatson, S. A., Paterson, D. L., & Walker, M. J. (2020). Antimicrobial resistance in ESKAPE pathogens. *Clinical Microbiology Reviews, 33*(3). https://doi.org/10.1128/cmr.00181-19

Do, N. T. T., Vu, H. T. L., Nguyen, C. T. K., Punpuing, S., Khan, W. A., Gyapong, M., Asante, K. P., Munguambe, K., Gómez-Olivé, F. X., John-Langba, J., Tran, T. K., Sunpuwan, M., Sevene, E., Nguyen, H. H., Ho, P. D., Matin, M. A., Ahmed, S., Karim, M. M., Cambaco, O., et al. (2021). Community-based antibiotic access and use in six low-income and middle-income countries: A mixed-method approach. *The Lancet Global Health, 9*(5), e610–e619. https://doi.org/10.1016/S2214-109X(21)00024-3

EcoAMR series. (2024). *Forecasting the fallout from AMR: Economic impacts of antimicrobial resistance in food-producing animals*. A report from the EcoAMR series. WOAH and World Bank. 10.20506/ecoAMR.3541

Elshobary, M. E., Badawy, N. K., Ashraf, Y., Zatioun, A. A., Masriya, H. H., Ammar, M. M., Mohamed, N. A., Mourad, S., & Assy, A. M. (2025). Combating antibiotic resistance: Mechanisms, multidrug-resistant pathogens, and novel therapeutic approaches: An updated review. *Pharmaceuticals, 18*(3), Article 3. https://doi.org/10.3390/ph18030402

Eshboev, F., Mamadalieva, N., Nazarov, P., Hussain, H., Katanaev, V., Egamberdieva, D., & Azimova, S. (2024). Antimicrobial action mechanisms of natural compounds isolated from endophytic microorganisms. *Antibiotics, 13*(3), 271. https://doi.org/10.3390/antibiotics13030271

Ferdiana, A., Liverani, M., Khan, M., Wulandari, L. P. L., Mashuri, Y. A., Batura, N., Wibawa, T., Yeung, S., Day, R., Jan, S., Wiseman, V., & Probandari, A. (2021). Community pharmacies, drug stores, and antibiotic dispensing in Indonesia: A qualitative study. *BMC Public Health, 21*(1), 1800. https://doi.org/10.1186/s12889-021-11885-4

Ferdiana, A., Mashuri, Y. A., Wulandari, L. P. L., Rahayu, I. D., Hasanah, M., Ayuningsih, Z., Batura, N., Khan, M., Liverani, M., Guy, R., Schierhout, G., Kaldor, J., Law, M., Day, R., Jan, S., Wibawa, T., Probandari, A., Yeung, S., & Wiseman, V. (2024). The impact of a multi-faceted intervention on non-prescription dispensing of antibiotics by urban community pharmacies in Indonesia: A mixed methods evaluation. *BMJ Global Health, 9*(10), e015620. https://doi.org/10.1136/bmjgh-2024-015620

Fergestad, M. E., Stamsås, G. A., Morales Angeles, D., Salehian, Z., Wasteson, Y., & Kjos, M. (2020). Penicillin-binding protein PBP2a provides variable levels of protection toward different β-lactams in Staphylococcus aureus RN4220. *MicrobiologyOpen, 9*(8), e1057. https://doi.org/10.1002/mbo3.1057

Gach, M. W., Lazarus, G., Simadibrata, D. M., Sinto, R., Saharman, Y. R., Limato, R., Nelwan, E. J., Doorn, H. R. van, Karuniawati, A., & Hamers, R. L. (2024). Antimicrobial resistance among common bacterial pathogens in Indonesia: A systematic review. The Lancet Regional Health—Southeast Asia, 26, 100414. https://doi.org/10.1016/j.lansea.2024.100414

Gandra, S., Alvarez-Uria, G., Turner, P., Joshi, J., Limmathurotsakul, D., & van Doorn, H. R. (2020). Antimicrobial resistance surveillance in low- and middle-income countries: Progress and challenges in eight South Asian and Southeast Asian countries. *Clinical Microbiology Reviews, 33*(3), e00048–e00019. https://doi.org/10.1128/cmr.00048-19

García-Sureda, L., Doménech-Sánchez, A., Barbier, M., Juan, C., Gascó, J., & Albertí, S. (2011). OmpK26, a novel porin associated with carbapenem resistance in Klebsiella pneumoniae. *Antimicrobial Agents and Chemotherapy, 55*(10), 4742–4747. https://doi.org/10.1128/aac.00309-11

Gong, Y., Jiang, N., Chen, Z., Wang, J., Zhang, J., Feng, J., Lu, Z., & Yin, X. (2020). Over-the-counter antibiotic sales in community and online pharmacies, China. *Bulletin of the World Health Organization, 98*(7), 449–457. https://doi.org/10.2471/BLT.19.242370

Halawa, E. M., Fadel, M., Al-Rabia, M. W., Behairy, A., Nouh, N. A., Abdo, M., Olga, R., Fericean, L., Atwa, A. M., El-Nablaway, M., & Abdeen, A. (2024). Antibiotic action and resistance: Updated review of mechanisms, spread, influencing factors, and alternative approaches for combating resistance. *Frontiers in Pharmacology, 14*, 1305294. https://doi.org/10.3389/fphar.2023.1305294

Hanna, N., Tamhankar, A. J., & Lundborg, C. S. (2023). Antibiotic concentrations and antibiotic resistance in aquatic environments of the WHO Western Pacific and South-East Asia regions: A systematic review and probabilistic environmental hazard assessment. *The Lancet Planetary Health, 7*(1), e45–e54. https://doi.org/10.1016/S2542-5196(22)00254-6

Harun, M. G. D., Sumon, S. A., Hasan, I., Akther, F. M., Islam, M. S., & Anwar, M. M. U. (2024). Barriers, facilitators, perceptions and impact of interventions in implementing antimicrobial stewardship programs in hospitals of low-middle and middle countries: A scoping review. *Antimicrobial Resistance & Infection Control, 13*(1), 8. https://doi.org/10.1186/s13756-024-01369-6

Hasan, C. M., Dutta, D., & Nguyen, A. N. T. (2022). Revisiting antibiotic resistance: Mechanistic foundations to evolutionary outlook. *Antibiotics, 11*(1), 40. https://doi.org/10.3390/antibiotics11010040

Hassen, B., & Jouini, A. (2025). Fluoroquinolone-resistant Escherichia coli: Mechanisms of resistance, environmental factors influencing resistance and clinical implications. *Infectious Microbes & Diseases, 7*(2), 84–91. https://doi.org/10.1097/IM9.0000000000000181

Ho, C. S., Wong, C. T. H., Aung, T. T., Lakshminarayanan, R., Mehta, J. S., Rauz, S., McNally, A., Kintses, B., Peacock, S. J., de la Fuente-Nunez, C., Hancock, R. E. W., & Ting, D. S. J. (2024). Antimicrobial resistance: A concise update. *The Lancet Microbe*, 100947. https://doi.org/10.1016/j.lanmic.2024.07.010

Hocking, L., Ali, G.-C., d'Angelo, C., Deshpande, A., Stevenson, C., Virdee, M., & Guthrie, S. (2021). A rapid evidence assessment exploring whether antimicrobial resistance complicates non-infectious health conditions and healthcare services, 2010–20. *JAC-Antimicrobial Resistance, 3*(4), dlab171. https://doi.org/10.1093/jacamr/dlab171

Huang, Y.-C., Kuo, S.-C., Fang, C.-T., & Lauderdale, T.-L. (2024). Changing epidemiology and antimicrobial resistance of bacteria causing bacteremia in Taiwan: 2002–2020. *Microbiology Spectrum, 12*(8), e00608–e00624. https://doi.org/10.1128/spectrum.00608-24

Ifedinezi, O. V., Nnaji, N. D., Anumudu, C. K., Ekwueme, C. T., Uhegwu, C. C., Ihenetu, F. C., Obioha, P., Simon, B. O., Ezechukwu, P. S., & Onyeaka, H. (2024). Environmental antimicrobial resistance: Implications for food safety and public health. *Antibiotics, 13*(11), 1087. https://doi.org/10.3390/antibiotics13111087

Islam, M. R., Yoshida, N., Tsuboi, H., Sovannarith, T., Dararath, E., Bun Kiet, H., Sokchamroeun, U., Keila, T., Tanimoto, T., & Kimura, K. (2017). Four-year survey of the quality of antimicrobial medicines in Cambodia. *Journal of International Health, 32*(4), 233–242. https://doi.org/10.11197/jaih.32.233

Jian, Z., Zeng, L., Xu, T., Sun, S., Yan, S., Yang, L., Huang, Y., Jia, J., & Dou, T. (2021). Antibiotic resistance genes in bacteria: Occurrence, spread, and control. *Journal of Basic Microbiology, 61*(12), 1049–1070. https://doi.org/10.1002/jobm.202100201

Jimenez, C. E. P., Keestra, S. M., Tandon, P., Pickering, A. J., Moodley, A., Cumming, O., & Chandler, C. I. R. (2023). One Health WASH: An AMR-smart integrative approach to preventing and controlling infection in farming communities. *BMJ Global Health, 8*(3), e011263. https://doi.org/10.1136/bmjgh-2022-011263

Kardos, N. (2017). Overuse of antibiotics and antibiotic resistance in medical applications featuring Carbapenemase Resistant Enterobacteriaceae (CRE). *SOJ Microbiology & Infectious Diseases, 5*(5), 1–21. https://doi.org/10.15226/sojmid/5/5/00183

Karvanen, M., & Cars, O. (2024). The language of antimicrobial and antibiotic resistance is blocking global collective action. *Infectious Diseases, 56*(6), 487–495. https://doi.org/10.1080/23744235.2024.2332455

La Rosa, M. C., Maugeri, A., Favara, G., La Mastra, C., Magnano San Lio, R., Barchitta, M., & Agodi, A. (2025). The impact of wastewater on antimicrobial resistance: A scoping review of transmission pathways and contributing factors. *Antibiotics, 14*(2), 131. https://doi.org/10.3390/antibiotics14020131

Lee, J.-Y., & Ko, K. S. (2012). OprD mutations and inactivation, expression of efflux pumps and AmpC, and metallo-β-lactamases in carbapenem-resistant Pseudomonas aeruginosa isolates from South Korea. *International Journal of Antimicrobial Agents, 40*(2), 168–172. https://doi.org/10.1016/j.ijantimicag.2012.04.004

Liebenberg, D., Gordhan, B. G., & Kana, B. D. (2022). Drug resistant tuberculosis: Implications for transmission, diagnosis, and disease management. *Frontiers in Cellular and Infection Microbiology, 12*, 943545. https://doi.org/10.3389/fcimb.2022.943545

Lim, C., Ashley, E. A., Hamers, R. L., Turner, P., Kesteman, T., Akech, S., Corso, A., Mayxay, M., Okeke, I. N., Limmathurotsakul, D., & van Doorn, H. R. (2021). Surveillance strategies using routine microbiology for antimicrobial resistance in low- and middle-income countries. *Clinical Microbiology and Infection, 27*(10), 1391–1399. https://doi.org/10.1016/j.cmi.2021.05.037

Limato, R., Broom, A., Nelwan, E. J., & Hamers, R. L. (2022). A qualitative study of barriers to antimicrobial stewardship in Indonesian hospitals: Governance, competing interests, cost, and structural vulnerability. *Antimicrobial Resistance & Infection Control, 11*(1), 85. https://doi.org/10.1186/s13756-022-01126-7

Low, C. X., Tan, L. T.-H., Ab Mutalib, N.-S., Pusparajah, P., Goh, B.-H., Chan, K.-G., Letchumanan, V., & Lee, L.-H. (2021). Unveiling the impact of antibiotics and alternative methods for animal husbandry: A review. *Antibiotics, 10*(5), 578. https://doi.org/10.3390/antibiotics10050578

Maeda, M., Muraki, Y., Kosaka, T., Yamada, T., Aoki, Y., Kaku, M., Seki, M., Tanabe, Y., Fujita, N., Niki, Y., Morita, K., Yanagihara, K., Yoshida, K., & Kawaguchi, T. (2021). Impact of health policy on structural requisites for antimicrobial stewardship: A nationwide survey conducted in Japanese hospitals after enforcing the revised reimbursement system for antimicrobial stewardship programs. *Journal of Infection and Chemotherapy, 27*(1), 1–6. https://doi.org/10.1016/j.jiac.2020.09.015

Maffioli, E. M., Montás, M. C., & Anyakora, C. (2024). Excessive active pharmaceutical ingredients in substandard and falsified drugs should also raise concerns in low-income countries. *Journal of Global Health, 14*, 03029. https://doi.org/10.7189/jogh.14.03029

Maffioli, E. M., Lu, Y., & Anyakora, C. (2025). Substandard and falsified antibiotics are associated with antimicrobial resistance: A retrospective country-level analysis. *BMJ Global Health, 10*(6), e017078. https://doi.org/10.1136/bmjgh-2024-017078

Mardalisa, M., Wang, R., Honda, R., Chiemchaisri, W., & Chiemchaisri, C. (2023). Mitigation of antimicrobial resistance during wastewater treatment by membrane technologies. *Journal of Applied Membrane Science & Technology, 27*(1), 79–88. https://doi.org/10.11113/amst.v27n1.263

Mathew, P., Thomas, S. A., & Chandy, S. J. (2022). The role of Schedule H1 and Red Line campaign in improving antibiotic use in India. *Journal of Family Medicine and Primary Care, 11*(6), 2656–2661. https://doi.org/10.4103/jfmpc.jfmpc_1811_21

McNeil, J. C. (2014). Staphylococcus aureus—Antimicrobial resistance and the immunocompromised child. *Infection and Drug Resistance, 7*, 117–127. https://doi.org/10.2147/IDR.S39639

Miller, W. R., & Arias, C. A. (2024). ESKAPE pathogens: Antimicrobial resistance, epidemiology, clinical impact and therapeutics. *Nature Reviews Microbiology, 22*(10), 598–616. https://doi.org/10.1038/s41579-024-01054-w

Mohanty, S., Ye, G., Sheets, C., Cossrow, N., Yu, K. C., White, M., Klinker, K. P., & Gupta, V. (2024). Association between social vulnerability and Streptococcus pneumoniae antimicrobial resistance in US adults. *Clinical Infectious Diseases, 79*(2), 305–311. https://doi.org/10.1093/cid/ciae138

Msemakweli, J., Mzuka, K., & Osward, A. (2024). One Health approach to antimicrobial resistance: Integrating human, animal, and environmental perspectives. *Journal of Public Health and Community Medicine*, 1. https://doi.org/10.5455/JPHCM.20240918103501

Murray, P. R., Rosenthal, K. S., & Pfaller, M. A. (2025). *Medical microbiology* (10th ed.). Elsevier.

Naghavi, M., Vollset, S. E., Ikuta, K. S., Swetschinski, L. R., Gray, A. P., Wool, E. E., Robles Aguilar, G., Mestrovic, T., Smith, G., Han, C., Hsu, R. L., Chalek, J., Araki, D. T., Chung, E., Raggi, C., Gershberg Hayoon, A., Davis Weaver, N., Lindstedt, P. A., Smith, A. E., et al. (2024). Global burden of bacterial antimicrobial resistance 1990–2021: A systematic analysis with forecasts to 2050. *The Lancet, 404*(10459), 1199–1226. https://doi.org/10.1016/S0140-6736(24)01867-1

Nava, A. R., Daneshian, L., & Sarma, H. (2022). Antibiotic resistant genes in the environment-exploring surveillance methods and sustainable remediation strategies of antibiotics and ARGs. *Environmental Research, 215*, 114212. https://doi.org/10.1016/j.envres.2022.114212

Nguyen, T. T. P., Do, T. X., Nguyen, H. A., Nguyen, C. T. T., Meyer, J. C., Godman, B., Skosana, P., & Nguyen, B. T. (2022). A national survey of dispensing practice and customer knowledge on antibiotic use in Vietnam and the implications. *Antibiotics, 11*(8), 1091. https://doi.org/10.3390/antibiotics11081091

Nguyen, M.-K., Lin, C., Bui, X.-T., Rakib, M. R. J., Nguyen, H.-L., Truong, Q.-M., Hoang, H.-G., Tran, H.-T., Malafaia, G., & Idris, A. M. (2024). Occurrence and fate of pharmaceutical pollutants in wastewater: Insights on ecotoxicity, health risk, and state–of–the-art removal. *Chemosphere, 354*, 141678. https://doi.org/10.1016/j.chemosphere.2024.141678

Nomoto, H., Saito, H., Ishikane, M., Gu, Y., Ohmagari, N., Pittet, D., Kunishima, H., Allegranzi, B., & Yoshida, M. (2022). First nationwide survey of infection prevention and control among healthcare facilities in Japan: Impact of the national regulatory system. *Antimicrobial Resistance & Infection Control, 11*(1), 135. https://doi.org/10.1186/s13756-022-01175-y

O'Neil, J. (2016). *Tackling drug-resistant infections globally: Final report and recommendations*. The Review on Antimicrobial Resistance.

Okeke, I. N., De Kraker, M. E. A., Van Boeckel, T. P., Kumar, C. K., Schmitt, H., Gales, A. C., Bertagnolio, S., Sharland, M., & Laxminarayan, R. (2024). The scope of the antimicrobial resistance challenge. *The Lancet, 403*(10442), 2426–2438. https://doi.org/10.1016/S0140-6736(24)00876-6

Padma, K. (2022). Overuse and misuse of antibiotics. *Journal of Biomedical and Pharmaceutical Research, 11*(1). https://doi.org/10.32553/jbpr.v11i1.899

Painter, C., Limmathurotsakul, D., Roberts, T., Doorn, H. R. V., Mayxay, M., Lubell, Y., Day, N. P. J., Turner, P., & Ashley, E. A. (2025). Sustainable antimicrobial resistance surveillance: Time for a global funding mechanism. *The Lancet Infectious Diseases, 25*(2), e99–e103. https://doi.org/10.1016/S1473-3099(24)00649-2

Pitt, S. J., & Gunn, A. (2024). The One Health concept. *British Journal of Biomedical Science, 81*, 12366. https://doi.org/10.3389/bjbs.2024.12366

Prestinaci, F., Pezzotti, P., & Pantosti, A. (2015). Antimicrobial resistance: A global multifaceted phenomenon. *Pathogens and Global Health, 109*(7), 309–318. https://doi.org/10.1179/2047773215Y.0000000030

Prinzi, A., & Rohde, R. E. (2023). *The role of bacterial biofilms in antimicrobial resistance*. American Society for Microbiology. https://asm.org:443/articles/2023/march/the-role-of-bacterial-biofilms-in-antimicrobial-re

Rhys-Davies, L., & Ogden, J. (2020). Vets' and pet owners' views about antibiotics for companion animals and the use of phages as an alternative. *Frontiers in Veterinary Science, 7*, 513770. https://doi.org/10.3389/fvets.2020.513770

Robles-Jimenez, L. E., Ghavipanje, N., Hernandez, J. C. A., & Gonzalez-Ronquillo, M. (2025). Recent developments in antibiotic contamination of animal products, soil, and water worldwide—A review. *Annals of Animal Science, 25*(1), 83–102. https://doi.org/10.2478/aoas-2024-0047

Roope, L. S. J., Smith, R. D., Pouwels, K. B., Buchanan, J., Abel, L., Eibich, P., Butler, C. C., Tan, P. S., Walker, A. S., Robotham, J. V., & Wordsworth, S. (2019). The challenge of antimicrobial resistance: What economics can contribute. *Science, 364*(6435), eaau4679. https://doi.org/10.1126/science.aau4679

Salam, M. A., Al-Amin, M. Y., Salam, M. T., Pawar, J. S., Akhter, N., Rabaan, A. A., & Alqumber, M. A. A. (2023). Antimicrobial resistance: A growing serious threat for global public health. *Healthcare, 11*(13), 1946. https://doi.org/10.3390/healthcare11131946

Samreen, Ahmad, I., Malak, H. A., & Abulreesh, H. H. (2021). Environmental antimicrobial resistance and its drivers: A potential threat to public health. *Journal of Global Antimicrobial Resistance, 27*, 101–111. https://doi.org/10.1016/j.jgar.2021.08.001

Shamas, N., Kariuki, J., Balasa, E., Kinamon, T., Liauw, F., Charles, S., Jaka, B., Purdie, R., Chavan, B., Lawal, M. O., Darcovich, A., & Carter, V. (2024). Antimicrobial resistance survivors: Calling the world to action. *The Lancet, 403*(10442), 2355–2357. https://doi.org/10.1016/S0140-6736(24)01030-4

Siahaan, S., Herman, M. J., & Fitri, N. (2022). Antimicrobial Resistance Situation in Indonesia: A Challenge of Multisector and Global Coordination. Journal of tropical medicine, 2022, 2783300. https://doi.org/10.1155/2022/2783300

Skandalis, N., Maeusli, M., Papafotis, D., Miller, S., Lee, B., Theologidis, I., & Luna, B. (2021). Environmental spread of antibiotic resistance. *Antibiotics, 10*(6), 640. https://doi.org/10.3390/antibiotics10060640

Sugden, R., Kelly, R., & Davies, S. (2016). Combatting antimicrobial resistance globally. *Nature Microbiology, 1*(10), 16187. https://doi.org/10.1038/nmicrobiol.2016.187

Sulis, G., & Gandra, S. (2021). Access to antibiotics: Not a problem in some LMICs. *The Lancet Global Health, 9*(5), e561–e562. https://doi.org/10.1016/S2214-109X(21)00085-1

Sumpradit, N., Wongkongkathep, S., Malathum, K., Janejai, N., Paveenkittiporn, W., Yingyong, T., Chuxnum, T., Vijitleela, A., Boonyarit, P., Akaleephan, C., Manosuthi, W., Thienthong, V., Srinha, J., Wongsrichai, S., Laoprasert, T., Athipunyakom, P., Kriengchaiyaprug, N., Intarukdach, K., Numsawad, S., et al. (2021). Thailand's national strategic plan on antimicrobial resistance: Progress and challenges. *Bulletin of the World Health Organization, 99*(9), 661–673. https://doi.org/10.2471/BLT.20.280644

Sundram, P., Lloyd, C., & Eri, R. (2024). Addressing residue and resistance in food animals: A policy imperative in Southeast Asia. *International Journal of Food Science and Technology, 59*(10), 6746–6757. https://doi.org/10.1111/ijfs.17063

Tahmasebi, H., Arjmand, N., Monemi, M., Babaeizad, A., Alibabaei, F., Alibabaei, N., Bahar, A., Oksenych, V., & Eslami, M. (2025). From cure to crisis: Understanding the evolution of antibiotic-resistant bacteria in human microbiota. *Biomolecules, 15*(1), 93. https://doi.org/10.3390/biom15010093

Tang, K. W. K., Millar, B. C., & Moore, J. E. (2023). Antimicrobial Resistance (AMR). *British Journal of Biomedical Science, 80*, 11387. https://doi.org/10.3389/bjbs.2023.11387

The World Bank. (2024). *Antimicrobial Resistance (AMR)* [Text/HTML]. World Bank. https://www.worldbank.org/en/topic/health/brief/antimicrobial-resistance-amr

Theodorakis, N., Feretzakis, G., Hitas, C., Kreouzi, M., Kalantzi, S., Spyridaki, A., Boufeas, I. Z., Sakagianni, A., Paxinou, E., Verykios, V. S., & Nikolaou, M. (2024). Antibiotic resistance in the elderly: mechanisms, risk factors, and solutions. *Microorganisms, 12*(10), 1978. https://doi.org/10.3390/microorganisms12101978

Tillotson, G. S., & Zinner, S. H. (2017). Burden of antimicrobial resistance in an era of decreasing susceptibility. *Expert Review of Anti-Infective Therapy, 15*(7), 663–676. https://doi.org/10.1080/14787210.2017.1337508

Uddin, T. M., Chakraborty, A. J., Khusro, A., Zidan, B. R. M., Mitra, S., Emran, T. B., Dhama, K., Ripon, M. K. H., Gajdács, M., Sahibzada, M. U. K., Hossain, M. J., & Koirala, N. (2021). Antibiotic resistance in microbes: History, mechanisms, therapeutic strategies and future prospects. *Journal of Infection and Public Health, 14*(12), 1750–1766. https://doi.org/10.1016/j.jiph.2021.10.020

Uruén, C., Chopo-Escuin, G., Tommassen, J., Mainar-Jaime, R. C., & Arenas, J. (2020). Biofilms as promoters of bacterial antibiotic resistance and tolerance. *Antibiotics, 10*(1), 3. https://doi.org/10.3390/antibiotics10010003

van Doorn, H. R., Miliya, T., Douangnouvong, A., Ta Thi Dieu, N., Soputhy, C., Lem, M., Chommanam, D., Keoluangkhot, V., Soumphonphakdy, B., Rassavong, K., Thanadabouth, K., Sayarath, M., Chansamouth, V., Vu, M. D., Dong, P. K., Dang, V. D., Tran, V. B., Do, T. K. Y., Ninh, T. N., et al. (2022). A Clinically Oriented antimicrobial Resistance surveillance Network (ACORN): Pilot implementation in three countries in Southeast Asia, 2019–2020. *Wellcome Open Research, 7*, 309. https://doi.org/10.12688/wellcomeopenres.18317.1

Wang, Z.-X. (2025). Generation and transmission of antibiotic resistance genes in livestock and poultry breeding environments. *Theoretical and Natural Science, 81*(1), 45–51. https://doi.org/10.54254/2753-8818/2025.20465

Warrier, A., Thanusubramanian, H., Routray, A., & Mane, A. (2023). Clinical and economic impact of antimicrobial resistance: Role of antimicrobial stewardship programs in Indian hospitals. *Journal of Academy of Hospital Administration, 35*(2), 60–70. https://doi.org/10.4103/jaha.jaha_7_24

Wen, B., & Lei, F. (2024). Transmission routes and prevention strategies of multidrug-resistant organism infections in hospitals. *Journal of Modern Medicine and Nursing, 1*(2). https://doi.org/10.70767/jmmn.v1i2.282

World Health Organization. (2023). *Antimicrobial resistance*. https://www.who.int/news-room/fact-sheets/detail/antimicrobial-resistance

Wozniak, T. M., Cuningham, W., Ledingham, K., & McCulloch, K. (2022). Contribution of socio-economic factors in the spread of antimicrobial resistant infections in Australian primary healthcare clinics. *Journal of Global Antimicrobial Resistance, 30*, 294–301. https://doi.org/10.1016/j.jgar.2022.06.005

Wulandari, L. P. L., Khan, M., Liverani, M., Ferdiana, A., Mashuri, Y. A., Probandari, A., Wibawa, T., Batura, N., Schierhout, G., Kaldor, J., Guy, R., Law, M., Day, R., Hanefeld, J., Parathon, H., Jan, S., Yeung, S., & Wiseman, V. (2021). Prevalence and determinants of inappropriate antibiotic dispensing at private drug retail outlets in urban and rural areas of Indonesia: A mixed methods study. *BMJ Global Health, 6*(8), e004993. https://doi.org/10.1136/bmjgh-2021-004993

Zabala, G. A., Bellingham, K., Vidhamaly, V., Boupha, P., Boutsamay, K., Newton, P. N., & Caillet, C. (2022). Substandard and falsified antibiotics: Neglected drivers of antimicrobial resistance? *BMJ Global Health, 7*(8). https://doi.org/10.1136/bmjgh-2022-008587

Zay Ya, K., Lambiris, M. J., Levine, G. A., Tediosi, F., & Fink, G. (2024). Coverage of policies to improve antimicrobial stewardship in human medicine in low and middle income countries: Results from the Global Survey of Experts on Antimicrobial Resistance. *BMC Public Health, 24*(1), 2297. https://doi.org/10.1186/s12889-024-19542-2

Chapter 6
Nutrition and One Health

Siti Mei Saroh, Auliya Syifaa Urrahman, Muhammad Ilham Gibran, and Reza Hanifatus Aini

6.1 Challenges in Food Nutrition Security and Agriculture

The agriculture industry plays a vital role in the One Health concept. Crop, livestock, fisheries, and aquaculture serve as the pillars of food security by meeting the demand of growing populations. Ensuring food security is essential for achieving good health and nutrition. On the other hand, agricultural practices directly influence environmental and ecological health. Sustainable practices cooperate positively with nature, while unsustainable ones adversely affect the stability of ecosystems.

Food security is described through four dimensions: physical availability of food, economic and physical access to food, food utilization, and stability of these three dimensions (World Bank, 2025). In practice, the agriculture industry undergoes intensification as the population continues to grow. However, the current system remains unsustainable (Araújo et al., 2023). Therefore, there is an urgent need to achieve a sustainable food system in support of one health. Challenges, however,

S. M. Saroh (✉) · R. H. Aini
Master of Public Health Program, Faculty of Medicine, Public Health, and Nursing, Universitas Gadjah Mada, Yogyakarta, Indonesia
e-mail: sr.may09@gmail.com; rezahanifatus07@gmail.com

A. S. Urrahman
Department of Global Agricultural Sciences, Graduate School of Agricultural and Life Sciences, The University of Tokyo, Tokyo, Japan
e-mail: auliyasyifaa@g.ecc.u-tokyo.ac.jp

M. I. Gibran
Doctoral Program in Medical and Health Sciences, Faculty of Medicine, Public Health, and Nursing, Universitas Gadjah Mada, Yogyakarta, Indonesia
e-mail: ilhamgibran950@mail.ugm.ac.id

© The Author(s), under exclusive license to Springer Nature Singapore Pte Ltd. 2026
A. U. Rauf, T. Wibawa (eds.), *The One Health Concept in Asian Contexts*,
https://doi.org/10.1007/978-981-95-9880-9_6

appear from various sectors that require cooperation among all countries to mitigate negative impacts.

6.1.1 Population Growth

Asia is home to some of the most populous countries in the world, including China, India, and Indonesia. Demographic changes have been ongoing in this region, with the population projected to grow from 4.7 billion in 2023 to 5.2 billion in 2050. Growth rates vary across sub-regions or countries. For example, South and Southwest Asian countries, such as Afghanistan and Pakistan, are projected to undergo a significant increase by 2050, while East Asian countries, such as Japan and South Korea, face a negative trajectory due to the declining in the total fertility rate (Economic and Social Commission for Asia and the Pacific (ESCAP), 2023).

Population rise directly increases food demands. A study by van Dijk et al. (2021) showed that the total global food demand will grow by 35–56% between 2010 and 2050. This means the agriculture industry needs to increase production to feed more people and cater to the changing dietary patterns. A similar trend is observed in Asia. The urbanization and income growth, along with a demand for food diversification and higher dietary quality, influenced the food system. The digitalization of the food system emerges to increase the connectivity between buyers and sellers (Pingali & Abraham, 2022).

The dynamic population changes also affect dietary habits and food culture. For instance, Southeast Asia had a significant increase in food consumption per capita between 1961 and 2019. Hence, the demand for cultivated land doubled from the initial level. This region also underwent the shift toward greater food diversification, marked by the rising consumption of livestock-based foods (Qin et al., 2023). A similar trend occurred in China, where the consumption of animal-based foods rapidly increased between 2000 and 2020. Households with improved living standards and incomes were able to afford more food to meet nutritional requirements (Li et al., 2024). Therefore, each country needs to implement the most effective strategies to meet the rising food demand amidst other challenges.

6.1.2 Climate Change

As the population grow, Asia has seen significant transformations in land use. Many developing countries, such as Vietnam, Bhutan, and the United Arab Emirates, have expanded agricultural land through intensification. However, the industry still operates unsustainably in practice and affects the environment, such as the excessive fertilizers and pesticides usage, fossil fuel reliance, and deforestation (Prabhakar, 2021). For instance, the palm oil crops mainly used deforestation to open the land.

As the demand keeps increasing, the industry greatly contributes to pollutions (Chiriacò et al., 2024).

Unsustainable agricultural practices result in soil, air, and water pollution. Soil degradation manifests in erosion, acidification, salinization, loss of soil genetic diversity, loss of soil organic matter, and GHG emissions to the air (Kopittke et al., 2019). The water systems are also polluted. An analysis of the Amu Darya and Syr Darya Rivers in Central Asia found that the lower stream suffered severe pollution and land salinization. The ionic composition changes and the presence of pollutants, such as pesticides, were detected, bringing the water unsuitable for drinking. It is mainly caused by irrigation and production processes (Liu et al., 2021). These problems lead to climate change, which harms the agricultural system. The accumulation of GHG emissions from human activities is the leading cause of global warming. Wang et al. (2023) found that the yearly temperature increases were 0.015595 °C since 1951 and 0.019795 °C since 1971. This warming effect declines crop yields. Dong and Wang (2023) projected that a 1% increase in particulate matter and tropospheric ozone (O_3) concentration would lower total factor productivity (TFP) in the agriculture industry by 0.104% and 0.207%, respectively.

The unstable temperature also disrupts precipitation patterns. Floods can waterlog soil, hindering oxygen and nutrient uptake for plants. Meanwhile, drought accelerates evaporation and induces stress (Hong et al., 2025). Both extremes adversely affected crops across Asia. In Southeast Asia, rainfed crops were impacted by droughts in the Monsoon Climate Region (e.g., Thailand, Myanmar, Lao PDR, Cambodia) and floods in the Equatorial Climate Region (e.g., Indonesia, the Philippines, Malaysia) (Venkatappa et al., 2021). Meanwhile, a study in Bangladesh showed that monsoon floods also affected crops such as rice, maize, potato, and pepper. In 2019, floods resulted in a significant loss of 2.25 metric tons of rice (Rahman et al., 2025). Climate change also threatens fisheries and aquaculture. Fish are sensitive to temperature changes. Temperature fluctuations might result in prolonged stress that leads to mortality. Meanwhile, the ocean acidification from CO_2 uptake hinders the growth, development, and survival of some aquatic species. The rising sea levels might break coastal ecosystems, such as mangrove, which is a habitat for wild fish stocks. It also becomes a threat to production facilities in lowland regions, such as cages, tanks, and ponds, because of the saline water infiltration (Maulu et al., 2021).

Other climatic events also damage the food system. For example, El Niño, which brings a warm phase or long dry season, reduced rice production in Magelang, Central Java, Indonesia. Some farmers reported that drought occurred during the growth period, resulting in harvesting in the first cropping season because the huge potential of crop failure as the transition between dry and rainy seasons becomes uncertain (Dyah Rahma & Ludwig, 2024). Meanwhile, La Niña, which brings cold air and rainfall, reduced the percentage of cropland in China with a larger effect than El Niño. The cold temperature caused chill injury, frost damage, and poor plant germination (Li et al., 2020a).

6.1.3 Food Loss and Waste (FLW)

Food loss and waste (FLW) significantly affects food security. Food loss describes the reduction in the quantity of edible food along the supply chain, particularly during production, postharvest, and processing. When the loss happens at the retail or consumer level, it is referred to as food waste. Both terms apply to products originally intended for human consumption (Food and Agriculture Organization (FAO), 2011). Several factors drive FLW, including strict quality standards and aesthetic preferences, poor packaging, improper post-harvest facilities and transportation, insufficient market facilities, and, in some cases, the lower price for disposal compared to reuse (Chauhan et al., 2021).

Globally, around one-third of food produced for human consumption is lost or wasted each year, though each regions has different patterns. In medium- and high-income countries, large amounts of food are discarded at retail and consumer levels, even when still edible, with over 40% losses at these levels. By contrast, in low-income countries, most losses occur during early and middle stages, with over 40% of losses happening at these stages, with relatively little waste at the consumer level (Food and Agriculture Organization (FAO), 2011).

For example, in South and Southeast Asia, rice crops are affected by FLW in the production, post-harvest handling, and storage stages (Food and Agriculture Organization (FAO), 2011). Addressing FLW is crucial as it impacts food availability and market prices. Improving supply chain efficiency can increase the yield productivity, enhance the economic value of the products, and reduce the waste of resources, such as inputs, water, and energy.

6.1.4 Political Instability and Conflicts

Food crises are common in regions where violent and armed conflicts emerge from political, social, geopolitical, and economic tensions. Most conflicts occur in rural areas and affect the populations. Smallholder farming and livestock production are especially vulnerable to destruction, infrastructure damage, and contamination. Conflicts also induce displacement as people seek safety, including farmers who might abandon their crops or livestock. As a result, food availability and access will be disrupted, causing food insecurity and soaring prices (Kemmerling et al., 2022).

In some cases, armed groups directly rule and control the agricultural resources and livestock. Those targeting specific segments, such as ethnic and religious groups, often use food insecurity as a weapon of war. They block access to food in acts of ethnic cleansing or genocide (Kemmerling et al., 2022). Consequently, conflicts leave long-term impacts on the nutritional status, particularly in children and people with disabilities. Both acute and chronic malnutrition cases appear as the burden of hunger increases with the degree of fragility of the country (Food and Agriculture Organization (FAO), 2016). Le and Nguyen (2020) found that exposure to armed conflict during pregnancy in developing countries raised the low-birth-weight prevalence by 3.2%.

The Middle East remains prone to conflicts. The ongoing war in Palestine has become the main reason for hunger, food insecurity, and health problems. Even before October 2023, the prevalence of households' food insecurity in the Gaza Strip was 71.5%, due to the long-term conflict between Palestine and Israel (El Bilbeisi et al., 2022). The escalation since October 2023 has worsened the conditions. Between May and July 2024, around 84% of the children in the household showed symptoms of starvation, such as significant weight loss and weakened immunity. The current condition displays that around 16% of individuals were underweight (Faris et al., 2025).

The citizens in the Gaza Strip are constantly hungry due to the food shortages. The availability is disrupted by the armed conflicts, forcing families to share the limited food among all members, especially children. Adults need to dedicate time, effort, financial resources, and personal safety to secure food. Meanwhile, they can only rely on limited food ingredients, such as canned foods and wild edible plants, indicating the decline in the diet quality and variety. Furthermore, processing food is hindered as homes and kitchens are destroyed (Alnabih et al., 2024).

Conflicts also arise from the political instability within a country. Food security can be both a reason and an outcome of frictions. For instance, the Arab Spring, a pro-democracy protest against corrupt and oppressive regimes across the Middle East, broke out in 2011. In the case of Egypt, the availability of food depends heavily on imports, particularly wheat for bread production. However, in 2010, global cereal production was hindered by droughts in major grain supplier countries (e.g., China and Russia), which decreased imports. Hence, food inflation occurred the following year. Rising prices exceeded household purchasing power, increasing public dissatisfaction with the government (Soffiantini, 2020).

Meanwhile, the Tulip Revolution broke out in 2005 and caused food insecurity in Kyrgyzstan. This uprising within two cities, Bishkek and Osh, prompted sudden supply chain disruptions due to massive looting and ransacking. Shops were closed because they were destroyed by fire, affecting the market and food prices. After the restoration, demand sharply increased while food expenditures during the revolution dropped considerably. Residents of Bishkek and Osh underwent a more significant reduction in food spending due to the impact of looting (Kimsanova et al., 2024).

6.1.5 Economic and Global Trade Issues

Economic policy uncertainty (EPU) negatively affects food security and prices in both developed and developing countries. It creates turbulence in the market and international food trade, triggering inflation. In response, food-exporting countries may raise food export taxes or adjust their trade policies (Su et al., 2023). Furthermore, uncertainty in tax and regulatory policies heightens the risks tied to investments. Companies postpone entering new markets to avoid high initial startup costs, which reduces export activity. Trade policy uncertainty concerning tariffs, stockpiling, bound and applied tariff rates, and exchange rates further affects the trade flows (Gignarta et al., 2024).

Another effect of EPU on food supply is that transportation costs increase due to fluctuating oil prices. The cost rise also reduces purchasing power as uncertainty is typically linked to economic recession. The downturns are accompanied by inflation, which further limits food access (Su et al., 2023). In China, the price of agricultural commodities responds differently to shocks from EPU, depending on supply and demand elasticity, marketization, and agricultural policies in the region. Livestock and vegetables show a stronger sensitivity to policy shifts, marked by greater price volatility than cereals (Hao & Ki-Seong, 2024).

The example of EPU is the US tariff policy for countries around the world, including China and several Asian countries. This tariff policy is designed to improve the trade balance by reducing imports through higher tariffs. Even though the effect on Asian economies is less than on Canada and Mexico, it is worth noting that many countries responded with various actions, such as imposing retaliatory tariffs or redirecting their imports elsewhere (Kang et al., 2025).

The People's Republic of China (PRC) is the most affected. Its net exports fall under most scenarios, with trade surplus projected to shrink by 24% under high tariffs or 18% with retaliation. Nevertheless, the PRC maintains a large trade surplus by shifting exports to other partners (Kang et al., 2025). During the trade war between the USA and PRC in 2018, the latter imposed a 25% retaliatory tariff on US soybean exports and redirected purchases to Brazil (Adjemian et al., 2021). Between 2025 and 2028, the PRC's nominal income is expected to fall by 1.3–2.2%, with its trade surplus shrinking by up to 24%. Even so, its GDP experiences only a slight decline (Kang et al., 2025).

6.1.6 *Outbreak and Recurrent Health Crises*

The outbreaks of zoonoses, or animal-transmitted diseases, adversely affect the agriculture industry, particularly livestock. These crises disrupt the supply chain by increasing morbidity and mortality of domestic animals. The livestock yield falls short of initial expectations, while treatment costs and other expenditures rise (Martins et al., 2015). An analysis of the provincial data in China from 2002 to 2017 showed that zoonoses outbreaks reduced total factor productivity (TFP) for six livestock products, namely beef, hog, dairy, broiler, egg, and mutton, with the latter suffering the greatest loss. The impact will be worsened if outbreaks occur during the breeding season (Gong et al., 2021).

Asia is the place where zoonoses emerge and re-emerge in the twenty-first century, such as highly pathogenic avian influenza (HPAI). From January to June 2025, Cambodia reported a resurgence of HPAI with 11 laboratory-confirmed cases in humans, which is caused by direct contact with sick or dead poultry (World Health Organization (WHO), 2025). These new cases add to the list of avian influenza outbreaks in Southeast Asia since the first wave in 2003 (Hatta et al., 2025). Meanwhile, South Asia also has a long history of bird influenza outbreaks, with Bangladesh reporting the highest number of cases from January 2006 to June 2019. The cases were reported in domestic poultry (Chowdhury et al., 2019).

Control measures are implemented at all levels to prevent the wider spread of disease. From social distancing to the plant shutdowns, these actions lower labor productivity, disrupt transportation, and reduce communication and cooperation, which lead to efficiency losses and resource misallocation (Gong et al., 2021). Product recalls and stamping out are also implemented, adding further costs for the related institutions. As a result, the industry loses its domestic and export markets, while prices continue to rise (Martins et al., 2015; Hatta et al., 2025).

From the consumer perspective, the behavior toward the food chain changes from confidence to distrust. This shift is related to health consciousness. Consumers view health as a key factor in food choices and incorporate this belief into daily activities. It is reflected in intentionally avoiding the purchase of animal products, as those may present a threat to health during zoonotic outbreaks. Consumers also become more aware of the product origins and tend to prioritize safety and cleanliness before buying. Furthermore, media coverage is crucial in building or damaging trust, as it is the first source of information during outbreaks (Wen et al., 2019).

The emergence of COVID-19 also became a threat to food security in Asia. The pandemic resulted in lockdown and travel restrictions to prevent the transmission. These measures inhibit trades, including import and export, which limit the availability of food stock to a certain extent. On the other hand, restrictions on movement reduced access, affordability, and worker productivity, resulting in delays or slower progress in meeting the growing demands (Ma et al., 2021; Dixon et al., 2021).

6.2 One Health Strategies for Food Nutrition Security a Sustainable Agriculture

Health and nutrition are fundamental to human well-being, yet they are increasingly challenged by rapid urbanization, shifting dietary patterns, and the escalating impacts of climate change. The region of Asia, which is home to more than half of the global population, pressures on food systems, ranging from deforestation for palm oil and rice production to monoculture-driven ecosystem decline, high levels of food loss and waste, and erratic weather patterns disrupting agricultural stability. These interconnected problems cannot be addressed in isolation; they demand systemic, cross-sectoral solutions that integrate human, animal, and environmental health. The One Health approach provides a comprehensive framework to build resilient, sustainable food systems that safeguard both people and the planet.

Sustainable agriculture is one of the key strategies for addressing the urgent challenge of providing sufficient and nutritious food without compromising environmental. By integrating ecological principles into farming systems, sustainable agriculture seeks to balance productivity with the preservation of soil, water, biodiversity, and climate stability, ensuring that food production does not undermine the natural resources and ecosystem. Practical efforts in Southeast and East Asia—documented Ecohealth and One Health projects in Vietnam, Thailand, Indonesia, and China—illustrate co-developed, community-engaged measures that address zoonoses, crop health, and environmental drivers simultaneously, for example by integrating plant health management with livestock and human health surveillance to limit crop losses and food-safety risks (Nguyen-Viet et al., 2021; Rizzo et al., 2021). Such integrated strategies reframe food security as a multisectoral outcome requiring coordinated policy, monitoring, and local action across health, agriculture, and environment sectors (Nguyen-Viet et al., 2021). Sustainable agriculture serves as a critical nexus connecting human, animal, and environmental health through multiple interconnected pathways that exemplify the One Health approach (Ebenso et al., 2022). It functions not only as a method of food production but also as a framework for resilience, equity, and planetary health. By reducing reliance on synthetic pesticides and fertilizers, sustainable farming practices significantly lower human dietary and occupational exposures to toxic chemicals while simultaneously decreasing environmental contamination that harms wildlife and livestock (Tiwari, 2023).

The biodiversity conservation inherent in sustainable agricultural systems supports natural enemies of pests and dilutes pathogen transmission, creating ecosystem services that reduce disease risk across the human-animal-environment interface (Dainese et al., 2019). Agroecological practices such as crop rotation, intercropping, and agroforestry enhance structural diversity within landscapes, providing habitats for pollinators and predators of agricultural pests (Estrada-Carmona et al., 2022). This ecological balance reduces the need for chemical interventions and strengthens natural disease regulation. From a One Health perspective, maintaining biodiversity is also critical for buffering against zoonotic spillovers: diverse ecosystems act as filters that disrupt transmission pathways between wildlife, livestock, and humans. Practical innovations across Asia underscore the feasibility of these approaches. Crop diversification provides a pathway to resilience, with climate-smart staples such as millet, sorghum, cassava, and other tubers promoted as alternatives to water- and input-intensive crops (Davis et al., 2019; Sharma et al., 2025). India's campaigns to revive millet consumption illustrate how climate adaptation and nutritional improvement can be achieved together (Ajatasatru et al., 2024). Similarly, alternate wetting and drying techniques in rice cultivation in Vietnam and the Philippines demonstrate how farming practices can maintain yields while reducing greenhouse gas emissions (Bwire et al., 2024; Zhang et al., 2023). By linking ecological sustainability with human and animal well-being, sustainable agriculture offers not only a response to current pressures on Asian food systems but also a transformative pathway toward equitable, climate-resilient, and health-promoting futures.

Reducing food loss and waste is equally critical for strengthening food security and minimizing environmental impact. In Asia, large proportions of food are lost post-harvest or during distribution due to weak infrastructure, inadequate storage, and fragmented markets. Upgrading infrastructure, such as cold-chain systems, storage facilities, and logistics can significantly reduce these losses, especially in developing regions where spoilage remains a major challenge (Nicastro & Carillo, 2021; Porat et al., 2018). Technological innovations, including improved packaging and digital tracking, further minimize losses during transport and storage (Porat et al., 2018). At the retail and food service level, waste can be reduced through better inventory management, portion size adjustments, and donation of surplus food. Community-driven redistribution programs, such as food banks in Indonesia and Singapore, also show how surplus food can reach vulnerable populations (Putri et al., 2025; Aaron Rasya & Budiman, 2025). Incorporating spices enhances the sensory appeal of food, thereby reducing reliance on oil for palatability. Community-driven redistribution programs, such as food banks and collective resource management, have demonstrated the ability to deliver essential goods and services to vulnerable populations, especially where government capacity is limited. Community-driven redistribution programs, such as food banks and collective resource management, have demonstrated the ability to deliver essential goods and services to vulnerable populations. These programs can provide much-needed infrastructure and improve access to resources, leading to improved welfare and resilience in the face of challenges like poverty and disasters. These approaches have the potential to measurable improvements in health, sanitation, and economic. Redistribution of surplus food not only addresses food insecurity but can also reduce environmental burdens by diverting food waste from landfills.

Embracing local and traditional foods is another powerful strategy for aligning nutrition with sustainability. Indigenous diets in Asia often rely on herbs, spices, and plant-based preparations that are both nutritionally dense and environmentally friendly. Local and traditional diets are often rich in whole grains, legumes, vegetables, and fermented foods, providing high nutritional value and supporting public health. These diets are associated with lower rates of obesity and non-communicable diseases compared to westernized, ultra-processed diets (Borelli et al., 2020; Durazzo, 2019; Oniang'o et al., 2025). Traditional food preparation methods such as fermentation, boiling, and drying help preserve nutrients and enhance bioavailability (Oniang'o et al., 2025). In rural and indigenous communities, traditional foods contribute to food security and help maintain cultural identity (Durazzo, 2019; Oniang'o et al., 2025). Traditional and local foods typically rely on native crops and low-input agricultural practices, which are more adaptable to local climates and require fewer resources like water and fertilizers, reducing environmental impact. The cultivation and consumption of local foods support agrobiodiversity and resilience to climate change (Coelho et al., 2018). Moreover, culinary practices such as boiling, steaming, and the use of diverse preparation methods can reduce dependence on palm oil, which is commonly used for frying but is associated with large-scale deforestation and habitat loss. By promoting food cultures that emphasize plant-based recipes and cooking methods less reliant on added oils, communities can lessen the demand for palm oil and its environmental footprint, while still ensuring palatability and nutritional adequacy. Promoting food cultures that emphasize plant-based recipes and cooking methods less reliant on added oils, communities can lessen the demand for palm oil and its environmental footprint, while still ensuring palatability and nutritional adequacy. However, the sustainability of local foods depends on production methods; not all local foods are inherently more sustainable than global alternatives, as factors like farming practices and seasonality play significant roles.

Education is a key driver of healthier, more sustainable, and equitable food systems, improving food security, dietary quality, and community resilience. Education fosters healthier dietary patterns, with higher education levels associated with greater consumption of fruits, vegetables, and diverse foods, and lower intake of ultra-processed foods, sweets, and red meats (Coelho et al., 2018; Fard et al., 2021; Prescott et al., 2019). Nutrition education programs in schools and communities can reduce food insecurity and improve diet quality, particularly when they include practical skills like meal planning and food preparation (Fard et al., 2021; Andrianarison, 2022). Food systems education, especially when delivered through experiential and peer-to-peer learning, can significantly reduce food waste by teaching practical skills in food storage, creative use of leftovers, and appreciation for local ingredients (Sterling et al., 2021). Food systems education, particularly when designed around experiential and peer-to-peer learning, plays a vital role in reducing food waste. Rather than relying solely on theoretical instruction, hands-on activities such as cooking demonstrations, community kitchens, or school garden projects, equip individuals with practical skills for storing ingredients, managing household supplies, and making creative use of leftovers. Peer-to-peer learning adds another layer of effectiveness, as people often adopt new habits more readily when they see them modeled by friends, family, or community members. This approach also fosters a sense of shared responsibility, where food is valued not only as a personal resource but as part of a collective system that supports nutrition, livelihoods, and environmental sustainability. By teaching communities to appreciate local ingredients and seasonality, food systems education strengthens cultural ties while simultaneously building resilience against overreliance on imported or highly processed foods. In doing so, it cultivates both the skills and the mindset needed to minimize waste and support more sustainable patterns of consumption. Integrating food systems education in schools and communities builds awareness of the environmental impact of food choices, strengthens cultural appreciation for local foods, and empowers individuals to participate in sustainable and equitable food systems transformation. Education, especially when practical, community-based, and systems-oriented, plays a central role in making food systems more resilient, equitable, and sustainable. It improves food security, dietary quality, and waste reduction, while empowering individuals and communities to make informed, sustainable food choices.

6.3 Food Safety and the Role of Biotechnology in One Health

6.3.1 Introduction—Biotechnology Beyond Surveillance

Food safety is best understood as a system of interdependence in which human, animal, and environmental health jointly determine whether food nourishes or harms. Within a One Health frame, risk arises not only from pathogens but also from the social and ecological conditions of production, transport, and consumption. Where wildlife is hunted or traded alongside livestock, cross-species transmission risk rises (Antunes et al., 2020) because such practices are tied to livelihoods and culture, prevention must be both effective and context-sensitive. Foodborne zoonoses exemplify this interdependence, as pathogens move through livestock, wildlife, and human populations (Zinsstag et al., 2023). Hazards arising at the interfaces of production, processing, and consumption therefore demand coordinated rather than fragmented governance (Wu et al., 2021; Zhang et al., 2024).

Recognition is insufficient without interruption; ensuring food safety requires active control measures that interrupt hazards before they enter the food chain. Standards and regulations provide a baseline, but they falter where enforcement capacity is weak or norms conflict with rules. Many outbreaks stem not from rare pathogens but from routine lapses: an infected food handler, meat that is insufficiently cooked, or products stored outside safe temperature ranges (Antunes et al., 2020). Such routine lapses underline the practical message: biotechnology must move beyond surveillance to prevention, offering tools that detect, neutralize, and block contamination before it reaches consumers.

Asia's food systems make this shift urgent. Smallholder farming, wet markets, rapid aquaculture growth, and climate extremes open multiple entry points for hazards.

6.3.2 Food Safety Risks in Asia—Where Biotechnology Can Intervene Early

Asia's hazards span the entire chain, thereby making early intervention critical. Bacterial pathogens such as *Salmonella*, *Campylobacter*, *Listeria monocytogenes*, and pathogenic *E. coli* remain the leading causes of foodborne illness in settings dominated by informal markets and small-scale production (Antunes et al., 2020; Zinsstag et al., 2023; Wu et al., 2021). These risks are amplified by globalized food trade, which can quickly spread contamination, and by environmental changes such as land-use conversion and climate variability that influence pathogen survival (Antunes et al., 2020; Zinsstag et al., 2023). Persistent chemical hazards including pesticide and veterinary drug residues and mycotoxins like aflatoxins reflect gaps in monitoring and enforcement, while environmental contaminants such as microplastics, heavy metals, and polluted water pose growing concerns in coastal aquaculture regions (Wu et al., 2021). The analytic point is clear: early detection and upstream control deliver the highest returns.

Salmonella illustrates the challenge; how a single pathogen can exploit multiple entry points in the food chain. It persists in soil, water, wildlife, and food products, spreading directly or via cross-contamination (Habiba et al., 2023; Li et al., 2021a). In Singapore, surveillance found *Salmonella* in 0.08% of >21,000 cooked or ready-to-eat samples, with poultry and eggs having the highest risk; wild birds carrying the pathogen suggest possible spillover into retail spaces (Aung et al., 2019). These findings identify poultry and eggs as critical control points and spotlight the need to build smallholders' capacity for monitoring and risk management. Without such early interventions, *Salmonella* and similar pathogens will continue to impose heavy public health and economic costs.

Biotechnology offers a set of tools capable of shifting food safety management from reactive response to proactive prevention. Rapid detection, precision tracking, and source-targeted interventions reduce spread, losses, antimicrobial use, and public distrust. The following sections explore how these tools can be applied at two chokepoints: during production to stop hazards from entering the chain and post-harvest to ensure any remaining threats are swiftly controlled.

6.3.3 Biotechnology for Prevention in Food Production Systems

Preventing hazards at their source is the most strategic yet least realized approach in Asia. Vaccination, illustrated by *Salmonella enterica* control in poultry, has reduced human disease in high-income contexts, but its impact is maximized only when paired with hygiene and ecological management (Antunes et al., 2020; Zinsstag et al., 2023; Wu et al., 2021). This integration demonstrates a central lesson: prevention cannot rely on stand-alone tools, but on programs that link biomedical, behavioral, and environmental interventions.

Microbiome and genetic innovations broaden the toolkit, but their uptake reveals persistent inequities. By enhancing natural resistance, microbiome-based interventions reduce antibiotic use and slow antimicrobial resistance (Zinsstag et al., 2023; Wu et al., 2021). Genetically improved crops and disease-resistant livestock reduce chemical inputs and lower early-stage contamination risks (Wu et al., 2021). Yet adoption often stalls among smallholders due to high costs, limited awareness, and fragmented input markets. These barriers matter not just because they restrict access, but because they perpetuate dependence on chemical-intensive practices that biotechnology is designed to replace.

Genomic tools offer precision, but their promise depends on system-level capacity. Whole-genome sequencing (WGS) and metagenomics can pinpoint persistent serovars, map transmission pathways, and identify antimicrobial resistance genes (Habiba et al., 2023; Li et al., 2021a; Benedetti et al., 2024; Wielinga & Schlundt,

2012). For instance, the detection of identical *Salmonella Typhimurium* strains in both food and wild birds highlights how environmental spillover undermines farm-level interventions (Aung et al., 2019). Such insights show that genomics is not just a diagnostic upgrade but a strategic tool to reframe prevention across ecological boundaries. However, routine use remains constrained by cost and expertise, underscoring the need for regional reference laboratories and shared data platforms.

Aquaculture magnifies these challenges and thus tests the limits of prevention. Intensification fosters bacterial infections and heavy antimicrobial use (Vergis et al., 2021), creating resistant pathogens that traverse aquatic–terrestrial boundaries via water and waste. Here, biotechnology's preventive function must cross systems, not just species. Consistent with the call of One Health Action Collaborative (OHAC) for integrated ecological, biomedical, and social approaches, production-stage control should be prioritized to break chains of contamination before they reach human populations (Zhang et al., 2024).

6.3.4 Biotechnology for Post-harvest Food Safety

Post-harvest biotechnology is the final safeguard, and its value lies less in novelty than in speed and containment. Rapid molecular diagnostics and biosensors now allow near-real-time detection in fresh and processed foods (Antunes et al., 2020; Wu et al., 2021). When embedded in packaging or logistics, they can intercept contaminated products before retail, a decisive advantage for perishable goods (Wu et al., 2021; Li et al., 2021a). The weakness lies not in scientific promise but in affordability and supply-chain stability, which still limit uptake among small-scale operators.

Adjunct technologies broaden this protective layer, but they succeed only when embedded in systems, not as stand-alone fixes. Antimicrobial coatings, improved cold chains, and biocontrol agents extend shelf-life and curb microbial growth (Antunes et al., 2020; Wu et al., 2021). Yet without training and logistical support, these innovations underperform. The synthesis lesson is clear: post-harvest safety depends less on adopting new tools than on aligning technology with practices and institutions. In this respect, biotechnology mirrors One Health itself: its effectiveness rests on the integration of technical, social, and organizational components.

Governance capacity ultimately sets the ceiling for impact. Hazard Analysis Critical Control Points (HACCP) frameworks remain underused in aquaculture, leaving critical points exposed (Vergis et al., 2021). Output-based standards could make surveillance more adaptive by distinguishing endemic from emerging hazards (Benedetti et al., 2024), but they require reliable baselines that many countries lack. Genomic traceback through WGS brings precision by linking clinical, food, and environmental isolates (Li et al., 2021a). Findings of identical *Salmonella* sequence types in food and wild birds underscore why environmental monitoring must be integral, not optional (Aung et al., 2019).

The analytic point is unmistakable: post-harvest biotechnology cannot carry food safety alone. Without enabling systems (standards, training, and cross-sector coordination) even advanced tools will falter. What these interventions reveal is the need for a farm-to-fork prevention mindset, one that distributes responsibility across producers, processors, regulators, and consumers alike (Wielinga & Schlundt, 2012). The central question, then, is whether governance and investment can transform promising technologies into equitable, durable protections.

6.3.5 Barriers to Biotech Adoption for Food Safety in Asia

The barriers to biotechnology adoption in Asia are less about technology itself than about the systems meant to sustain it. High costs, limited technical skills, and weak regulatory frameworks constrain uptake in low-resource settings (Antunes et al., 2020; Zinsstag et al., 2023). Smallholders and SMEs, which anchor regional food systems, are most affected because they lack sustained funding and localized R&D (Zinsstag et al., 2023; Wu et al., 2021). The result is a structural inequity: cutting-edge tools remain confined to well-resourced laboratories, while the farmers most vulnerable to outbreaks are left with little more than conventional practices. Sequencing platforms and bioinformatics pipelines, priced beyond the reach of many, deepen divides between high- and low-/middle-income countries (Habiba et al., 2023; Li et al., 2021a). This inequity matters not only for fairness but for safety: in globalized trade, one weak link can destabilize regional food chains.

Yet financial and technical barriers explain only part of the gap; trust is just as decisive. Public skepticism toward genetically modified organisms (GMOs) and biotech-derived foods persists across many Asian contexts (Antunes et al., 2020; Zinsstag et al., 2023). Here, adoption stalls not because tools fail but because institutions are not trusted to safeguard their use. Weak or inconsistently enforced regulation (Wu et al., 2021) compounds the problem, feeding cycles of doubt in which consumers hesitate precisely because they suspect governments cannot guarantee safety. Trust, then, is not a by-product of adoption; it is a precondition.

Governance fragmentation amplifies these challenges, leaving even strong technologies brittle when institutions are weak. Professional silos, fragile coordination, and weak national-to-international collaboration make integration uneven (Zhang et al., 2024; Benedetti et al., 2024). Singapore illustrates this dependence on external cooperation: importing over 90% of its food, it cannot trace or control contamination without international collaboration (Aung et al., 2019). In such contexts, domestic innovation is necessary but insufficient; regional governance becomes the missing layer.

Aquaculture exposes the regulatory blind spots most clearly. Countries vary widely in antimicrobial use, frustrating harmonized surveillance and complicating oversight (Vergis et al., 2021). Risk assessments remain skewed toward bacterial hazards while neglecting viral threats such as norovirus or hepatitis viruses that circulate through aquatic chains (Vergis et al., 2021). At the same time, socioeconomic dependence on livestock and aquaculture renders drastic measures like culling politically and economically unfeasible (Vergis et al., 2021). These contradictions show how scientific knowledge can outpace regulatory readiness, leaving critical hazards unaddressed.

Even when systems adopt advanced tools, communication failures can recreate resistance. WGS exemplifies this paradox: while technically powerful, it risks sparking backlash if data sharing and uncertainty communication are not handled transparently (Benedetti et al., 2024; Allard et al., 2020). Just as GMO skepticism reflected unease with opaque decision-making, genomic surveillance may falter if experts cannot translate complexity into accessible terms. In this sense, barriers are not only structural but narrative: technologies fail as much in communication as in cost.

The pattern across these barriers in Asia is consistent: innovation collides with inequity, governance lags behind science, and mistrust turns opportunity into resistance. The implication is sobering. Unless cost, coordination, and communication are addressed together, biotechnology risks remaining powerful in theory but peripheral in practice; an unfulfilled promise rather than a transformative force in One Health.

6.3.6 Opportunities and Future Directions

The same interdependence that generates risk can be leveraged for resilience. Integrated surveillance that links veterinary, public health, and environmental systems amplifies the value of biotechnology, moving interventions from isolated pilots to coordinated strategies with regional impact. This is especially vital in Asia, where food systems are porous and a pathogen spillover in one sector can cascade quickly across borders.

The first opportunity lies in context-sensitive design. Regionally adapted vaccines and low-cost diagnostics increase uptake in low- and middle-income countries where resources are constrained (Antunes et al., 2020). Embedding such interventions within national food security programs creates "triple wins"—protecting health, supporting livelihoods, and conserving ecosystems. The pattern is instructive: technologies scale when they are framed not as stand-alone innovations, but as integral to broader policy priorities.

Governance and participation shape whether tools endure or fade. Top-down coordination ensures alignment with national and international goals, while bottom-up engagement fosters trust and legitimacy (Zhang et al., 2024). This dual strategy—global vision paired with local adaptation—reduces the risk that biotechnology is dismissed as a foreign imposition. Capacity-building becomes the hinge: without trained personnel and functioning institutions, even the most elegant tools will wither.

Technical opportunities are real but meaningful only if embedded in systems. Integrating multilocus sequence typing (MLST) with antimicrobial resistance

(AMR) profiling provides a pragmatic model for national programs, while wildlife monitoring extends One Health upstream by flagging zoonotic risks before they enter food chains (Aung et al., 2019). Regional genomic surveillance networks offer a second-order benefit: not only detecting transboundary *Salmonella* strains more quickly but also producing shared datasets that accelerate collective responses (Habiba et al., 2023; Li et al., 2021a). The tension here is pace: microbes evolve faster than regulation, making regional coordination essential if biotechnology is to keep up.

The forward challenge is normalization, not novelty. Post-pandemic, One Health surveillance must shift from being a conceptual aspiration to a routine preparedness practice (Benedetti et al., 2024). Emerging tools such as artificial intelligence and ontologies linked to WGS metadata can anticipate contamination risks and support climate-resilient food safety strategies (Allard et al., 2020). Economic modeling underscores the stakes: adoption of WGS could reduce national foodborne illness burdens by up to one-third, saving billions globally (Allard et al., 2020). This reframes biotechnology from a scientific aspiration into a fiscal imperative.

The analytic point is clear: opportunities are not scattered "add-ons" but levers to resolve the very tensions identified in Section 5. Local adaptation must be balanced with global alignment; technical innovation must be matched with governance capacity; and scientific desirability must be reinforced with fiscal prudence. The future of biotechnology in Asian food systems therefore depends less on discovering new tools than on weaving existing ones into a durable One Health fabric: policies, communities, laboratories, and ecosystems stitched together to create food systems that are safe, resilient, and future-ready.

6.4 Nutrition and One Health: Cross-Sector Surveillance of Foodborne Pathogens

6.4.1 The Urgency of Transforming Surveillance Systems

Asia is a region with high biodiversity, dense human and livestock populations, and rapid land use change. These factors make Asia one of the regions with a high risk of zoonotic diseases (Halton et al., 2013; Li et al., 2021b). Data from the European Union's Rapid Alert System for Food and Feed (RASFF) shows that many food products from the Asia-Pacific region have received warnings related to microbiological hazards, particularly *Salmonella* contamination. This indicates that food safety remains a serious challenge (Dada et al., 2021).

Asia has a long history of dealing with various disease outbreaks, from SARS to avian influenza. This history makes Asia an important location for developing and testing health monitoring systems. Southeast Asia is known as a region actively developing the One Health approach, supported by political interests and the need to address cross-border diseases or outbreaks (Lajaunie et al., 2025).

Advances in digital, genomic, and computational technologies are opening up significant opportunities to enhance health surveillance systems. Technology not only accelerates processes but also transforms the way monitoring is conducted, shifting from merely waiting for case reports to predicting outbreaks earlier and from isolated or separate data systems to interconnected data across sectors. The WHO's 2023 Joint External Evaluation (JEE) noted that Indonesia has made significant progress in implementing the International Health Regulations (IHR), although there is still room for improvement (World Health Organization, 2024).

6.4.2 *Utilization of Technology for Cross-Sectoral Detection and Response to Foodborne Pathogens*

The use of technology in the detection and response to foodborne pathogens from various countries in Asia, including China, Thailand, Japan, Cambodia, and others, has identified three main pillars of technological transformation in cross-sector surveillance systems. The three complementary pillars are (1) digital and mobile platforms that enable community participation in early monitoring of disease cases; (2) genomic and molecular technologies used to identify pathogens and track transmission with precision; and (3) integrated information and artificial intelligence (AI) that serves as a connector for all information and predictive modeling.

6.4.3 *Data Collection Through Digital Platforms and Community Participation*

The foundation of any surveillance system is the availability of timely and accurate data. Traditional survey methodologies are often constrained by costs, time, limited human resources, and the time lag between data collection and analysis. The proliferation of smartphones and the internet across Asia presents a significant opportunity to directly involve communities in monitoring. Various countries in Asia have implemented methods to involve the community in disease case monitoring.

A study in Cambodia on dengue fever case monitoring showed that village health volunteers were able to detect clusters of dengue fever cases not recorded in the health reporting system. This was because most infected individuals were treated at home and never sought examination at the nearest healthcare facility. Health volunteers in villages are crucial as a source of information for monitoring in the surveillance system (Halton et al., 2013). A study in Thailand involving a survey of health professionals from various sectors revealed that the main obstacle in the surveillance system is the lack of communication and data transfer systems across sectors (George et al., 2023). These findings indicate the need to develop an integrated digital platform to strengthen coordination and efficiency in cross-sectoral responses.

Cross-sector collaborative methods are being systematically implemented through Joint Risk Assessment activities. South Korea uses a combination of several monitoring models to maximize coverage and detection speed (Jang et al., 2025). The first model is the reporting of high-risk disease cases. The next model is sentinel surveillance through a network of selected laboratories or health facilities to monitor disease trends on a regular basis. Sentinel surveillance is also used to monitor foodborne pathogens in India through the ICMR-FoodNet network, which collects data from laboratories spread across various regions (Albert et al., 2024).

Although the potential for community involvement in monitoring is enormous, there are several challenges in its implementation. The digital divide and infrastructure issues such as internet access are obstacles in rural areas. Therefore, technology platforms need to be designed with offline-first capabilities or without using the internet for data collection, which can then be synchronized when an internet connection is available (Morris & Wang, 2024). The effectiveness of digital tools depends on the ability of human resources (HR) to operate them. Continuous training programs for health volunteers and responsive technical support are essential to ensure proper and effective use of the tools (Morris & Wang, 2024). The lack of incentives to participate discourages community involvement. Incentives are needed that are tailored to the local context, such as rewards, social recognition, and access to useful information (Halton et al., 2013). Overall, the use of this technology provides an opportunity to involve more people in data collection. Rather than relying solely on a top-down system, this approach encourages direct participation from the community (bottom up), so that the monitoring system can be faster and more widespread.

6.4.4 Genomic and Molecular Technologies for Pathogen Identification and Transmission Tracking with Precision

WGS has become the gold standard tool in foodborne pathogen surveillance by comparing the entire genomes of bacteria from various samples, enabling researchers to accurately determine whether their origin and source are the same (Shigemura et al., 2020). A study in China using WGS to track *Salmonella enterica* in livestock successfully mapped the distribution of serotypes, disease-causing genes, and antimicrobial resistance patterns. This information provides a comprehensive overview of the potential risks of pathogens in the food chain from a One Health perspective (Tang et al., 2023). China has also established the National Foodborne Disease Molecular Tracing Network to track the source of outbreaks nationally, thereby accelerating the intervention process and improving targeting accuracy (Li et al., 2020b). When genomic data is combined with location and time information, a genomic epidemiology approach is formed. This method enables detailed reconstruction of transmission chains and understanding of how diseases can spread (Morris & Wang, 2024). During the global pandemic, this method is crucial for tracking the transmission of new viruses between countries. PulseNet International has also recommended the use of WGS as a global standard for monitoring foodborne diseases. However, the adoption of this technology still faces challenges in low- and middle-income countries (LMICs), including high operational costs, a shortage of skilled personnel, and inadequate laboratory infrastructure (Davedow et al., 2022).

New molecular diagnostic technologies besides WGS are being developed to improve disease monitoring in the field. These technologies are designed to be faster, easier to use, portable, and cost-effective, making them suitable for implementation in areas with limited resources. CRISPR-based diagnostics uses enzymes such as Cas12 and Cas13 to specifically detect pathogenic nucleic acids. The detection process takes less than an hour and can be used in simple methods such as test strips (similar to pregnancy test kits). CRISPR is used to detect various bacterial and viral pathogens, as well as antimicrobial resistance (AMR) genes from food or clinical samples without extensive laboratory preparation (Borah et al., 2025; Liberty et al., 2025).

Advanced biosensors are currently being developed, such as biosensors based on magnetic relaxation switching (MRS) combined with CRISPR. This device can detect pathogens with high sensitivity without the need for complex amplification processes. Its principle of operation involves detecting changes in the magnetic field caused by interactions between magnetic nanoparticles and target pathogens. This technology is suitable for use in complex environments as it provides rapid results with high accuracy (Borah et al., 2025).

Although molecular technologies like WGS offer very strong analytical capabilities, their application in Asia still faces several obstacles (Davedow et al., 2022). The high costs of sequencing, reagents, and equipment pose barriers for laboratories. The lack of experts in bioinformatics means that many laboratories have adequate capabilities but lack the resources for genomic analysis and interpretation. The storage requirements and computational capacity needed to manage large amounts of genomic data necessitate advanced and expensive infrastructure. Finally, the absence of uniform standards for interpreting WGS results complicates data comparison between laboratories and countries, thereby hindering regional collaboration (Davedow et al., 2022).

6.4.5 Data Synthesis and Predictive Intelligence Through Information Systems and AI

Information collected through digital platforms and analyzed using genomic technology needs to be combined within an integrated analytical framework so that it can generate intelligence that can be used for real action in the field. The main challenge in the One Health approach is the fragmentation of data among various institutions (Morris & Wang, 2024; Li et al., 2020b). This issue is being addressed through the development of the Zoonosis and EID Information System (SIZE) in Indonesia. This platform is designed to connect data from various vertically integrated surveillance systems, such as EWARS for human health, iSIKHNAS for animal health, and SEHATSATLI for wildlife health (World Health Organization, 2024). Similar platforms, such as DHIS2, enable cross-sector data visualization and analysis so that anomalies indicating potential outbreaks can be detected more quickly. The success of such systems depends not only on technological sophistication but also on the willingness of institutions to share data and ensure good interoperability (Dwi Raharjo et al., 2022).

Artificial intelligence (AI) and machine learning (ML) offer significant opportunities to detect complex patterns in large datasets that are difficult to capture using traditional analytical methods. The application of AI in Asia includes epidemic intelligence, where algorithms scan non-traditional data sources such as news reports and social media to detect early signs of an outbreak—an approach known as digital epidemiology (Halton et al., 2013; Jang et al., 2025). Artificial intelligence is also used for predictive modeling, for example in China and Vietnam, where models are trained using historical outbreak data alongside variables such as climate, land cover, and population mobility to predict the risk of disease outbreaks (Morris & Wang, 2024). AI even has the potential to be integrated with CRISPR-based diagnostics, enabling it to help design optimal RNA guidelines and analyze results automatically. This integration will reduce the need for manual interpretation by experts and accelerate responses to health threats (Liberty et al., 2025).

Competing Interests The author(s) has no competing interests to declare that are relevant to the content of this manuscript.

References

Aaron Rasya, A., & Budiman, I. (2025). Policy brief: Scaling up food loss and waste reduction programs in Indonesia. *Cips, 26*, 14.

Adjemian, M. K., Smith, A., & He, W. (2021). Estimating the market effect of a trade war: The case of soybean tariffs. *Food Policy, 105*, 102152.

Ajatasatru, A., Prabhu, V., Pal, B., & Mukhopadhyay, K. (2024). Economy-wide impact of climate smart agriculture in India: A SAM framework. *Journal of Economic Structures, 13*, 1–30.

Albert, V., Ramamurthy, T., Das, M., Das, S., Ojha, A. K., Sarmah, P., et al. (2024). Surveillance of food and waterborne pathogens in North-East India: Protocol for a laboratory-based sentinel surveillance study. *JMIR Research Protocol*, 13.

Allard, M. W., Zheng, J., Cao, G., Timme, R., Stevens, E., & Brown, E. W. (2020). Food safety genomics and connections to One Health and the clinical microbiology laboratory. *Clinical Laboratory Medicine* [Internet], *40*(4), 553–563. Available from: https://linkinghub.elsevier.com/retrieve/pii/S0272271220300652

Alnabih, A., Alnabeh, N. A., Aljeesh, Y., & Aldabbour, B. (2024). Food insecurity and weight loss during wartime: A mixed-design study from the Gaza Strip. *Journal of Health, Population, and Nutrition, 43*(1), 222.

Andrianarison, F. (2022). Unravelling the linkage between food security, poverty reduction, and education for sustainable development. *Journal of Development Studies, 58*, 2198–2221.

Antunes, P., Novais, C., & Peixe, L. (2020). Food-to-humans bacterial transmission. *Microbiological Spectrum* [Internet], *8*(1). Available from: http://www.ncbi.nlm.nih.gov/pubmed/31950894

Araújo, R. G., Chavez-Santoscoy, R. A., Parra-Saldívar, R., Melchor-Martínez, E. M., & Iqbal, H. M. N. (2023). Agro-food systems and environment: Sustaining the unsustainable. *Current Opinions in Environmental Science and Health* [Internet] [cited 2025 Aug 20], *31*, 100413. Available from: https://www-sciencedirect-com.utokyo.idm.oclc.org/science/article/pii/S2468584422000885

Aung, K. T., Chen, H. J., Chau, M. L., Yap, G., Lim, X. F., Humaidi, M., et al. (2019). Salmonella in retail food and wild birds in Singapore—Prevalence, antimicrobial resistance, and sequence types. *International Journal of Environmental Research in Public Health* [Internet], *16*(21), 4235. Available from: https://www.mdpi.com/1660-4601/16/21/4235

Benedetti, G., Boisen, N., & Prada, J. M. (2024). Editorial: One Health surveillance in practice: experiences of integration among human health, animal health, environmental health, and food safety sectors. *Frontiers in Public Health* [Internet], *12*, 1384988. Available from: https://www.frontiersin.org/articles/10.3389/fpubh.2024.1384988/full

Borah, H., Bashir, O., Pawase, P. A., Mondal, I. U. H., Várallyay, S., Ungai, D., et al. (2025). Exploring the versatility of Magnetic Relaxation Switching (MRS) and CRISPR-based biosensors for the detection of foodborne pathogens; a comprehensive review. *Applied Food Research*, 101190.

Borelli, T., Hunter, D., Padulosi, S., Amaya, N., Meldrum, G., De Oliveira Beltrame, D. M., et al. (2020). Local solutions for sustainable food systems: The contribution of orphan crops and wild edible species. *Agronomy*.

Bwire, D., Saito, H., Sidle, R., & Nishiwaki, J. (2024). Water management and hydrological characteristics of paddy-rice fields under alternate wetting and drying irrigation practice as climate smart practice: A review. *Agronomy*.

Chauhan, C., Dhir, A., Akram, M. U., & Salo, J. (2021). Food loss and waste in food supply chains. A systematic literature review and framework development approach. *Journal of Cleaner Production, 295*, 126438.

Chiriacò, M. V., Galli, N., Santini, M., & Rulli, M. C. (2024). Deforestation and greenhouse gas emissions could arise when replacing palm oil with other vegetable oils. *Science of The Total Environment, 914*, 169486.

Chowdhury, S., Hossain, M. E., Ghosh, P. K., Ghosh, S., Hossain, M. B., Beard, C., et al. (2019). The pattern of highly pathogenic avian influenza H5N1 outbreaks in South Asia. *Tropical Medicine and Infectious Disease, 4*(4), 138.

Coelho, F., Coelho, E., & Egerer, M. (2018). Local food: Benefits and failings due to modern agriculture. *Science in Agriculture, 75*, 84–94.

Dada, A. C., Somorin, Y. M., Ateba, C. N., Onyeaka, H., Anyogu, A., Kasan, N. A., et al. (2021). Microbiological hazards associated with food products imported from the Asia-Pacific region based on analysis of the rapid alert system for food and feed (RASFF) notifications. *Food Control, 129*.

Dainese, M., Martin, E., Aizen, M., Albrecht, M., Bartomeus, I., Bommarco, R., et al. (2019). A global synthesis reveals biodiversity-mediated benefits for crop production. *Science Advances, 5*.

Davedow, T., Carleton, H., Kubota, K., Palm, D., Schroeder, M., Gerner-Smidt, P., et al. (2022). PulseNet international survey on the implementation of whole genome sequencing in low and middle-income countries for foodborne disease surveillance. *Foodborne Pathogens and Disease, 19*(5), 332–340.

Davis, K., Chhatre, A., Rao, N., Singh, D., Ghosh-Jerath, S., Mridul, A., et al. (2019). Assessing the sustainability of post-Green Revolution cereals in India. *Proceedings of the National Academy of Sciences of the United States of America, 116*, 25034–25041.

Dixon, J. M., Weerahewa, J., Hellin, J., Rola-Rubzen, M. F., Huang, J., Kumar, S., et al. (2021). Response and resilience of Asian agrifood systems to COVID-19: An assessment across twenty-five countries and four regional farming and food systems. *Agricultural Systems, 193*, 103168.

Dong, D., & Wang, J. (2023). Air pollution as a substantial threat to the improvement of agricultural total factor productivity: Global evidence. *Environment International, 173*, 107842.

Durazzo, A. (2019). The close linkage between nutrition and environment through biodiversity and sustainability: Local foods, traditional recipes, and sustainable diets. *Sustainability*.

Dwi Raharjo, U., Aditya Pratama, R., Ninda Sutriana, V., & Arsyam, R. M. A. (2022). Implementasi DHIS2 untuk Program Surveilans Kasus Gigitan Hewan Penyebab Rabies di Indonesia. *Journal of Information Systems for Public Health, 7*.

Dyah Rahma, A., & Ludwig, F. (2024). El Nino effects on water availability for agriculture: Case study of Magelang, Central Java, Indonesia. *Applied Environmental Research, 46*(2).

Ebenso, B., Otu, A., Giusti, A., Cousin, P., Adetimirin, V., Razafindralambo, H., et al. (2022). Nature-based One Health approaches to urban agriculture can deliver food and nutrition security. *Frontiers in Nutrition, 9*.

Economic and Social Commission for Asia and the Pacific (ESCAP). (2023). *Asia-Pacific Population and Development Report 2023* [Internet]. [cited 2025 Aug 19]. Available from: https://www.un.org/development/desa/pd/sites/www.un.org.development.desa.pd/files/undesa_pd_2024_escap-report-population-development-17.pdf

El Bilbeisi, A. H., Al-Jawaldeh, A., Albelbeisi, A., Abuzerr, S., Elmadfa, I., & Nasreddine, L. (2022). Households' food insecurity and its association with demographic and socioeconomic factors in Gaza Strip, Palestine: A cross- sectional study. *Ethiopian Journal of Health Sciences, 32*(2).

Estrada-Carmona, N., Sánchez, A., Remans, R., & Jones, S. (2022). Complex agricultural landscapes host more biodiversity than simple ones: A global meta-analysis. *Proceedings of the National Academy of Sciences of the United States of America, 119*.

Fard, N. A., Morales, G., Mejova, Y., & Schifanella, R. (2021). On the interplay between educational attainment and nutrition: A spatially-aware perspective. *EPJ Data Science, 10*, 1–21.

Faris, M., Abutair, A. S., Elfarra, R. M., Barqawi Nida, A., Firwana, A. M., Firwana, R. M., et al. (2025). Catastrophic famine in Gaza: Unprecedented levels of hunger post-October 7th. A real population-based study from the Gaza Strip. *PLoS One, 20*(5), e0309854.

Food and Agriculture Organization (FAO). (2011). *Global food losses and food waste—Extent, causes and prevention* [Internet]. [cited 2025 Aug 19]. Available from: https://www.fao.org/4/mb060e/mb060e.pdf

Food and Agriculture Organization (FAO). (2016). *Peace conflict and food security: What do we know about the linkages?* [Internet]. [cited 2025 Aug 19]. Available from: https://openknowledge.fao.org/server/api/core/bitstreams/3fc73834-753a-469b-8580-1edf00e875bd/content

George, S. E., Smink, M., Sangkachai, N., Wiratsudakul, A., Sakcamduang, W., Suwanpakdee, S., et al. (2023). Stakeholder attitudes and perspectives on wildlife disease surveillance as a component of a One Health approach in Thailand. *One Health, 17*.

Gignarta, T. S., Borojo, D. G., & Guan, Z. (2024). The impacts of economic policy uncertainties on agriculture export. *Cogent Economics & Finance, 12*(1).

Gong, B., Zhang, S., Liu, X., & Chen, K. Z. (2021). The Zoonotic diseases, agricultural production, and impact channels: Evidence from China. *Global Food Security, 28*, 100463.

Habiba, U. E., Khan, A., Mmbaga, E. J., Green, I. R., & Asaduzzaman, M. (2023). Use of antibiotics in poultry and poultry farmers- a cross-sectional survey in Pakistan. *Frontiers in Public Health* [Internet], *11*, 1154668. Available from: https://www.frontiersin.org/articles/10.3389/fpubh.2023.1154668/full

Halton, K., Sarna, M., Barnett, A., Leonardo, L., & Graves, N. (2013). A systematic review of community-based interventions for emerging zoonotic infectious diseases in Southeast Asia.

Hao, L., & Ki-Seong, L. (2024). The impact of economic policy uncertainty on agricultural prices: Evidence from China. *Asia and the Global Economy, 4*(2), 100100.

Hatta, M. N. A., Nga, Y. X., Amirnuddin, E. N., Muzafar, S. N., & Khairat, J. E. (2025). Landscape of H5 infections in ASEAN region: Past insights, present realities, & future strategies. *Viruses, 17*(4), 535.

Hong, C., Zhong, R., Xu, M., He, P., Mo, H., Qin, Y., et al. (2025). Interactions among food systems, climate change, and air pollution: A review. *Engineering, 44*, 215–233.

Jang, Y., Lee, H., & Park, H. (2025). Surveillance system for infectious disease prevention and management: Direction of Korea's infectious disease surveillance system. *Journal of Korean Medical Science. Korean Academy of Medical Science, 40.*

Kang, J. W., Kim, Y. G., & Tayag, M. (2025). *Potential impact of higher United States tariffs on Asian economies* [Internet] [cited 2025 Aug 19]. Available from: https://www.adb.org/sites/default/files/publication/1023516/adb-brief-332-us-tariffs-asian-economies.pdf

Kemmerling, B., Schetter, C., & Wirkus, L. (2022). The logics of war and food (in)security. *Global Food Security, 33*, 100634.

Kimsanova, B., Sanaev, G., & Herzfeld, T. (2024). Dynamics of food demand during political instability: Evidence from Kyrgyzstan. *Agricultural Economics, 55*(1), 41–53.

Kopittke, P. M., Menzies, N. W., Wang, P., McKenna, B. A., & Lombi, E. (2019). Soil and the intensification of agriculture for global food security. *Environment International, 132*, 105078.

Lajaunie, C., Morand, S., & Hinjoy, S. (2025). Southeast Asia at the heart of the implementation of the One Health approach. *Discoveries in Public Health, 22*(1).

Le, K., & Nguyen, M. (2020). Armed conflict and birth weight. *Economics and Human Biology, 39*, 100921.

Li, Y., Strapasson, A., & Rojas, O. (2020a). Assessment of El Niño and La Niña impacts on China: Enhancing the early warning system on food and agriculture. *Weather and Climate Extremes, 27*, 100208.

Li, W., Pires, S. M., Liu, Z., Ma, X., Liang, J., Jiang, Y., et al. (2020b). Surveillance of foodborne disease outbreaks in China, 2003–2017. *Food Control, 118.*

Li, R., Li, Y., Peng, K., Yin, Y., Liu, Y., He, T., et al. (2021a). Comprehensive genomic investigation of tigecycline resistance gene *tet* (X4)-bearing strains expanding among different settings. In J. Kovac (Ed.), *Microbiology in spectrum* (Vol. 9, Issue 3, pp. e01633–21) [Internet. Available from: https://journals.asm.org/doi/10.1128/spectrum.01633-21

Li, H., Chen, Y., Machalaba, C. C., Tang, H., Chmura, A. A., Fielder, M. D., et al. (2021b). *Wild animal and zoonotic disease risk management and regulation in China: Examining gaps and One Health opportunities in scope, mandates, and monitoring systems* (Vol. 13). One Health. Elsevier B.V..

Li, S., Chen, X., Ren, Y., & Glauben, T. (2024). The impact of demographic dynamics on food consumption and its environmental outcomes: Evidence from China. *Journal of Integrative Agriculture, 23*(2), 414–429.

Liberty, J. T., Bromage, S., Peter, E., Ihedioha, O. C., Alsalman, F. B., & Odogwu, T. S. (2025). CRISPR revolution: Unleashing precision pathogen detection to safeguard public health and food safety. *Methods, 240*, 180–194.

Liu, Y., Wang, P., Gojenko, B., Yu, J., Wei, L., Luo, D., et al. (2021). A review of water pollution arising from agriculture and mining activities in Central Asia: Facts, causes and effects. *Environmental Pollution, 291*, 118209.

Ma, N. L., Peng, W., Soon, C. F., Noor Hassim, M. F., Misbah, S., Rahmat, Z., et al. (2021). Covid-19 pandemic in the lens of food safety and security. *Environmental Research, 193*, 110405.

Martins, S. B., Häsler, B., & Rushton, J. (2015). Economic aspects of zoonoses: Impact of zoonoses on the food industry. In *Zoonoses—Infections affecting humans and animals* (pp. 1107–1126). Springer.

Maulu, S., Hasimuna, O. J., Haambiya, L. H., Monde, C., Musuka, C. G., Makorwa, T. H., et al. (2021). Climate change effects on aquaculture production: Sustainability implications, mitigation, and adaptations. *Frontiers in Sustainable Food Systems, 12*, 5.

Morris, R., & Wang, S. (2024). Building a pathway to One Health surveillance and response in Asian countries. *Science in One Health, 3*. Elsevier B.V.

Nguyen-Viet, H., Pham, G., Lam, S., Pham-Duc, P., Dinh-Xuan, T., Jing, F., et al. (2021). International, transdisciplinary, and ecohealth action for sustainable agriculture in Asia. *Frontiers in Public Health, 9.*

Nicastro, R., & Carillo, P. (2021). Food loss and waste prevention strategies from farm to fork. *Sustainability (Switzerland), 13*(10).

Oniang'o, R., Maingi, Z., Jaika, S., & Konyole, S. (2025). Africa's contribution to global sustainable and healthy diets: A scoping review. *Frontiers in Nutrition*, 12.

Pingali, P., & Abraham, M. (2022). Food systems transformation in Asia—A brief economic history. *Agricultural Economics, 53*(6), 895–910.

Porat, R., Lichter, A., Terry, L. A., Harker, R., & Buzby, J. (2018). Postharvest losses of fruit and vegetables during retail and in consumers' homes: Quantifications, causes, and means of prevention. *Postharvest Biology and Technology, 139*, 135–149.

Prabhakar, S. V. R. K. (2021). A succinct review and analysis of drivers and impacts of agricultural land transformations in Asia. *Land Use Policy, 102*, 105238.

Prescott, M., Burg, X., Metcalfe, J., Lipka, A., Herritt, C., & Cunningham-Sabo, L. (2019). Healthy planet, healthy youth: A food systems education and promotion intervention to improve adolescent diet quality and reduce food waste. *Nutrients*, 11.

Putri, I., Dwiartama, A., & Rosmiati, M. (2025). Exploring grassroots initiatives in food waste reduction—A case study of two Indonesian food banks. *Food Security*.

Qin, Y., Tang, J., Li, T., Qi, X., Zhang, D., Wang, S., et al. (2023). Cultivated land demand and pressure in Southeast Asia from 1961 to 2019: A comprehensive study on food consumption. *Food, 12*(19), 3531.

Rahman, M. A., Alam, M. S., Sultana, R., & Sultana, R. (2025). Assessing the interrelationship between monsoon flood disasters and major crop production in Bangladesh. *International Journal of Disaster Risk Reduction, 121*, 105401.

Rizzo, D. M., Lichtveld, M., Mazet, J. A. K., Togami, E., & Miller, S. A. (2021). Plant health and its effects on food safety and security in a One Health framework: Four case studies. *One Health Outlook, 3*(1).

Sharma, A., Ceasar, S., Pandey, H., Devadas, V., Kesavan, A. K., Heisnam, P., et al. (2025). Millets: Nutrient-rich and climate-resilient crops for sustainable agriculture and diverse culinary applications. *Journal of Food Composition and Analysis*.

Shigemura, H., Sakatsume, E., Sekizuka, T., Yokoyama, H., Hamada, K., Etoh, Y., et al. (2020). Food workers as a reservoir of extended-spectrum-cephalosporin-resistant salmonella strains in Japan.

Soffiantini, G. (2020). Food insecurity and political instability during the Arab Spring. *Global Food Security, 26*, 100400.

Sterling, E., Betley, E., Ahmed, S., Akabas, S., Clegg, D., Downs, S., et al. (2021). Centering equity in sustainable food systems education. 5.

Su, F., Liu, Y., Chen, S. J., & Fahad, S. (2023). Towards the impact of economic policy uncertainty on food security: Introducing a comprehensive heterogeneous framework for assessment. *Journal of Cleaner Production, 386*, 135792.

Tang, B., Siddique, A., Jia, C., Ed-Dra, A., Wu, J., Lin, H., et al. (2023). Genome-based risk assessment for foodborne Salmonella enterica from food animals in China: A One Health perspective. *International Journal of Food Microbiology, 390*.

Tiwari, A. K. (2023). The role of organic farming in achieving agricultural sustainability: Environmental and socio-economic impacts. *Acta Biology Forum*.

van Dijk, M., Morley, T., Rau, M. L., & Saghai, Y. (2021). A meta-analysis of projected global food demand and population at risk of hunger for the period 2010–2050. *Nature Food, 2*(7), 494–501.

Venkatappa, M., Sasaki, N., Han, P., & Abe, I. (2021). Impacts of droughts and floods on croplands and crop production in Southeast Asia—An application of Google Earth Engine. *Science of The Total Environment, 795*, 148829.

Vergis, J., Rawool, D. B., Singh Malik, S. V., & Barbuddhe, S. B. (2021) Food safety in fisheries: Application of One Health approach. *Indian Journal of Medical Research* [Internet], *153*(3), 348–357. Available from: https://ijmr.org.in/food-safety-in-fisheries-application-of-one-health-approach/

Wang, L., Wang, L., Li, Y., & Wang, J. (2023). A century-long analysis of global warming and earth temperature using a random walk with drift approach. *Decision Analytics Journal, 7*, 100237.

Wen, X., Sun, S., Li, L., He, Q., & Tsai, F. S. (2019). Avian influenza—Factors affecting consumers' purchase intentions toward poultry products. *International Journal of Environmental Research and Public Health, 16*(21), 4139.

Wielinga, P. R., & Schlundt, J. (2012). Food safety: At the center of a One Health approach for combating zoonoses. In J. S. Mackenzie, M. Jeggo, P. Daszak, & J. A. Richt (Eds.), *One Health: The human-animal-environment interfaces in emerging infectious diseases* (pp. 3–17) [Internet]. Springer. Available from: http://link.springer.com/10.1007/978-3-662-45791-7_238

World Bank. (2025). *What is food security?* [Internet]. [cited 2025 Aug 20]. Available from: https://www.worldbank.org/en/topic/agriculture/brief/food-security-update/what-is-food-security

World Health Organization. (2024) Joint external evaluation of the International Health Regulations (2005) core capacities of Indonesia.

World Health Organization (WHO). (2025). *Avian Influenza A(H5N1)—Cambodia* [cited 2025 Aug 19]. Available from: https://www.who.int/emergencies/disease-outbreak-news/item/2025-DON575

Wu, D., Elliott, C., & Wu, Y. (2021). Food safety strategies: The One Health approach to global challenges and China's actions. *China CDC Weekly* [Internet], *3*(24), 507–513. Available from: files/419/Wu et al. - 2021 - Food Safety Strategies The One Health Approach to Global Challenges and China's Actions.pdf

Zhang, Y., Wang, W., Li, S., Zhu, K., Hua, X., Harrison, M., et al. (2023). *Integrated management approaches enabling sustainable rice production under alternate wetting and drying irrigation*. Agric Water Manag.

Zhang, X. X., Lederman, Z., Han, L. F., Schurer, J. M., Xiao, L. H., Zhang, Z. B., et al. (2024). Towards an actionable One Health approach. *Infectious Disease Poverty* [Internet], *13*(1):28. Available from: https://idpjournal.biomedcentral.com/articles/10.1186/s40249-024-01198-0

Zinsstag, J., Kaiser-Grolimund, A., Heitz-Tokpa, K., Sreedharan, R., Lubroth, J., Caya, F., et al. (2023). Advancing One human–animal–environment Health for global health security: What does the evidence say? *The Lancet, 401*(10376), 591–604.

Chapter 7
Climate Change and Health

Intan Rosenanda Sofiany, Fitri Revita Nurannisa, Nurendah Ratri Azhar Rusprayunita, Andang Evrilianto, and Yudhi Ratna Nugraheni

7.1 The Impact of Climate Change on Human Health

7.1.1 Overview of Climate Change and Global Health Threats

Climate change refers to long-term variations in heat levels, rainfall patterns, and other climatic conditions. The current global average earth's temperature has risen by 1.29 °C in comparison to the twentieth-century average (Costello et al., 2009). This significant increase highlights climate change as one of the major and urgent challenges to human health in this century (Buttke et al., 2023; Campbell-Lendrum et al., 2023; Kjellstrom & McMichael, 2013). The World Health Organization (WHO) notes that climate change influences not only the environment but also the social, economic, and health sectors, with its widespread effects expected to reach populations around the world (Costello et al., 2009). According to the Intergovernmental Panel on Climate Change (IPCC), in the Sixth Assessment

I. R. Sofiany (✉) · F. R. Nurannisa · N. R. A. Rusprayunita
Master of Public Health Program, Faculty of Medicine, Public Health, and Nursing, Universitas Gadjah Mada, Yogyakarta, Indonesia
e-mail: intanrosenandasofiany@mail.ugm.ac.id; fitrirevitanuarnnisa@mail.ugm.ac.id; nurendahratriazharrusprayunita@mail.ugm.ac.id

A. Evrilianto
Department of Health Administration and Policy, Faculty of Public Health, University of Indonesia, Depok, Indonesia
e-mail: andang.evrilianto@ui.ac.id

Y. R. Nugraheni
Department of Parasitology, Faculty of Veterinary Medicine, Universitas Gadjah Mada, Yogyakarta, Indonesia

One Health Centre of Excellence, Universitas Gadjah Mada, Yogyakarta, Indonesia
e-mail: yudhi.ratna.n@mail.ugm.ac.id

© The Author(s), under exclusive license to Springer Nature Singapore Pte Ltd. 2026
A. U. Rauf, T. Wibawa (eds.), *The One Health Concept in Asian Contexts*, https://doi.org/10.1007/978-981-95-9880-9_7

Report (AR6), climate risks are emerging more quickly and severely than anticipated (Calvin et al., 2023).

Climate change is a *"threat multiplier,"* not only creating new risks but also exacerbating existing vulnerabilities and inequalities, which may reverse the progress in global health over the years (Baxter et al., 2022). The health consequences are not uniform but vary by population group, region, and the responsiveness of the public health system. In its findings, the US Global Change Research Program (USGCRP) recognized seven main health risks resulting from climate change and emphasized the need for ongoing surveillance and research in these priority areas: extreme heat, poor outdoor air quality, flooding, water, vector, and food-borne disease, and mental health impact (Parums, 2024). As global heating intensifies, adaptation will become increasingly challenging, particularly for vulnerable populations and fragile health systems.

7.1.2 Direct and Indirect Impact of Climate Change on Human Health

The multifaceted nature of climate change, along with its environmental and social impacts, gives rise to a broad spectrum of global health risks via both direct and indirect mechanisms (Agache et al., 2022).

7.1.2.1 Direct Impact

Heat-Related Disorders The most immediate consequence of a warming planet is the burden of heat stress and its health complications. When temperatures rise beyond the body's physiological tolerance, they can disrupt organ function, alter mood, and influence behavior (Kjellstrom, 2009; Kjellstrom & McMichael, 2013; Shapira et al., 2025). Furthermore, the ongoing rise in global temperatures contributes to more frequent and intense heatwaves, resulting in heat exhaustion, heatstroke, and the worsening of cardiovascular and respiratory diseases (Dianati Tilaki et al., 2021; Kim et al., 2014; Kjellstrom, 2009; Malhotra, 2024).

Extreme Weather Events Climate change drives extreme weather, with regional weather patterns expected to become more erratic and unpredictable, resulting in extreme rainfall, flood events, and prolonged droughts (Calvin et al., 2023; Dianati Tilaki et al., 2021). These events cause injuries, loss of life, and population displacement, leading to long-term consequences.

Sea-Level Rise Rising sea levels present both direct and indirect risks to human health. The immediate dangers include physical threats from coastal inundation, frequent flooding, and more intense storm surges, particularly when coinciding with high tides. Destruction of coastal infrastructure such as roadways, residential areas, and sanitation facilities further heightens immediate risks. Accelerate photochemical reactions involving volatile organic compounds from vehicle emissions, thereby increasing ozone concentrations, a key component of urban smog. These pollutants are associated with adverse respiratory outcomes, including asthma exacerbations, reduced pulmonary function, and an increased risk of respiratory infections.

7.1.2.2 Indirect Impact

Disease Transmission Rising temperatures enhance the life cycles of vectors and pathogens, thereby increasing the potential for disease spread. Variations in temperature and rainfall distribution also affect the spread and reproductive cycles of vectors such as mosquitoes and ticks. Consequently, malaria, dengue fever, and Lyme disease are spreading into previously unaffected areas (Hime et al., 2018; Kim et al., 2014; Patz et al., 2014). Changing rainfall patterns also provide suitable environments for vector proliferation. Excessive rainfall generates stagnant water that serves as a breeding site for mosquitoes, while periods of drought concentrate water sources and increase contact between humans and vectors. Extreme weather events, including storms and floods, disrupt ecosystems and human settlements, heightening the risk of vector exposure. In addition, population displacement due to climate disasters can accelerate the transmission of vector-borne diseases across different regions (McMichael & Lindgren, 2011).

Food Insecurity Climate change affects agricultural productivity through various mechanisms, posing a challenge to global food security. Uncertainty in both the intensity and distribution of rainfall, particularly in regions dependent on rain-fed agriculture, has led to sharp declines in crop yields. Reduced agricultural productivity not only increases the risk of malnutrition from undernutrition to other related health problems but also contributes to weakened immune systems and shifting disease landscapes (Kim et al., 2014; McMichael & Lindgren, 2011).

Water Insecurity Water scarcity is closely linked to climate change, as higher global temperatures coupled with variations in precipitation exacerbate droughts, reduce access to clean water, and lower agricultural productivity (Kim et al., 2014; McMichael & Lindgren, 2011). These conditions heighten the likelihood of waterborne diseases, malnutrition, and social vulnerability. In the long term, water scarcity may also trigger conflicts and forced migration, further worsening the public health burden both physically and mentally.

Mental Health Disorders The effects of climate change extend to mental health, where extreme climatic events and population displacement potentially cause anxiety, depression, and post-traumatic stress disorder (PTSD). Individuals who survive disasters, including tropical storms, floods, and wildfires, frequently experience long-lasting trauma. In addition, chronic stressors like prolonged droughts and sea-level rise generate feelings of helplessness and uncertainty. This has led to the emergence of *eco-anxiety*, a persistent fear of environmental catastrophe, particularly prevalent among younger generations aware of climate change's long-term consequences (Kjellstrom, 2009; McMichael & Lindgren, 2011; Wan et al., 2023).

Social Disruption and Population Displacement Climate change is driving large-scale human displacement due to declining food yields, reduced freshwater availability, and coastal flooding (McMichael & Lindgren, 2011). The impacts are particularly severe for poor communities in developing countries living in areas prone to floods, storms, or landslides, where public health resources are limited. Migration driven by climate change increases risks of malnutrition, communicable diseases, social tension, mental health disorders, and risky behaviors, including alcohol use, tobacco use, and transactional sex. Children are among the most vulnerable, facing threats to mental well-being, emotional development, and physical safety, as evidenced by increases in child abuse following major disasters.

7.1.3 Vulnerable Populations in These Challenges

7.1.3.1 Children and the Elderly

The elderly and children represent groups at heightened risk of health consequences associated with climate change. In older adults, declining thermoregulatory capacity due to reduced skin blood vessel dilation, decreased sweat production, and weakened cardiovascular function, combined with physical frailty, chronic medical conditions, and sometimes dependence on others, increases susceptibility to heat stress, malnutrition, and communicable diseases. Children, due to underdeveloped immune systems, show greater vulnerability to water-borne diseases and nutritional deficiencies resulting from disruptions in food systems. These groups are also prone to mental health consequences, such as anxiety, depression, and post-traumatic stress disorder (PTSD) (Dianati Tilaki et al., 2021; Kjellstrom & McMichael, 2013; McMichael & Lindgren, 2011).

7.1.3.2 Community in Poverty

Low-income groups face heightened vulnerability to climate change as they often have limited financial and social resources needed to cope with extreme heat. Socioeconomic disadvantages such as limited access to heat-adapted housing, cooling systems, and healthcare heighten the potential for heat-induced illness and fatalities. Poor baseline health, common among disadvantaged populations, further increases susceptibility (Bennett et al., 2015; Saha et al., 2024; Shapira et al., 2025).

7.1.3.3 Geographically Vulnerable Areas

Populations living in coastal regions and small islands are particularly exposed to the consequences of climate change, including higher sea levels and recurrent extreme weather events like cyclones and storm surges (Calvin et al., 2023). In arid areas, prolonged droughts threaten water availability and agricultural productivity, intensifying food insecurity and related medical conditions. High-altitude communities are vulnerable to glacial melt and changes in precipitation patterns, which disrupt freshwater supplies and traditional livelihoods. Limited access to healthcare, infrastructure, and emergency resources in these regions further exacerbates the vulnerability (McMichael & Lindgren, 2011; Shapira et al., 2025).

7.1.3.4 People with Chronic Conditions

People with underlying medical conditions are at increased risk from climate change impacts (Bennett et al., 2015; Saha et al., 2024; Shapira et al., 2025). Chronic diseases, such as cardiovascular, pulmonary, kidney, and mental health problems, are linked to higher morbidity and mortality during heatwaves. This vulnerability can stem from the underlying disease mechanisms or from medications used in treatment, which may impair the body's capacity to cope with extreme heat.

7.1.3.5 Outdoor Workers

Occupational heat exposure is an increasing health risk as global temperatures rise, reducing the number of safe working hours and potentially lowering productivity (Bennett et al., 2015; Buttke et al., 2023; Shapira et al., 2025; Tsakonas et al., 2025). Workers in tropical low- and middle-income countries, particularly those performing outdoor labor, are most at risk due to direct sun exposure, heavy physical activity, and the need for protective clothing. Adequate hydration is crucial but often challenging, especially when high temperatures persist during rest periods or at night. Vulnerability is heightened among populations in precarious employment, with limited social protection and low income.

7.2 Extreme Weather Events and Their Health Consequences

7.2.1 Overview and Types of Extreme Weather Events

Over time, human activities such as industrial emissions, transformation in land use, and the overexploitation of ecological resources have contributed to a steady increase in global temperatures and the destabilization of long-standing weather patterns (Shivanna, 2022; Hausfather et al., 2020). Consequently, extreme climatic conditions ranging from prolonged droughts and unprecedented rainfall to intensified heatwaves and wildfires are becoming more frequent, intense, and less predictable (Upadhyay, 2020).

7.2.1.1 Heatwaves

One of the most notable manifestations of these shifting climate patterns in Southeast Asia is the increasing occurrence of heatwaves. Once considered rare in equatorial regions, extreme heat events are now becoming a significant public health concern across several countries in the region (Sharma et al., 2022). These extreme heat events are largely attributed to rising global temperatures caused by human-driven activities, including fossil fuel combustion, deforestation, and urban heat island effects (Stott, 2016; Elmarakby & Elkadi, 2024). Although heatwaves are widely recognized as a consequence of anthropogenic climate change, their formation is also underpinned by complex interactions across the Earth's atmospheric, geospherical, and geospatial systems. At the atmospheric level, increased greenhouse gas emissions have disrupted the planet's energy balance, leading to the accumulation of heat in the lower layers of the atmosphere and the development of persistent high-pressure systems that inhibit air circulation (Nunes, 2023). From a geospherical perspective, land degradation and deforestation reduce natural cooling processes such as evapotranspiration, resulting in greater heat absorption and diminished surface resilience (Takahashi et al., 2017). Furthermore, geospatial changes and remarkably rapid urbanization have intensified the urban heat island effect (EPA, 2025; Takahashi et al., 2017).

7.2.1.2 Heavy Rainfall and Floods

Another frequently reported extreme weather event in Southeast Asia is heavy rainfall, often followed by flash floods. In recent years, numerous flooding incidents have been recorded across the region, affecting both urban and rural populations (Torti, 2012). While these events are partially caused by anthropogenic activities, such as poor land-use planning, deforestation, and inadequate civil infrastructure, they are also largely determined by shifting meteorological and climatological patterns (Wang et al., 2019; Elsner et al., 2010). The intensification of the hydrological cycle, influenced by higher atmospheric moisture content and warmer sea surface temperatures, has resulted in greater intensity and less predictable precipitation patterns (Greve et al., 2014; Olsson et al., 2016). From a hydrogeological perspective, reduced infiltration capacity due to soil compaction, erosion, and impermeable surfaces in rapidly urbanized areas contributes to faster surface runoff and overwhelmed drainage systems. The recurrence of La Niña conditions in the region further amplifies the risk, bringing above-average rainfall and saturated ground conditions that increase the likelihood of landslides and prolonged flooding (Yang & Zhang, 2011; Feng et al., 2021; Vega et al., 2024).

7.2.1.3 Tropical Cyclones and Typhoons

The tropical cyclone is another extreme weather event commonly observed across the Asia-Pacific region. Meteorologically, tropical cyclones form over warm ocean waters, where sustained sea surface temperatures above 26.5 °C supply the heat and moisture needed to fuel convective activity. Climatologically, their frequency and distribution are influenced by large-scale ocean-atmosphere interactions (Wang et al., 2025; Camargo et al., 2023). While anthropogenic factors are not directly responsible for their genesis, anthropogenic climate change, particularly global warming and ocean heat content increase, has been linked to the intensification of these storms (Fudeyasu et al., 2014).

7.2.1.4 Droughts

Droughts are among the most complex climate-induced disasters to address due to their slow onset, widespread impact, and the high economic and technological demands of mitigation, especially in remote areas with limited infrastructure. Countries such as Indonesia, Cambodia, and Thailand have reported recurrent droughts in recent years, which are closely linked to shifting meteorological, climatological, and hydrogeological dynamics (Ha et al., 2022; Kim et al., 2020).

Droughts often arise from a convergence of meteorological and climatological factors. Meteorologically, they are commonly associated with persistent high-pressure systems that inhibit cloud formation and suppress precipitation over extended periods. Such atmospheric anomalies are often amplified by large-scale climate patterns like the El Niño–Southern Oscillation (ENSO), which can delay or weaken the monsoon season in Southeast Asia (Phan-Van et al., 2022; Kim et al., 2020). Climatologically, increasing global temperatures have altered rainfall distribution and intensified evapotranspiration, leading to significant moisture deficits in soils and vegetation. Additionally, precipitation has become increasingly erratic, occurring in shorter and more intense bursts, thereby limiting groundwater recharge and exacerbating surface water scarcity (Zhang et al., 2023; Green, 2016).

7.2.1.5 Air Pollution and Haze

As anthropogenic climate change drives the increase in global temperatures, the occurrence and severity of wildfires have escalated, especially across tropical and subtropical regions. One of the most pervasive environmental consequences of these fires is transboundary haze, a recurring phenomenon in Southeast Asia. Indonesia's Sumatra, Kalimantan, Nusa Tenggara, and parts of Eastern Indonesia are particularly vulnerable due to their peat-rich soils, prolonged dry spells, and complex interactions among land use, climate variability, and atmospheric circulation (Choy & Onuma, 2025; Davies-Barnard et al., 2023). From a hydro-meteorological standpoint, wildfires in these regions are typically triggered by a combination of extreme heat, low humidity, and extended periods without precipitation, often intensified by El Niño–Southern Oscillation (ENSO) events. The geological characteristics of peatlands, organic-rich and waterlogged soils, make them highly flammable when dried, resulting in fires that can smolder underground for weeks and release vast quantities of particulate matter and greenhouse gases (Yulianti & Hayasaka, 2023).

Once fires are ignited, meteorological forces are important in the dispersion of haze. Seasonal wind structures, such as the southwesterly monsoon, facilitate the transboundary movement of particulate matter (PM2.5 and PM10), which often travels hundreds of kilometers across national borders. This air-borne pollution regularly affects neighboring countries like Singapore, Malaysia, and Brunei, causing regional diplomatic tensions and public health crises (Hayasaka & Usup, 2023; Wooster et al., 2018).

7.2.2 Health Outcomes from Extreme Weather

Extreme weather conditions present major risks to public health through direct exposures and indirect pathways that are often less visible but equally harmful. Among these events, heatwaves stand out as particularly dangerous. When temperatures rise significantly, the human body experiences difficulty in regulating its core temperature. Prolonged exposure to high heat can result in exhaustion, heatstroke, and severe dehydration, which in turn may trigger cardiovascular and pulmonary complications (Paravantis et al., 2017; Cheng et al., 2019). Vulnerable groups experience these effects more severely, including the elderly, whose thermoregulatory responses are often impaired. In Europe, for example, many heatwave-related deaths occur among older adults living alone or in poorly ventilated housing. Low humidity further compounds the problem by accelerating fluid loss, thereby disrupting essential physiological functions (D'Ippoliti et al., 2010; Rikkert et al., 2009).

Floods, another increasingly frequent extreme event, bring their own set of direct health consequences. Drowning remains one of the most immediate and fatal risks, especially in areas with rapid water rise or poor evacuation infrastructure. The force of moving water can cause traumatic injuries from collisions with debris or collapsing structures. Exposure to standing water and electrical hazards, such as downed power lines or submerged appliances, may lead to electrocution. In colder conditions, prolonged exposure to floodwaters can also result in hypothermia, particularly in children and the elderly (Lowe et al., 2013; Paterson et al., 2018).

Natural disasters such as storms, hurricanes, and typhoons frequently occur in many regions across the globe, especially in regions like the United States and the Asia-Pacific. These disasters can have an immediate and devastating impact on human health. High-speed winds often carry debris that can strike individuals, causing blunt force injuries and trauma. Lightning strikes, though rare, are another deadly consequence (Bartholdson & von Schreeb, 2018; Hawkins et al., 2024; Goldman et al., 2014).

Wildfires are another pressing threat, especially during dry seasons. These fires not only damage property and ecosystems but also have serious respiratory consequences. Smoke and haze from wildfires irritate the eyes and impair vision, creating discomfort for entire communities. Among people with underlying pulmonary conditions, including asthma, the risk of exacerbation and even the progression of chronic obstructive pulmonary disease (COPD) significantly increases. In severe cases, wildfires that approach residential areas can result in burn injuries, particularly among vulnerable populations (Mkorombindo & Balkissoon, 2021; Wilgus & Merchant, 2024).

Landslides, while often triggered by tectonic activity, are increasingly driven by anthropogenic activities, including deforestation. The health impacts of landslides can be immediate and life-threatening, including burial injuries, severe trauma, and death (Kennedy et al., 2015; Petrucci, 2022; Pollock & Wartman, 2020). The consequences of drought are wide-ranging and interlinked, affecting sectors from agriculture to public health. Crop failures due to water stress impair food production, threatening food security and driving up prices. This can lead to hunger and undernutrition, particularly among low-income populations (Lin et al., 2022; Amondo et al., 2023). Malnutrition weakens the immune system, increasing vulnerability to infectious diseases. Moreover, water scarcity undermines sanitation and hygiene practices, contributing to the spread of water-borne illnesses (Hepatology, 2022; Morales et al., 2023).

Extreme weather events cause direct and indirect consequences that significantly impact human health. Among the most prominent impacts is the growing risk of infectious diseases. Floods and rising temperatures create a favorable environment for the distribution of vector-borne illnesses, including malaria and dengue fever. Additionally, water-borne diseases, including cholera, leptospirosis, and hepatitis A, commonly increase following flood events, when water sources become contaminated. Food-borne illnesses also tend to rise due to disrupted cold chains, food spoilage, and poor sanitation, all of which are exacerbated during and after these incidents (Balta et al., 2024; Saatchi et al., 2024).

In addition to physical illnesses, extreme weather also significantly impacts psychological conditions. Individuals who experience disasters may suffer from psychological conditions, such as post-traumatic stress disorder (PTSD), anxiety, depression, and suicidal thoughts, especially when they have lost loved ones or their homes and livelihoods. Furthermore, the disruption of food supply chains can lead to malnutrition and micronutrient deficiencies, particularly in vulnerable populations (Crane et al., 2022; Wang et al., 2023).

7.2.3 Impact of Extreme Weather on Health Infrastructure

Beyond direct and indirect health outcomes, extreme climate conditions also give rise to a range of non-health-specific consequences that significantly affect population health. Infrastructure damage represents one of the most immediate and tangible impacts. Roads may become impassable, buildings may be structurally compromised, and power outages are frequently reported. These disruptions can hinder emergency response efforts, delay medical treatment, and exacerbate the health conditions of affected populations, particularly those requiring continuous care or access to life-saving medications (Chang et al., 2025; Bell et al., 2018).

On a broader population health level, the displacement of residents and the resulting pressures on temporary shelters can have serious implications. Overcrowded and poorly resourced shelters are hotspots for the transmission of infectious diseases, face shortages of essential supplies such as clean water and contraceptives, and may lack the infrastructure necessary to protect vulnerable groups (Romano et al., 2025). The health risks extend beyond infection; limited access to sanitation and reproductive health services, for example, can disproportionately affect women and girls, particularly with respect to menstrual hygiene management in crisis settings (Conzatti et al., 2022; Hirani, 2024).

7.2.4 Case Study in Asia

Typhoons and tropical cyclones are common occurrences in Asia, particularly in countries like the Philippines, Vietnam, China, and Japan. These weather events are often triggered by the interaction between warm sea surface temperatures that are typically above 27 °C and low subtropical atmospheric pressure, creating ideal conditions for cyclonic activity (Tory & Dare, 2015). One of the most recent typhoons, Typhoon Yagi, struck in September 2024 and affected Southeast Asian countries, such as the Philippines, Vietnam, Myanmar, Lao PDR, and Thailand. Although it caused widespread disruptions, the damage it inflicted was not as severe as that of Typhoon Haiyan in 2013. Haiyan remains among the most devastating and deadly typhoons ever recorded, claiming over 6200 lives in the Philippines alone and resulting in an estimated loss of USD 13 billion (Hugelius et al., 2017).

Japan is often regarded as a model for disaster mitigation, especially in managing typhoons. The country developed a highly effective early warning system that integrated into mobile phones and broadcast widely through media channels. Japanese technology plays a key role in ensuring timely alerts and collective preparedness

(Bean et al., 2025; Cao et al., 2024). The Philippines in contrast, despite being geographically prone to typhoons due to its location near the equator, continues to face challenges in disaster mitigation. The country's vulnerability is exacerbated by inadequate infrastructure and significant social disparities, making it difficult to respond effectively to large-scale disasters (Lloyd et al., 2022; Ignacio, 2025).

Wildfires and the resulting transboundary haze are a recurrent environmental and public health issue in Southeast Asia, particularly affecting Indonesia. Regions such as Sumatra, Kalimantan, and Nusa Tenggara are frequently impacted during the dry season (typically June to September), with haze often spreading to neighboring countries like Malaysia, Singapore, and Brunei. In 2015, the haze crisis led to nearly 900,000 reported cases of acute respiratory infections (ARI), reflecting the severe health toll of this event. Despite having mitigation strategies in place, Indonesia's response mechanisms remain suboptimal compared to high-income neighboring countries. The absence of a well-integrated early warning system and real-time hotspot alerts for citizens, along with persistent issues in land governance and weak law enforcement, continues to hinder effective management of wildfire-related air pollution (Fitriany et al., 2021; Noviarini et al., 2024; Widyastuti et al., 2020).

Drought is another increasingly prevalent extreme weather event in Southeast Asia, particularly in Thailand, Vietnam, Indonesia, and Cambodia. These countries often share similar vulnerabilities, including limited economic capacity, political instability, and underdeveloped water management infrastructure (Krishna Prabhakar, 2022). Prolonged droughts are exacerbated by shifting atmospheric pressure systems, increased rates of evaporation due to rising temperatures, and a decline in aquifer recharge. Furthermore, human activities such as excessive groundwater extraction contribute to water scarcity. Mitigation efforts in these countries are often fragmented, lacking both regional coordination and long-term sustainability planning (Stanke et al., 2013; Soliman dan Amin, 2025).

In contrast to droughts, extreme flooding is frequently reported across Asia, with China, Indonesia, and Japan among the most affected countries. One of the most recent and catastrophic events occurred in Hebei, China, in July 2025, displacing over 80,000 people. Apart from the immediate threat to human life, floods also trigger secondary disasters such as landslides in mountainous areas and widespread contamination or shortages of clean water. While countries like Japan have developed advanced flood forecasting and disaster response systems, others continue to struggle with early warning dissemination and coordinated evacuation planning.

Heatwaves have become increasingly common in East and Southeast Asia, particularly in China, Japan, South Korea, and Vietnam. In August 2025, Chongqing, China, recorded an unprecedented temperature of over 44 °C, leading to surges in electricity consumption and a spike in heat-related hospital admissions. Similar patterns of health system strain and increased mortality have been reported in South Korea and Japan, with hundreds of medical emergencies and several mortality cases (Chan et al., 2018; Wang et al., 2014). While some countries have implemented integrated early warning systems to alert citizens of heatwave conditions, others lack such infrastructure.

7.3 Climate Change-Related Diseases

7.3.1 Vector-Borne Disease

Various studies have demonstrated that climate change, particularly driven by polluted air, has an immediate impact on mortality rates and the increased transmission of vector-borne diseases (Gao et al., 2021; Poursafa & Kelishadi, 2011). Air pollution and the increasing frequency of heatwaves, which damage habitats and disrupt ecosystem balance, are largely caused by releases of greenhouse gases, with carbon dioxide from fossil fuels being a primary contributor. Climate is one of the key environmental factors influencing disease transmission patterns. Ongoing climate variability is forecasted to influence the emergence and spread of pathogens, particularly as a result of shifts in temperature and rainfall patterns (Gao et al., 2021).

Increasing environmental temperatures enhance the proliferation of pests, disease-causing agents, and infectious vectors in the farming industry (McDermott-Levy et al., 2021). A vector is an organism that plays a role in spreading disease-causing agents, namely by transferring pathogens from one host to another (Cheng et al., 2020; Carnes et al., 2014). The reservoir itself can be a human, animal, or insect, which serves as the primary habitat for pathogens to survive and reproduce. Various vector-borne diseases, including malaria, dengue fever, Chagas disease, leishmaniasis, trypanosomiasis, schistosomiasis, and yellow fever, are generally spread through the bite of contaminated arthropods and constitute a large part of the worldwide infectious disease challenges (Ewing et al., 2021; Yaghoobi-Ershadi, 2016).

Vector-borne diseases are widely regarded as an important public health challenge in various regions across the globe. In Southern Europe, the warm Mediterranean climate allows disease vectors, including mosquitoes, ticks, and sandflies, to survive and thrive. Its geographical proximity to Africa further facilitates the cross-continental spread of diseases. In January 2022, Northern Italy reported its first case of African swine fever virus (ASFV) in the Piedmont region, detected in a wild boar found dead in Ovada, Alessandria Province. Climate change has expanded the distribution of these ticks, therefore elevating the likelihood of disease transmission (Ostfeld & Brunner, 2015; Artigas et al., 2021).

7.3.2 Water-Borne Disease

Climate change triggers alterations in precipitation patterns, increasing sea levels, and changes in salinity, all of which influence air temperature and the survival of pathogens in aquatic environments (Berry et al., 2018; Kendrovski & Gjorgjev, 2012). These conditions increase the risk of diseases such as cholera, typhoid, and *Salmonella*, with each 1 °C rise in global temperature potentially increasing the risk of *Salmonella* infection by 5–10% (Kendrovski & Gjorgjev, 2012). Water-borne diseases (WBDs) can infect humans through activities such as washing, personal hygiene, or consuming pathogen-contaminated water. Climate change impacts the habitat and survival behavior of pathogens, elevating the likelihood of transmission (Khan et al., 2019; Wu et al., 2016). Examples of WBDs include cholera, salmonellosis, typhoid, hepatitis A and E, diarrhea, leptospirosis, amoebiasis, cryptosporidiosis, *Campylobacter enteritis*, and poliomyelitis (Wu et al., 2016; Khan et al., 2019; Murphy et al., 2014; Cheesbrough, 2005).

Water-borne diseases (WBDs) are becoming an increasingly serious concern due to insufficient access to safe water for consumption (Bidhuri et al., 2018). Children are more vulnerable than adults because their immune systems and self-regulation abilities are not yet fully developed (Jones, 2013). Water-borne diseases associated with extreme weather events tend to impact vulnerable groups more severely, worsening health inequalities. One of the pathogens most frequently associated with extreme climate change is *Vibrio cholerae*, the bacterium responsible for cholera (Cann et al., 2013). Climate change further heightens the likelihood of WBDs by degrading water source quality and raising the occurrence of natural disasters that can pollute water supplies.

According to the WHO, approximately 1.1 billion people still consume drinking water contaminated with feces, and around 1.8 million people pass away annually due to diarrhea and water-borne diseases (Bain et al., 2014; Organization, 2005). The climate change impacts on WBD vary across countries and regions. Two major diseases that present a major health challenge are typhus and cholera. Developing countries, particularly in the ASEAN region, are at high risk of WBD outbreaks and climate disasters, including intense rainfall, floods, rising temperatures, and droughts. These risks are exacerbated by densely populated areas, widespread poverty, underdevelopment, and limited adaptive capacity (McMichael, 2003).

7.3.3 Heat-Related Disease

Heatwaves contribute to more deaths than any other extreme weather event, with their global frequency, intensity, and duration having escalated under the influence of climate change (Greene et al., 2011; Smith et al., 2015). Heat-related diseases include heat cramps, heat fatigue, and heat stroke. They can further heighten the severity of chronic diseases, such as pulmonary disorders, cardiovascular diseases, diabetes, and stroke. Extreme heat also poses significant risks to mental health, increasing the risk of suicide and violence, while reducing learning ability, productivity, and cognitive functioning (Schwartz et al., 2015; Schulte et al., 2021; Thompson et al., 2018).

The elderly population is at a higher likelihood of heat waves (Sarofim et al., 2016). During extreme weather, they are at risk of dehydration and hypernatremia, which can lead to kidney failure and cardiovascular problems. This risk is further increased if they take medications that interfere with body temperature regulation, have underlying health conditions, live alone, or are socially isolated (Flynn et al., 2005; Luber & McGeehin, 2008).

7.4 Adapting to Climate Change and Mitigating Its Health Risks

7.4.1 Urgency to Mitigate Climate Change and Its Health Risks

The World Health Organization (WHO) reported that around 3.6 billion people worldwide inhabit areas that are particularly vulnerable to climate change (World Health Organization, 2023). Without serious intervention, climate change is projected to contribute to an additional 250,000 annual mortality from malnutrition, malaria, diarrhea, and heat-related stress (World Health Organization, 2023). Given its wide-ranging impacts, there is an urgent need to develop adaptive measures to mitigate the worst consequences of climate change, especially for vulnerable groups (Kinney et al., 2023).

Climate change mitigation involves measures implemented by governments, the private sector, and individuals to decrease greenhouse gas emissions and increase carbon sinks through ecosystems (United Nations Development Programme, 2024). Conversely, adaptation aims at enhancing resilience against the health effects of climate change, addressing both existing and anticipated obstacles. These strategies may consist of behavioral changes, infrastructure improvements, and technological innovations (Kinney et al., 2023). Climate change mitigation can further create opportunities to improve global health by reducing disease burdens, enhancing community resilience, alleviating poverty, and narrowing global inequalities (Tong et al., 2016). Intervention can be implemented at multiple scales; however, local-level strategies are particularly important because climate exposures, vulnerabilities, and health impacts are usually location-specific. Adaptation must also take into consideration the vulnerable populations, comprising of children, the elderly, people with comorbidities, and people with limited economic capacity (Kinney et al., 2023). Effective planning also relies on continuously updating knowledge about climate-related health risks, projecting future impacts, and ensuring policymakers have access to accurate evidence to design appropriate and evidence-based interventions (Tong et al., 2016).

7.4.2 *Strategies to Mitigate Climate Change and Its Health Risks*

7.4.2.1 Strengthening Climate-Adaptive Health Surveillance Systems

Over time, health risks due to climate change are projected to continue increasing, and no country is exempt from this threat (Tong et al., 2016). To anticipate this, public health systems need to adopt climate-adaptive disease surveillance, which can predict and manage outbreaks more effectively. This surveillance should integrate climate data, prevention measures, vector control programs, and public education on preventing infectious diseases influenced by climate change (Walimah et al., 2024). Furthermore, surveillance is fundamental in monitoring, evaluating, and improving adaptation policies implemented at the local, regional, and national levels (Toloo et al., 2014).

7.4.2.2 Strengthening Health Infrastructure and Facilities

Climate change is projected to increase the frequency, severity, duration, and spatial extent of extreme weather events, including tropical storms, heat waves, floods, wildfires, and droughts worldwide (Tong et al., 2016). Therefore, building climate-adaptive health systems is essential to prepare for emergencies (Tong et al., 2016). This includes developing climate-resilient healthcare facilities, such as ambulances, hospitals, emergency units, and community health centers (Walimah et al., 2024). Moreover, support for mental health should be incorporated into emergency response and disaster recovery systems (Tong & Ebi, 2019).

7.4.2.3 Developing Climate Change Early Warning Systems

Addressing climate change threats requires holistic approaches that integrate technology with health systems (Walimah et al., 2024). One current strategy is the development of early warning systems that integrate climate data with technological innovations (Tong et al., 2016). Such systems enable faster responses and more efficient resource allocation, using real-time data and predictive models to strengthen public health resilience. Examples include alerts for heat waves, floods, or air pollution (Tong et al., 2016). During periods of poor air quality, alerts can advise the public to limit outdoor activity or wear masks to reduce exposure to air pollutants (Kinney et al., 2023). They can also provide facilities like cooling centers to reduce heat stress risks. Such systems must be cost-effective, easy to maintain, and adapted to local needs and resources (Kinney et al., 2023).

7.4.2.4 Promoting Sustainable Climate Change Education

Public education on climate threats and their health impacts is essential to reduce risks through behavior change (Tong & Ebi, 2019). Communities can learn practical measures, such as staying hydrated, limiting outdoor activities, and using fans, air conditioning, or water sprays to prevent heat stress (Kinney et al., 2023). Education should also promote the use of protective masks against air pollutants (Kinney et al., 2023). Furthermore, the public should be informed about vulnerable groups, such as the older adults, children, women during pregnancy, and individuals with cardiovascular or respiratory diseases, along with strategies to strengthen their resilience (Tong & Ebi, 2019).

7.4.2.5 Developing Climate-Resilient Infrastructure

Amid the increasing climate change effects, cities around the world are acknowledging the necessity of adapting their infrastructure to protect public health (Walimah et al., 2024). Urban infrastructure must be resilient to climate pressures at all spatial scales. Infrastructure resilient to climate change must be planned, designed, constructed, and managed to predict, get ready for, and react to evolving climate conditions, which requires careful long-term planning. For example, housing standards should withstand extreme temperatures through thermal insulation or cooling systems (Tong & Ebi, 2019). Infrastructure planning should also protect biodiversity, preserve ecological continuity, and consider advantages for human and environmental health. Nature-based options, such as reforestation, expanding floodplains, protecting wetlands, and incorporating urban green spaces and permeable pavements, reduce flood risks while improving environmental quality. Importantly, adaptation planning must address equity to ensure vulnerable groups are not further marginalized (Kinney et al., 2023).

7.4.2.6 Strengthening Research and Technological Innovations

The rising burden of morbidity and mortality from climate change requires in-depth research on its health consequences to develop public health measures relevant to different patterns of extreme climate (Tong et al., 2016). Studies linking climate change and infectious disease transmission, including identification of vulnerable groups, must be strengthened as part of risk assessment and management planning (Tong et al., 2016). The work of epidemiologists is vital for developing and improving research and monitoring schemes to evaluate the magnitude and urgency of climate threats and to guide actions at local to global levels. Furthermore, research on vaccine development for climate-sensitive diseases, such as Zika virus, is essential to reduce public health burdens (Paz & Semenza, 2016; Tong et al., 2016). Such research must be interdisciplinary, policy-oriented, and involve policymakers throughout to ensure findings directly support decision-making (Tong et al., 2016).

7.4.2.7 Reforming Climate Change Policies at Multiple Levels

Mitigating climate change requires strong, evidence-based policies that guide interventions (Tong et al., 2016). Policies should prioritize evidence-based science over political will. Developing effective public health policies is important for dealing with the impacts of climate change (Tong et al., 2016). Collaboration between scientists and policymakers is essential for creating public policies that address climate change impacts, not only for current but also for future generations (Tong et al., 2016). For example, the Paris Agreement exemplifies global efforts to reduce emissions while also protecting vulnerable populations from climate-related health risks (Walimah et al., 2024). These policies ensure that health and climate risks are addressed in an integrated manner. Policy reform is key to ensuring a coherent approach between health and climate that includes community engagement (Walimah et al., 2024).

7.4.2.8 Strengthening Cross-Sectoral Collaboration

The impacts of climate change transcend borders, making cross-sectoral collaboration crucial in developing public health strategies. Climate change mitigation is a shared responsibility among governments, the private sector, health systems, and local communities. Individuals can contribute through sustainable lifestyles and advocacy for change. Governments play a central role in formulating regulations and facilitating interventions, while the private sector can drive innovation in responding to climate change (United Nations Development Programme, 2024). Such collaboration allows the exchange of resources, knowledge, and technology to improve the adaptive capacity of the health system against extreme weather, rising temperatures, and other climate risks (Walimah et al., 2024).

7.4.3 Case Study in Asia

7.4.3.1 Saudi Arabia

Saudi Arabia faces climate change challenges due to high CO_2 emissions, which heighten the risk of infectious diseases (Al Khatib et al., 2025). To address this, the government emphasizes adaptation and mitigation through public awareness campaigns, involving healthcare workers and health promotion specialists. The campaigns focus on disseminating information about the importance of green spaces as natural CO2 absorbers and encouraging community participation in addressing climate-related health impacts (Al Khatib et al., 2025).

7.4.3.2 Lebanon

In Lebanon, climate change has driven increases in food-borne and vector-borne diseases. One of the strategies adopted is the utilization of hydropower as a major energy source to reduce emissions from fossil fuel combustion, which aggravates the climate emergency. Currently, five hydropower plants operate across Lebanon, particularly in the western mountain region. Moreover, the adoption of solar energy is also expanding in the country (Al Khatib et al., 2025).

7.4.3.3 India

India has integrated the climate change issue by developing the National Action Plan on Climate Change and Human Health (NAPCCHH) (Kaladharan et al., 2025). The government supports states in preparing action plans in collaboration with local stakeholders. This decentralization enables interventions to target local health risks while empowering local actors and communities in climate and health adaptation decisions (Asia Pacific Malaria Elimination Network, 2025).

In Kerala, one of the states with the highest level of decentralization, the State Action Plan on Climate Change and Human Health (SAPCCHH) was developed to build climate-resilient healthcare services via decentralized primary care that enables timely decision-making, as well as the establishment of community groups, such as *Jagaratha Samithi* (Vigilance committees), to ensure grassroots participation (Kaladharan et al., 2025). In Odisha, a cross-sectoral task force coordinates the meteorology, health, and environment sectors using an early warning system with machine learning to predict dengue outbreaks and enable timely interventions (Asia Pacific Malaria Elimination Network, 2025). Additionally, in Bhor, Maharashtra, a participatory community-based project involves local healthcare workers in identifying risks and interventions (Asia Pacific Malaria Elimination Network, 2025).

7.4.3.4 Japan

Over 90% of Japan's population lives in urban areas, making them highly vulnerable to extreme heat. In response, the government enacted the Climate Change Adaptation Act in December 2018, which outlines the climate-related health risks and adaptation measures. One initiative is the Action Plan for Heatstroke Prevention, which focuses on protecting the elderly and strengthening collaboration with local communities and industries. The Japan Meteorological Agency has also introduced the Heat Stroke Alert, when daily temperatures are forecasted to reach or surpass 35 °C, to encourage public preparedness. The National Institute for Environmental Studies (NIES) developed the Climate Change Adaptation Information Platform (A-PLAT) to disseminate government and private sector interventions. Locally, Yokohama distributes Heatstroke Prevention Notification Postcards in collaboration with post offices and fire departments to raise awareness about heatstroke (Kim et al., 2023). In Saitama prefecture, the Cool Oasis Campaign provides around 9000 cooling shelters in multiple locations, comprising minimarkets, pharmacies, mailing centers, and car outlets (Kim et al., 2023). Beyond extreme heat, the government also enhances adaptation to infectious diseases through outbreak monitoring, vector-borne disease prevention, and infection risk surveillance related to climate change (Health and Global Policy Institute, 2024).

7.4.3.5 Thailand

Thailand faces significant challenges from global warming, worsened by rising air pollution. Since 2019, PM2.5 levels have steadily increased, and in 2023, over 10 million people suffered from pollution-related lung diseases (Macnab, 2025). In response, the Ministry of Health developed a climate change adaptation roadmap emphasizing cross-sector collaboration and a stronger healthcare system. One of the initiatives is the GREEN and CLEAN Hospital program to improve waste management and promote renewable energy in healthcare facilities (Asia Pacific Malaria Elimination Network, 2025; Macnab, 2025). In collaboration with the WHO, the Ministry also introduced the Smart Energy and Climate Action (SECA) policy to lower greenhouse gas emissions through the expansion of solar power utilization and the enhancement of energy efficiency (Asia Pacific Malaria Elimination Network, 2025).

7.4.3.6 Bangladesh

The government of Bangladesh has developed Health National Adaptation Plans (HNAPs) to prioritize actions addressing climate-related health risks to strengthen responses that are more coordinated, resilient, and inclusive (United Nations Development Programme, 2025). One strategy is the introduction of new national standards for WASH (Water, Sanitation, and Hygiene) in healthcare centers and training health workers, from village nurses to officials at the central ministry on climate and health-related topics. Bangladesh also formulated climate and health curricula for health educators to support capacity building for health professionals. A climate-adapted disease surveillance system, based on WHO's Early Warning, Alert, and Response System (EWARS), was also piloted in Bangladesh. The program was implemented across 10 sentinel hospitals (designated hospitals that monitor key disease trends), focusing on dengue, cholera, diarrhea, and rotavirus (United Nations Development Programme, 2025). EWARS combines climate information, such as temperature, precipitation, and sea surface temperature, utilizing real-time monitoring to forecast and prepare for outbreaks. During the 2023 dengue outbreak, EWARS enabled authorities to track disease trends both spatially and temporally, allowing for more targeted response measures (Asia Pacific Malaria Elimination Network, 2025).

7.4.3.7 Singapore

To tackle heatwaves, Singapore launched the Cooling Singapore Project in 2017. This initiative explores potential measures to cool urban areas, including greening, city geometry design, the use of water elements, material and surface selection, shading structures, and transport and energy strategies (Aik et al., 2023). The Ministry of Sustainability and the Environment released the Heat Stress Advisory Framework, using the Wet Bulb Globe Temperature (WBGT) index to guide public actions during extreme heat. In 2023, the National University of Singapore (NUS), in collaboration with the Ministry of Manpower (MOM) and the Singapore Armed Forces (SAF), established the Heat Resilience and Performance Center to integrate laboratory and field research to strengthen adaptability to rising temperatures (Aik et al., 2023).

Another initiative, Project Heat Safe, was designed to understand climate-related health risks and identify sustainable preventive policies. Adaptation measures, including regulation, education, workplace safety, and training, have reduced cases of heat-related injuries from approximately 200 cases annually in the 1990s to 20 cases annually in the 2000s, despite rising ambient temperatures (Aik et al., 2023). Beyond heat resilience, Singapore developed an early warning system integrating disease data, meteorology, and vector surveillance to predict dengue outbreaks. First applied in 2013, the system effectively enhanced outbreak preparedness and response. Healthcare professionals have also contributed to sustainability initiatives by implementing recycling programs for single-use medical items, including IV fluid bags, oxygen tubing, and oxygen masks (Zain et al., 2024).

7.4.3.8 Taiwan

Taiwan is experiencing increasingly frequent extreme weather events and an ongoing rise in sea levels due to global warming. Over the past two years, average temperatures have been the highest in the last century, leading to water shortages, economic losses, threats to community well-being, and reduced hydropower capacity (Ministry of Foreign Affairs Republic of China (Taiwan), 2018). A 1 °C rise in average temperature is reported to elevate the likelihood of heat illness by up to 71% (Yang et al., 2024). In response, Taiwan has developed climate policies to reduce carbon emissions (Yang et al., 2024). In August 2018, the Air Pollution Control Act was revised to curb air pollution and enhance energy transition by restricting transportation and industry emissions, improving air quality, and strengthening pollution source management (Ministry of Foreign Affairs Republic of China (Taiwan), 2018). In 2023, the Climate Change Response Act required every ministry and local authority to examine climate impacts and enhance the adaptive capacity of vulnerable groups (Yang et al., 2024). Taiwan is also shifting to energy-efficient technologies and clean energy to reduce respiratory diseases caused by air pollution (Amnuaylojaroen & Parasin, 2024). Additionally, the country developed a synchronous epidemiological monitoring and early warning system to track heat-related diseases (Yang et al., 2024).

7.5 Conclusion

The increasingly unpredictable nature of climate change has made it a major threat to global health in this century. One of its clearest manifestations is the escalating frequency and severity of extreme weather conditions, including heatwaves, heavy precipitation and floods, tropical cyclones and typhoons, droughts, as well as air pollution and haze. These events have immediate consequences on human health by increasing the risk of heatstroke, cardiovascular diseases, infectious diseases, and respiratory disorders. Beyond its immediate effects, climate change also presents indirect risks to human health. Altered weather patterns can accelerate disease transmission, worsen food and water shortage, increase the prevalence of mental health disorders, and trigger social disruption and population displacement. The growing frequency of natural disasters also threatens the integrity of health infrastructure, which can hinder the delivery of primary health services. While the entire population experiences the consequences of climate change, certain groups remain disproportionately vulnerable, including children, the elderly, low-income populations, geographically vulnerable areas, people with chronic illnesses, and outdoor workers.

The impacts of climate change extend beyond the health sector, creating a domino effect across environmental, social, and economic systems. Although all countries face similar threats, the degree of impact varies depending on the capacity of public health systems to respond. Countries including the Philippines, Japan, and China frequently experience typhoons and tropical cyclones. During dry seasons, large-scale wildfires in Indonesia often cause transboundary haze affecting neighboring countries such as Malaysia, Singapore, and Brunei. Meanwhile, Thailand and Cambodia face recurring droughts, while Indonesia and Japan often report severe flooding. These patterns highlight the critical need to strengthen both adaptation and mitigation actions across the region.

Adaptation and mitigation efforts aim to safeguard global health by reducing disease burdens, enhancing community resilience, alleviating poverty, and narrowing global inequalities. A range of strategies can be implemented, including strengthening climate-adaptive health surveillance systems, improving health infrastructure and facilities, developing early warning systems, promoting climate education and public awareness, advancing research and technological innovation, reforming climate policies at multiple levels, and reinforcing cross-sectoral collaboration. Saudi Arabia has promoted public awareness campaigns involving health promotion specialists. Lebanon has invested in hydropower development as a major energy source to reduce emissions from fossil fuel combustion. Japan has launched the *Heat Stroke Alert* system to enhance public preparedness during periods of extreme heat. Singapore has established the *Heat Resilience and Performance*

Center to integrate laboratory and field research in adaptation to rising temperatures. Similarly, the Taiwanese government continues to develop national climate policies focused on reducing carbon emissions.

Competing Interests The author(s) has no competing interests to declare that are relevant to the content of this manuscript.

References

Agache, I., Sampath, V., Aguilera, J., Akdis, C. A., Akdis, M., Barry, M., Bouagnon, A., Chinthrajah, S., Collins, W., Dulitzki, C., Erny, B., Gomez, J., Goshua, A., Jutel, M., Kizer, K. W., Kline, O., LaBeaud, A. D., Pali-Schöll, I., Perrett, K. P., et al. (2022). Climate change and global health: A call to more research and more action. *Allergy: European Journal of Allergy and Clinical Immunology, 77*(5), 1389–1407. https://doi.org/10.1111/all.15229. John Wiley and Sons Inc.

Aik, J., et al. (2023). Climate change and population health in Singapore: A systematic review. *The Lancet Regional Health—Western Pacific, 40*(100947), 1–11. https://doi.org/10.1016/j.lanwpc.2023.100947

Al Khatib, A., et al. (2025). Mitigating climate change impacts on health: A comparative analysis of strategies in Saudi Arabia and Lebanon. *Frontiers in Public Health, 13*(1551559). https://doi.org/10.3389/fpubh.2025.1551559

Amnuaylojaroen, T., & Parasin, N. (2024). Human health adaptation strategies to climate induced extreme weather events: A systematic review. *Earth, 5*, 724–742. https://doi.org/10.3390/earth5040038

Amondo, E. I., Nshakira-Rukundo, E., & Mirzabaev, A. (2023). The effect of extreme weather events on child nutrition and health. *Food Security, 15*, 571–596.

Artigas, P., Reguera-Gomez, M., Valero, M. A., Osca, D., da Silva Pacheco, R., Rosa-Freitas, M. G., Fernandes Silva-do-Nascimento, T., Paredes-Esquivel, C., Lucientes, J., & Mas-Coma, S. (2021). Aedes albopictus diversity and relationships in south-western Europe and Brazil by rDNA/mtDNA and phenotypic analyses: ITS-2, a useful marker for spread studies. *Parasites & Vectors, 14*(1), 333.

Asia Pacific Malaria Elimination Network. (2025). *Adapting strategies to mitigate the impact of climate and environmental changes on vector-borne diseases in the Asia-Pacific region*.

Bain, R., Cronk, R., Hossain, R., Bonjour, S., Onda, K., Wright, J., Yang, H., Slaymaker, T., Hunter, P., & Prüss-Ustün, A. (2014). Global assessment of exposure to faecal contamination through drinking water based on a systematic review. *Tropical Medicine & International Health, 19*(8), 917–927.

Balta, I., Lemon, J., Murane, C., Pet, I., Vintila, T., McCcleery, D., Callaway, T., Douglas, A., Stef, L., & Corcionivoschi, N. (2024). The One Health aspect of climate events with impact on foodborne pathogens transmission. *One Health, 19*, 100926.

Bartholdson, S., & Von Schreeb, J. (2018). Natural disasters and injuries: What does a surgeon need to know? *Current Trauma Reports, 4*, 103–108.

Baxter, L., McGowan, C. R., Smiley, S., Palacios, L., Devine, C., & Casademont, C. (2022). The relationship between climate change, health, and the humanitarian response. *The Lancet, 400*(10363), 1561–1563. https://doi.org/10.1016/S0140-6736(22)01991-2. Elsevier B.V.

Bean, H., Takenouchi, K., & Cruz, A. M. (2025). Mobile public warning in Japan and the United States: A sister cities collaboration. *Frontiers in Communication, 10*, 1518729.

Bell, J. E., Brown, C. L., Conlon, K., Herring, S., Kunkel, K. E., Lawrimore, J., Luber, G., Schreck, C., Smith, A., & Uejio, C. (2018). Changes in extreme events and the potential impacts on human health. *Journal of the Air & Waste Management Association, 68*, 265–287.

Bennett, N. J., Dearden, P., & Peredo, A. M. (2015). Vulnerability to multiple stressors in coastal communities: A study of the Andaman coast of Thailand. *Climate and Development, 7*(2), 124–141. https://doi.org/10.1080/17565529.2014.886993

Berry, H. L., Waite, T. D., Dear, K. B. G., Capon, A. G., & Murray, V. (2018). The case for systems thinking about climate change and mental health. *Nature Climate Change, 8*(4), 282–290.

Bidhuri, S., Taqi, M., & Khan, M. M. A. (2018). Water-borne disease: Link between human health and water use in the Mithepur and Jaitpur area of the NCT of Delhi. *Journal of Public Health, 26*(1), 119–126.

Buttke, D. E., Raynor, B., & Schuurman, G. W. (2023). Predicting climate-change induced heatrelated illness risk in Grand Canyon National Park visitors. *PLoS ONE, 18*(8 August). https://doi.org/10.1371/journal.pone.0288812

Calvin, K., Dasgupta, D., Krinner, G., Mukherji, A., Thorne, P. W., Trisos, C., Romero, J., Aldunce, P., Barret, K., Blanco, G., Cheung, W. W. L., Connors, S. L., Denton, F., Diongue-Niang, A., Dodman, D., Garschagen, M., Geden, O., Hayward, B., Jones, C., et al. (2023). *IPCC, 2023: Climate change 2023: synthesis report, summary for policymakers.* Contribution of Working Groups I, II and III to the Sixth Assessment Report of the Intergovernmental Panel on Climate Change [Core Writing Team, H. Lee and J. Romero (Eds.)]. IPCC. https://doi.org/10.59327/IPCC/AR6-9789291691647.001

Camargo, S. J., Murakami, H., Bloemendaal, N., Chand, S. S., Deshpande, M. S., Dominguez-Sarmiento, C., Gonzales-Aleman, J. J., Knutson, T. R., Lin, I.-I., & Moon, I.-J. (2023). An update on the influence of natural climate variability and anthropogenic climate change on tropical cyclones. *Tropical Cyclone Research and Review, 12*, 216–239.

Campbell-Lendrum, D., Neville, T., Schweizer, C., & Neira, M. (2023). Climate change and health: Three grand challenges. *Nature Medicine*, *29*(7), 1631–1638). https://doi.org/10.1038/s41591-023-02438-w. Nature Research.

Cann, K., Thomas, D. R., Salmon, R., Wyn-Jones, A., & Kay, D. (2013). Extreme water-related weather events and waterborne disease. *Epidemiology and Infection, 141*(4), 671–686.

Cao, A., Nakamura, S., Otsuyama, K., Namba, M., & Yoshimura, K. (2024). Current status and challenges in operating flood early warning systems at the local level in Japan. *International Journal of Disaster Risk Reduction, 112*, 104802.

Carnes, B. A., Staats, D., & Willcox, B. J. (2014). Impact of climate change on elder health. *The Journals of Gerontology. Series A, Biological Sciences and Medical Sciences, 69*(9), 1087–1091.

Chan, E. Y., Lam, H. C., So, S. H., Goggins, W. B., III, Ho, J. Y., Liu, S., & Chung, P. P. (2018). Association between ambient temperatures and mental disorder hospitalizations in a subtropical city: A time-series study of Hong Kong special administrative region. *International Journal of Environmental Research and Public Health, 15*.

Chang, K., Hirsch, J. A., Clay, L., & Michael, Y. L. (2025). Healthcare access in the aftermath: A longitudinal analysis of disaster impact on US communities. *International Journal of Environmental Research and Public Health, 22*, 733.

Cheesbrough, M. (2005). *District laboratory practice in tropical countries, part 2.* Cambridge University Press.

Cheng, J., Xu, Z., Bambrick, H., Prescott, V., Wang, N., Zhang, Y., Su, H., Tong, S., & Hu, W. (2019). Cardiorespiratory effects of heatwaves: A systematic review and meta-analysis of global epidemiological evidence. *Environmental Research, 177*, 108610.

Cheng, J., Bambrick, H., Yakob, L., Devine, G., Frentiu, F. D., Toan, D. T. T., Thai, P. Q., Xu, Z., & Hu, W. (2020). Heatwaves and dengue outbreaks in Hanoi, Vietnam: New evidence on early warning. *PLoS Neglected Tropical Diseases, 14*(1), e0007997.

Choy, Y. K., & Onuma, A. (2025). The tropical peatlands in Indonesia and global environmental change: A multi-dimensional system-based analysis and policy implications. *Regional Science and Environmental Economics, 2*, 17.

Conzatti, A., Kershaw, T., Copping, A., & Coley, D. (2022). A review of the impact of shelter design on the health of displaced populations. *Journal of International Humanitarian Action, 7*, 18.

Costello, A., Abbas, M., Allen, A., Ball, S., Bell, S., Bellamy, R., Friel, S., Groce, N., Johnson, A., Kett, M., Lee, M., Levy, C., Maslin, M., Mccoy, D., Mcguire, B., Montgomery, H., Napier, D., Pagel, C., Patel, J., et al. (2009). The Lancet Commissions Executive summary. *www.thelancet.com, 373*. www.thelancet.com

Crane, K., Li, L., Subramanian, P., Rovit, E., & Liu, J. (2022). Climate change and mental health: a review of empirical evidence, mechanisms and implications. *Atmosphere, 13*, 2096.

D'ippoliti, D., Michelozzi, P., Marino, C., De'donato, F., Menne, B., Katsouyanni, K., Kirchmayer, U., Analitis, A., Medina-Ramon, M., & Paldy, A. (2010). The impact of heat waves on mortality in 9 European cities: Results from the EuroHEAT project. *Environmental Health, 9*, 37.

Davies-Barnard, T., Catto, J. L., Harper, A. B., Imron, M. A., & Van Veen, F. F. (2023). Future fire risk under climate change and deforestation scenarios in tropical Borneo. *Environmental Research Letters, 18*, 024015.

Dianati Tilaki, R. A., Zazouli, M. A., & Ala, A. R. (2021). Climate change and its consequences on human health: A review study. *Journal of Advances in Environmental Health Research, 9*(1), 1–6. https://doi.org/10.32598/JAEHR.9.1.1188. Kurdistan University of Medical Sciences.

Elmarakby, E., & Elkadi, H. (2024). Prioritising urban heat island mitigation interventions: Mapping a heat risk index. *Science of the Total Environment, 948*, 174927.

Elsner, M. M., Cuo, L., Voisin, N., Deems, J. S., Hamlet, A. F., Vano, J. A., Mickelson, K. E., Lee, S.-Y., & Lettenmaier, D. P. (2010). Implications of 21st century climate change for the hydrology of Washington State. *Climatic Change, 102*, 225–260.

EPA. (2025). *Urbanization—Temperature* [Online].

Ewing, D. A., Purse, B. V., Cobbold, C. A., & White, S. M. (2021). A novel approach for predicting risk of vector-borne disease establishment in marginal temperate environments under climate change: West Nile virus in the UK. *Journal of the Royal Society Interface, 18*(178), 20210049.

Feng, B., Zhang, Y., & Bourke, R. (2021). Urbanization impacts on flood risks based on urban growth data and coupled flood models. *Natural Hazards, 106*, 613–627.

Fitriany, A. A., Flatau, P. J., Khoirunurrofik, K., & Riama, N. F. (2021). Assessment on the use of meteorological and social media information for forest fire detection and prediction in Riau, Indonesia. *Sustainability, 13*.

Flynn, A., McGreevy, C., & Mulkerrin, E. (2005). Why do older patients die in a heatwave? *QJM, 98*(3), 227–229.

Fudeyasu, H., Hirose, S., Yoshioka, H., Kumazawa, R., & Yamasaki, S. (2014). A global view of the landfall characteristics of tropical cyclones. *Tropical Cyclone Research and Review, 3*, 178–192.

Gao, H., Wang, L., Ma, J., Gao, X., Xiao, J., & Wang, H. (2021). Modeling the current distribution suitability and future dynamics of Culicoides imicola under climate change scenarios. *PeerJ, 9e12308*.

Goldman, A., Eggen, B., Golding, B., & Murray, V. (2014). The health impacts of windstorms: A systematic literature review. *Public Health, 128*, 3–28.

Green, T. R. (2016). Linking climate change and groundwater. In *Integrated groundwater management: Concepts, approaches and challenges*. Springer.

Greene, S., Kalkstein, L. S., Mills, D. M., & Samenow, J. (2011). An examination of climate change on extreme heat events and climate–mortality relationships in large US cities. *Weather, Climate, and Society, 3*(4).

Greve, P., Orlowsky, B., Mueller, B., Sheffield, J., Reichstein, M., & Seneviratne, S. I. (2014). Global assessment of trends in wetting and drying over land. *Nature Geoscience, 7*, 716–721.

Ha, T. V., Huth, J., Bachofer, F., & Kuenzer, C. (2022). A review of earth observation-based drought studies in Southeast Asia. *Remote Sensing, 14*, 3763.

Hausfather, Z., Drake, H. F., Abbott, T., & Schmidt, G. A. (2020). Evaluating the performance of past climate model projections. *Geophysical Research Letters, 47*, e2019GL085378.

Hawkins, E., Gostigian, G., & Diurba, S. (2024). Lightning strike injuries. *Emergency Medicine Clinics, 42*.

Hayasaka, H., & Usup, A. (2023). Air pollution caused by peatland fires in Central Kalimantan. In *Vegetation fires and pollution in Asia*. Springer.

Health and Global Policy Institute. (2024). *Developing a national health and climate strategy for Japan: Recommendations for building a climate resilient, decarbonized health system.*

Hepatology, T. L. G. (2022). Water and sanitation for all.

Hime, N., Vyas, A., Lachireddy, K., Wyett, S., Scalley, B., & Corvalan, C. (2018). Climate change, health and wellbeing: Challenges and opportunities in NSW, Australia. In *Public health research and practice* (Vol. 28, Issue 4). Sax Institute. https://doi.org/10.17061/phrp2841824

Hirani, S. A. A. (2024). Barriers to women's menstrual hygiene practices during recurrent disasters and displacement: A qualitative study. *International Journal of Environmental Research and Public Health, 21*.

Hugelius, K., Gifford, M., Örtenwall, P., & Adolfsson, A. (2017). Health among disaster survivors and health professionals after the Haiyan Typhoon: A self-selected Internet-based web survey. *International Journal of Emergency Medicine, 10*, 13.

Ignacio, J. A. F. (2025). Mapping and assessing high-resolution typhoon exposure and vulnerability in the Philippines: A scoping review. *Journal of Management for Global Sustainability, 12*, 8.

Jones, P. B. (2013). Adult mental health disorders and their age at onset. *The British Journal of Psychiatry, 202*(s54), s5–s10.

Kaladharan, S., et al. (2025). Mitigating human health impacts of climate change: A case of Kerala state in India. *Global Transitions, 7*, 383–386. https://doi.org/10.1016/j.glt.2025.06.006

Kendrovski, V., & Gjorgjev, D. (2012). Climate change: Implication for food-borne diseases (Salmonella and food poisoning among humans in R. Macedonia). *Structure and Function of Food Engineering*.

Kennedy, I. T., Petley, D. N., Williams, R., & Murray, V. (2015). A systematic review of the health impacts of mass earth movements (landslides). *PLoS Currents, 7*, ecurrents. dis. 1d49e84c8bbe678b0e70cf7fc35d0b77.

Khan, M. D., Thi Vu, H. H., Lai, Q. T., & Ahn, J. W. (2019). Aggravation of human diseases and climate change nexus. *International Journal of Environmental Research and Public Health, 16*(15), 2799.

Kim, K. H., Kabir, E., & Ara Jahan, S. (2014). A review of the consequences of global climate change on human health. *Journal of Environmental Science and Health—Part C Environmental Carcinogenesis and Ecotoxicology Reviews, 32*(3), 299–318. https://doi.org/10.1080/10590501.2014.941279

Kim, J.-B., So, J.-M., & Bae, D.-H. (2020). Global warming impacts on severe drought characteristics in Asia monsoon region. *Water, 12*, 1360.

Kim, Y., et al. (2023). Enhancing health resilience in Japan in a changing climate. *The Lancet Regional Health—Western Pacific, 40*(100970), 1–17. https://doi.org/10.1016/j.lanwpc.2023.100970

Kinney, P. L., et al. (2023). Health-based strategies for overcoming barriers to climate change adaptation and mitigation. *The Journal of Allergy and Clinical Immunology, 152*(5), 1053–1059. https://doi.org/10.1016/j.jaci.2023.09.012

Kjellstrom, T. (2009). Climate change, direct heat exposure, health and well-being in low and middle-income countries. *Global Health Action, 2*(1). https://doi.org/10.3402/gha.v2i0.1958

Kjellstrom, T., & McMichael, A. J. (2013). Climate change threats to population health and well-being: The imperative of protective solutions that will last. *Global Health Action, 6*(1). https://doi.org/10.3402/gha.v6i0.20816

Krishna Prabhakar, S. V. R. (2022). Implications of regional droughts and transboundary drought risks on drought monitoring and early warning: A review. *Climate, 10*, 124.

Lin, H.-I., Yu, Y.-Y., Wen, F.-I., & Liu, P.-T. (2022). Status of food security in East and Southeast Asia and challenges of climate change. *Climate, 10*, 40.

Lloyd, S., Gray, J., Healey, S., & Opdyke, A. (2022). Social vulnerability to natural hazards in the Philippines. *International Journal of Disaster Risk Reduction, 79*, 103103.

Lowe, D., Ebi, K. L., & Forsberg, B. (2013). Factors increasing vulnerability to health effects before, during and after floods. *International Journal of Environmental Research and Public Health, 10*, 7015–7067.

Luber, G., & McGeehin, M. (2008). Climate change and extreme heat events. *American Journal of Preventive Medicine, 35*(5), 429–435.

Macnab, A. J. (2025). Climate change: The urgent need for global health strategies to counter adverse impacts on human health. *Global Health Management Journal, 8*(1), 39–42. https://doi.org/10.35898/ghmj-811205

Malhotra, N. (2024). Climate change and health-a global perspective. *International Journal of Research and Analytical Reviews, 766*. www.ijrar.org

McDermott-Levy, R., Scolio, M., Shakya, K. M., & Moore, C. H. (2021). Factors that influence climate change-related mortality in the United States: An integrative review. *International Journal of Environmental Research and Public Health, 18*(15), 8220.

McMichael, A. J. (2003). *Climate change and human health: Risks and responses*. World Health Organization.

McMichael, A. J., & Lindgren, E. (2011). Climate change: Present and future risks to health, and necessary responses. *Journal of Internal Medicine, 270*(5), 401–413. https://doi.org/10.1111/j.1365-2796.2011.02415.x

Ministry of Foreign Affairs Republic of China (Taiwan). (2018). *Combating climate change-Taiwan can help, Ministry of Foreign Affairs Republic of China (Taiwan)*. Available at: https://en.mofa.gov.tw/News_Content.aspx?n=1575&s=34810. Accessed 18 Aug 2025.

Mkorombindo, T., & Balkissoon, R. (2021). Journal club: Respiratory impact of wildfire smoke. *Chronic Obstructive Pulmonary Diseases: Journal of the COPD Foundation, 8*, 408.

Morales, F., Montserrat-De La Paz, S., Leon, M. J., & Rivero-Pino, F. (2023). Effects of malnutrition on the immune system and infection and the role of nutritional strategies regarding improvements in children's health status: A literature review. *Nutrients, 16*, 1.

Murphy, H., Pintar, K., McBean, E., & Thomas, M. (2014). A systematic review of waterborne disease burden methodologies from developed countries. *Journal of Water and Health, 12*(4), 634–655.

Noviarini, D., Delina, M., & Yamani, A. (2024). The development of early warning system for fire catcher in rain forest of Sumatera. In *AI in business: Opportunities and limitations: Volume 2*. Springer.

Nunes, L. J. (2023). The rising threat of atmospheric CO_2: A review on the causes, impacts, and mitigation strategies. *Environments, 10*, 66.

Olsson, J., Arheimer, B., Borris, M., Donnelly, C., Foster, K., Nikulin, G., Persson, M., Perttu, A.-M., Uvo, C. B., & Viklander, M. (2016). Hydrological climate change impact assessment at small and large scales: Key messages from recent progress in Sweden. *Climate, 4*, 39.

Organization, W. H. (2005). *Guidelines for laboratory and field testing of mosquito larvicides*.

Ostfeld, R. S., & Brunner, J. L. (2015). Climate change and Ixodes tick-borne diseases of humans. *Philosophical Transactions of the Royal Society, B: Biological Sciences, 370*(1665), 20140051.

Paravantis, J., Santamouris, M., Cartalis, C., Efthymiou, C., & Kontoulis, N. (2017). Mortality associated with high ambient temperatures, heatwaves, and the urban heat island in Athens, Greece. *Sustainability, 9*, 606.

Parums, D. V. (2024). A review of the increasing global impact of climate change on human health and approaches to medical preparedness. In *Medical science monitor* (Vol. 30). International Scientific Information, Inc. https://doi.org/10.12659/MSM.945763

Paterson, D. L., Wright, H., & Harris, P. N. (2018). Health risks of flood disasters. *Clinical Infectious Diseases, 67*, 1450–1454.

Patz, J. A., Frumkin, H., Holloway, T., Vimont, D. J., & Haines, A. (2014). Climate change: Challenges and opportunities for global health. *JAMA : The Journal of the American Medical Association, 312*(15), 1565–1580. https://doi.org/10.1001/jama.2014.13186

Paz, S., & Semenza, J. C. (2016). El Niño and climate change—contributing factors in the dispersal of Zika virus in the Americas? *Lancet, 387*. https://doi.org/10.1016/S0140-6736(16)00256-7

Petrucci, O. (2022). Landslide fatality occurrence: A systematic review of research published between January 2010 and March 2022. *Sustainability, 14*, 9346.

Phan-Van, T., Nguyen-Ngoc-Bich, P., Ngo-Duc, T., Vu-Minh, T., Le, P. V., Trinh-Tuan, L., Nguyen-Thi, T., Pham-Thanh, H., & Tran-Quang, D. (2022). Drought over Southeast Asia and its association with large-scale drivers. *Journal of Climate, 35*, 4959–4978.

Pollock, W., & Wartman, J. (2020). Human vulnerability to landslides. *GeoHealth, 4*, e2020GH000287.

Poursafa, P., & Kelishadi, R. (2011). What health professionals should know about the health effects of air pollution and climate change on children and pregnant mothers. *Iranian Journal of Nursing and Midwifery Research, 16*(3), 257.

Rikkert, M. G. O., Melis, R. J., & Claassen, J. A. (2009). *Heat waves and dehydration in the elderly*. British Medical Journal Publishing Group.

Romano, A., Bianchi, G., De Luca, M., Ricci, L., & Greco, A. (2025). Epidemiology of infectious disease outbreaks in displacement settings: Surveillance gaps and community-based solutions in refugee camps. *International Journal of Hygiene and Environmental Health, 264*, 52–61.

Saatchi, M., Khankeh, H. R., Shojafard, J., Barzanji, A., Ranjbar, M., Nazari, N., Mahmodi, M. A., Ahmadi, S., & Farrokhi, M. (2024). Communicable diseases outbreaks after natural disasters: A systematic scoping review for incidence, risk factors and recommendations. *Progress in Disaster Science, 23*, 100334.

Saha, M. K., Biswas, A. A. A., & Faisal, M. (2024). Livelihood vulnerability of coastal communities in context of the climate change: A index-based assessment. *World Development Sustainability, 4*. https://doi.org/10.1016/j.wds.2024.100152

Sarofim, M. C., Saha, S., Hawkins, M. D., Mills, D. M., Hess, J., Horton, R., Kinney, P., Schwartz, J., & St Juliana, A. (2016). *Temperature-related death and illness*. US Global Change Research Program.

Schulte, F., Röösli, M., & Ragettli, M. S. (2021). Heat-related cardiovascular morbidity and mortality in Switzerland: A clinical perspective. *Swiss Medical Weekly, 151*(3738), w30013.

Schwartz, J. D., Lee, M., Kinney, P. L., Yang, S., Mills, D., Sarofim, M. C., Jones, R., Streeter, R., Juliana, A. S., & Peers, J. (2015). Projections of temperature-attributable premature deaths in 209 US cities using a cluster-based Poisson approach. *Environmental Health, 14*(1), 85.

Shapira, S., Rosenthal, A., Singer, M., Natour, S., & Negev, M. (2025). Direct and indirect pathways of climate-related impacts on vulnerable populations: Insights from a nationwide study in the Eastern Mediterranean. *International Journal of Disaster Risk Reduction, 128*. https://doi.org/10.1016/j.ijdrr.2025.105750

Sharma, A., Andhikaputra, G., & Wang, Y.-C. (2022). Heatwaves in South Asia: Characterization, consequences on human health, and adaptation strategies. *Atmosphere, 13*, 734.

Shivanna, K. R. (2022). Climate change and its impact on biodiversity and human welfare. *Proceedings of the Indian National Science Academy, 88*, 160–171.

Smith, K. R., Chafe, Z., Woodward, A., Campbell-Lendrum, D., Chadee, D., Honda, Y., Liu, Q., Olwoch, J., Revich, B., & Sauerborn, R. (2015) Human health: Impacts, adaptation, and co-benefits. In *Climate change 2014 impacts, adaptation and vulnerability: Part A: Global and sectoral aspects*.

Soliman, K., & Amin, D. (2025). Vulnerability of groundwater quantity for an arid coastal aquifer under the climate change and extensive exploitation. *Applied Water Science, 15*, 1–19.

Stanke, C., Kerac, M., Prudhomme, C., Medlock, J., & Murray, V. (2013). Health effects of drought: A systematic review of the evidence. *PLoS Currents, 5*, ecurrents. dis. 7a2cee9e980 f91ad7697b570bcc4b004.

Stott, P. (2016). How climate change affects extreme weather events. *Science, 352*, 1517–1518.

Takahashi, A., Kumagai, T. O., Kanamori, H., Fujinami, H., Hiyama, T., & Hara, M. (2017). Impact of tropical deforestation and forest degradation on precipitation over Borneo Island. *Journal of Hydrometeorology, 18*, 2907–2922.

Thompson, R., Hornigold, R., Page, L., & Waite, T. (2018). Associations between high ambient temperatures and heat waves with mental health outcomes: A systematic review. *Public Health*, 161171–161191.

Toloo, G. S., FitzGerald, G., & Tong, S. (2014). Managing health risks of extreme weather events: Need for a systematic approach. *Australian and New Zealand Journal of Public Health, 38*(1), 90–91. https://doi.org/10.1111/1753-6405.12151

Tong, S., & Ebi, K. (2019). Preventing and mitigating health risks of climate change. *Environmental Research, 174*, 9–13. https://doi.org/10.1016/j.envres.2019.04.012

Tong, S., et al. (2016). Managing and mitigating the health risks of climate change: Calling for evidence-informed policy and action. *Environmental Health Perspectives, 124*(10), 176–179. https://doi.org/10.1289/EHP555

Torti, J. (2012). Floods in Southeast Asia: A health priority. *Journal of Global Health, 2*, 020304.

Tory, K. J., & Dare, R. A. (2015). Sea surface temperature thresholds for tropical cyclone formation. *Journal of Climate, 28*, 8171–8183.

Tsakonas, K., Badyal, S., Takaro, T., & Buse, C. (2025). Occupational health impacts of climate-related emergency events on health system workers in British Columbia. *International Journal of Disaster Risk Reduction, 118*. https://doi.org/10.1016/j.ijdrr.2025.105227

United Nations Development Programme. (2024). *What is climate change mitigation and why is it urgent? UNDP climate promise*. Available at: https://climatepromise.undp.org/news-and-stories/what-climate-change-mitigation-and-why-it-urgent

United Nations Development Programme. (2025). *How health systems in Asia are adapting to climate change impacts, UNDP climate promise*. Available at: https://climatepromise.undp.org/news-and-stories/how-health-systems-asia-are-adapting-climate-change-impacts. Accessed 18 Aug 2025.

Upadhyay, R. K. (2020). Markers for global climate change and its impact on social, biological and ecological systems: A review. *American Journal of Climate Change*.

Vega, J., Barco, J., & Hidalgo, C. (2024). Space-time analysis of the relationship between landslides occurrence, rainfall variability and ENSO in the Tropical Andean Mountain region in Colombia. *Landslides, 21*.

Walimah, E., et al. (2024). Mitigating the impact of climate change on public health: Strategies for resilience. *Global International Journal of Innovative Research, 2*(9), 2231–2244.

Wan, Z., Liu, Y., Jiang, Y., Chen, J., & Wang, Z. (2023). Burnout and work ability: A study on mental health of Chinese seafarers from the job demand resource model perspective. *Ocean and Coastal Management, 237*. https://doi.org/10.1016/j.ocecoaman.2023.106517

Wang, X., Lavigne, E., Ouellette-Kuntz, H., & Chen, B. E. (2014). Acute impacts of extreme temperature exposure on emergency room admissions related to mental and behavior disorders in Toronto, Canada. *Journal of Affective Disorders, 155*, 154–161.

Wang, X., He, K., & Dong, Z. (2019). Effects of climate change and human activities on runoff in the Beichuan River Basin in the northeastern Tibetan Plateau, China. *Catena, 176*, 81–93.

Wang, Z., Jiang, B., Wang, X., Wang, D., & Xue, H. (2023). Psychological challenges and related factors of ordinary residents after "7.20" heavy rainstorm disaster in Zhengzhou: A cross-sectional survey and study. *BMC Psychology, 11*, 3.

Wang, Y., Satoh, M., Zhan, R., Zhao, J., & Xie, S.-P. (2025). Tropical sea surface warming patterns and tropical cyclone activity: A review. *Advances in Atmospheric Sciences*, 1–22.

Widyastuti, K., Imron, M. A., Pradopo, S. T., Suryatmojo, H., Sopha, B. M., Spessa, A., & Berger, U. (2020). PeatFire: An agent-based model to simulate fire ignition and spreading in a tropical peatland ecosystem. *International Journal of Wildland Fire, 30*, 71–89.

Wilgus, M.-L., & Merchant, M. (2024). Clearing the air: understanding the impact of wildfire smoke on asthma and COPD. *Healthcare. MDPI, 307*.

Wooster, M. J., Gaveau, D. L., Salim, M. A., Zhang, T., Xu, W. C., Green, D., Huijnen, V., Murdiyarso, D., Gunawan, D., & Borchard, N. (2018). New tropical peatland gas and particulate emissions factors indicate 2015 Indonesian fires released far more particulate matter (but less methane) than current inventories imply. *Remote Sensing, 10*, 495.

World Health Organization. (2023). *Climate change*, *World Health Organization*. Available at: https://www.who.int/news-room/fact-sheets/detail/climate-change-and-health

Wu, X., Lu, Y., Zhou, S., Chen, L., & Xu, B. (2016). Impact of climate change on human infectious diseases: Empirical evidence and human adaptation. *Environment International*, 8614–8623.

Yaghoobi-Ershadi, M. R. (2016). Control of phlebotomine sand flies in Iran: A review article. *Journal of Arthropod-Borne Diseases, 10*(4), 429.

Yang, J.-L., & Zhang, G.-L. (2011). Water infiltration in urban soils and its effects on the quantity and quality of runoff. *Journal of Soils and Sediments, 11*, 751–761.

Yang, H.-Y., Wu, C.-F., & Tsai, K.-H. (2024). Projections of climate change impact on acute heat illnesses in Taiwan: Case-crossover study. *JMIR Public Health and Surveillance, 10*. https://doi.org/10.2196/57948

Yulianti, N., & Hayasaka, H. (2023). Recent active fires in Indonesia's Southern Papua province caused by El Niño conditions. *Remote Sensing, 15*, 2709.

Zain, A., et al. (2024). Climate change and its impact on infectious diseases in Asia. *Singapore Medical Journal, 65*, 211–219. https://doi.org/10.4103/singaporemedj.SMJ-2023-180

Zhang, W., Koch, J., Wei, F., Zeng, Z., Fang, Z., & Fensholt, R. (2023). Soil moisture and atmospheric aridity impact spatio-temporal changes in evapotranspiration at a global scale. *Journal of Geophysical Research: Atmospheres, 128*, e2022JD038046.

Chapter 8
Biodiversity Loss and Health

Annisa Firdaus Winta Damarsya, Yuliana Fashani, Mukhlish Jamal Musa Holle, Denis Oxy Handika, Sandy Nurvianto, and Abdul Rahman Siregar

8.1 The Importance of Biodiversity for Human, Animals, and Environment

Human life will always have a close connection with nature. Since the dawn of history, humans have depended on the diversity of living creatures to fulfill their needs for food, clothing, shelter, and medicine. Humanity's ability to domesticate plants and animals triggered the agricultural revolution, which was only possible because of the diversity of species (Diamond, 1997). Even today, crops such as rice, corn, and wheat, domesticated thousands of years ago, along with animals like cattle, chickens, and goats, continue to provide staple food and essential resources for billions of people worldwide (Diamond, 1997; Larson & Fuller, 2014; Zeder, 2008). Many customs and cultures that deeply understand their communities' dependence on nature pass on their knowledge to their descendants, emphasizing that human welfare cannot be separated from ecosystem health (Gadgil et al., 1993). Beyond meeting basic needs, biodiversity also shapes cultural identity and inspiration, from traditionally used medicinal plants to sacred landscapes that remain central to spiritual traditions (Posey, 1999).

A. F. W. Damarsya (✉) · Y. Fashani · D. O. Handika
Master of Public Health Program, Faculty of Medicine, Public Health, and Nursing, Universitas Gadjah Mada, Yogyakarta, Indonesia
e-mail: annisafirdauswintada@mail.ugm.ac.id; yulianafashani@mail.ugm.ac.id; denisoxyhandika@mail.ugm.ac.id

M. J. M. Holle · A. R. Siregar
Faculty of Biology, Universitas Gadjah Mada, Yogyakarta, Indonesia
e-mail: holle@ugm.ac.id; ar.siregar@ugm.ac.id

S. Nurvianto
Faculty of Forestry, Universitas Gadjah Mada, Yogyakarta, Indonesia
e-mail: sandy_nuvi@ugm.ac.id

© The Author(s), under exclusive license to Springer Nature Singapore Pte Ltd. 2026

A. U. Rauf, T. Wibawa (eds.), *The One Health Concept in Asian Contexts*,
https://doi.org/10.1007/978-981-95-9880-9_8

By the mid-twentieth century, people had begun to realize more clearly that biodiversity was in grave danger. Rapid industrial growth, deforestation, and rising pollution pushed many species to the brink of extinction and weakened the ecosystems that people depended on for their daily lives (McCormick, 1991; Carson, 1962). These impacts were not distant or theoretical. People could feel them directly. The decline of pollinators, such as bees and butterflies, reduced food production worldwide, while the loss of wetlands stripped away natural defenses that once protected communities from floods and storms (Klein et al., 2007; Potts et al., 2010; Mitsch & Gosselink, 2015).

Faced with these risks, the global community began to take action. One of the earliest milestones in global conservation came in 1948 with the founding of the International Union for Conservation of Nature (IUCN), which brought together scientists and policymakers to safeguard biodiversity (Holdgate, 1999; IUCN, 2008). Building on this foundation, the World Wildlife Fund (WWF) was established in 1961, mobilizing public attention and international fundraising for the protection of iconic species such as the giant panda and the tiger (Adams, 2004; WWF, 2021). These initiatives set the stage for the 1972 Stockholm Conference, which gave rise to the United Nations Environment Programme (UNEP) and marked a decisive moment that placed biodiversity firmly on the global policy agenda (UNEP, 2012; Strong, 1973; Soroos, 1997).

The Earth Summit held in Rio de Janeiro in 1992 marked another turning point in global conservation. At this meeting, 156 nations and the European Community signed the Convention on Biological Diversity (CBD) (UN, 1992; CBD, 2011). For the first time, countries committed to a legally binding framework to conserve biodiversity, to use it sustainably, and to share its benefits fairly among all people (Glowka et al., 1994). The agreement made clear that biodiversity is not only about protecting rare species but also about maintaining the systems that sustain human life. The term biodiversity itself had only recently entered international debates. Coined in the mid-1980s as a contraction of "biological diversity" (Wilson, 1988), it quickly gained traction because it captured the richness of life in a single word. By the time of the Earth Summit, biodiversity had become a powerful unifying concept that framed global discussions and guided policy responses (Takacs, 1996).

Countries then began to translate these global commitments into national policies and programs, including Costa Rica, Namibia, and Indonesia. Costa Rica, which ratified the CBD in 1994, became a pioneer by linking forest protection with payments for ecosystem services. This approach restored large tracts of forest while creating a sustainable base for ecotourism (Pagiola, 2008; Sanchez-Azofeifa et al., 2007; CBD, 2024a). Namibia ratified the CBD in 1997 and used it as a foundation for expanding its community conservancy program, granting rural communities rights over wildlife and demonstrating how conservation could also improve livelihoods (Jones, 2010; NACSO, 2013; CBD, 2024b). Indonesia, which ratified in 1994, integrated biodiversity goals into community forestry and coastal management. Mangrove rehabilitation in Java and Sumatra, for instance, has supported both ecosystems and local economies (Moeliono et al., 2017; Arifanti et al., 2019; FAO, 2020; CBD, 2024c).

Biodiversity refers to the variety and variability of all forms of life on Earth, encompassing genetic, species, and ecosystem levels. According to the Convention on Biological Diversity, biodiversity includes diversity within species, between species, and among ecosystems. The World Health Organization (WHO) emphasizes that biodiversity is the foundation of ecosystem services that are crucial to human well-being, such as the provision of clean air, water, food, and disease regulation (WHO, 2022a). Similarly, the Millennium Ecosystem Assessment highlights that biodiversity involves not only the number of species but also the functional diversity and complex relationships among organisms in a given environment (Mace et al., 2005). Therefore, biodiversity is not merely an ecological concept; it is a fundamental determinant of public health, human survival, and sustainable development (Linhares et al., 2023; Marselle et al., 2021). It is a dynamic and constantly evolving phenomenon, shaped by natural processes such as evolution as well as human activities like habitat destruction. Thus, safeguarding biodiversity is inseparable from efforts to promote global health, ensure food and water security, and maintain ecosystem resilience in the face of environmental change (Linhares et al., 2023; WHO, 2022a).

Biodiversity preservation constitutes one of the most critical foundations for achieving the United Nations' 17 Sustainable Development Goals (SDGs). Its relevance is evident in goals such as Zero Hunger (SDG 2), Climate Action (SDG 13), Life Below Water (SDG 14), and Life on Land (SDG 15), while also underpinning broader objectives including Good Health and Well-being (SDG 3), Reduced Inequalities (SDG 10), and Responsible Consumption and Production (SDG 12). Ensuring biodiversity across diverse landscapes and habitats is essential not only for ecological balance but also for fostering human understanding of life systems and sustaining human well-being (Neergheen-Bhujun et al., 2017). Crucially, biodiversity preservation directly benefits humanity, particularly in drug discovery. Wild species provide indispensable molecular diversity for medical innovation, prevention, and treatment (Scannell & Bosley, 2016). However, accelerating biodiversity loss driven by extinction rates estimated to be 100–1000 times higher than historical norms threatens this resource (Pimm et al., 2014). Current estimates suggest that at least one potential therapeutic compound is lost every 2 years, alongside the erosion of irreplaceable traditional knowledge and molecular diversity. These parallel losses jeopardize biomedical research and, ultimately, human survival (Pimm et al., 1995).

To address these challenges, interdisciplinary research that integrates evolutionary ecology, biochemistry, and ethnopharmacology offers promising pathways for pharmacological innovation, reframing medicinal plants as synergistic partners rather than merely as chemical reservoirs (Davis & Choisy, 2024). Supporting this, a comprehensive analysis notes that over 30% of new drugs derive from natural molecules sourced from plants and microbes, and more than 70% of cancer therapeutics are "bioinspired," underscoring biodiversity's critical role in disease treatment (Anitha et al., 2024; Omidian et al., 2023; Sabu et al., 2018). The World Health Organization further quantifies this, reporting that over 40% of modern medicines originate from natural sources such as fungi and other plants, and it is estimated that 60% of the world's population utilizes traditional medicines (Dias et al., 2012;

WHO, 2022b). More recently, innovations in biodigital applications like environmental DNA (eDNA) sequencing have expanded the molecular discovery toolbox; for example, Basecamp Research exploits rich environmental samples to fuel AI-driven drug discovery, identifying millions of novel genetic sequences with high therapeutic potential (Woodie, 2024). These developments highlight how biodiversity, combined with emerging technologies, continues to offer vast opportunities for discovering life-saving treatments.

Biodiversity plays a critical role in regulating disease and protecting human health. Biodiversity loss is the single most significant environmental driver of infectious disease outbreaks, even surpassing climate change and species invasions. For instance, loss of habitats through deforestation has also been linked to severe zoonotic disease transmission (Barbier, 2021; Keesing & Ostfeld, 2021; Weston, 2024). Moreover, a study featured in *Philosophical Transactions B* explains that diminishing local biodiversity and shifts in host–vector communities in anthropogenic landscapes can reshape disease ecology, often escalating disease burden and transmission potential (Gibb et al., 2025; Wood et al., 2017). Collectively, these findings affirm that preserving biodiversity is not only an environmental imperative but also a powerful strategy for disease prevention and safeguarding public health.

As civilization advances, evidence highlighting the importance of biodiversity in supporting human mental health has increasingly accumulated. A study in Canada where 65,000 Canadians are interviewed each year on various aspects of their health and lifestyle found that neighborhoods with higher bird and tree species diversity were associated with improved self-reported mental health; specifically, a one-standard-deviation increase in bird diversity raised the likelihood of good mental health by approximately 7% and tree diversity by about 5% (Buxton, 2024). Complementing this, research from King's College London using real-time mobile assessments revealed that environments rich in natural features (trees, birds, waterways) led to stronger improvements in mental well-being compared to less diverse areas (Hammoud et al., 2024). Mechanistic insights further reinforce these findings: a study emphasizes that biodiversity enhances mental restoration through established frameworks like Attention Restoration Theory and Stress Recovery Theory, where perceived biodiversity amplifies cognitive recovery and stress reduction pathways (Rozario et al., 2024). Additionally, a large-scale study in China indicated that people's perceived biodiversity in greenspaces shaped by psychological and physiological restoration and satisfaction strongly predicted improved mental health, suggesting that the subjective experience of biodiversity may matter more than objective measures (Ma & Wu, 2025). Moreover, practical mental health interventions such as nature prescriptions have shown promise where prescribing nature through structured activities in green settings yields lower depression, reduced anxiety, and improved blood pressure outcomes (Lemieux et al., 2025; Ma & Wu, 2025).

The One Health approach underscores the intrinsic connection among human, animal, and environmental health. Biodiversity conservation emerges as a pivotal strategy in this context, safeguarding against disease emergence originating from wildlife–human interactions. The One Health framework is increasingly recognized in transformative biodiversity governance as essential for mitigating disease risks linked to human-wildlife interfaces (Assmuth et al., 2020). Moreover, IUCN has issued policy guidelines emphasizing the indispensable role of biodiversity stakeholders in identifying and proactively reducing disease risks under a One Health paradigm (IUCN, 2025). Several countries offer compelling examples of biodiversity-health policy integration:

France has been actively developing a "Biodiversity/Health nexus" approach, incorporating it into the National Health-Environment Plan and local government agendas. This includes initiatives to understand the links between biodiversity and infectious disease prevention, demonstrating a proactive approach to integrating these issues (Gautier et al., 2023).

The EU's Common Agricultural Policy (CAP), while serving as a central instrument for biodiversity conservation, continues to face significant challenges in fully realizing its biodiversity objectives due to competing agricultural, economic, and environmental interests. Recognizing these limitations, the EU has also introduced the Biodiversity Strategy for 2030, a comprehensive framework designed to halt biodiversity loss while simultaneously addressing its far-reaching implications for human health, ecosystem resilience, and economic sustainability (CIRAD, 2022).

Colombia's approach places particular emphasis on the health impacts of extractive industries, with a strong focus on mercury contamination resulting from mining activities. This perspective underscores the complex interplay between environmental degradation and public health, illustrating how biodiversity loss not only disrupts ecosystems but also generates tangible and often severe consequences for human well-being. By framing extractive industries as a critical driver of both ecological and health crises, Colombia highlights the urgent need for integrated policies that address biodiversity conservation alongside the protection of community health (Anderson, 2024).

In Costa Rica, the implementation of the Payment for Ecosystem Services (PES) program provides direct financial incentives to landowners for engaging in activities such as forest conservation, the establishment of timber plantations, and the promotion of agroforestry systems. This approach not only secures ecological benefits, such as carbon sequestration, watershed protection, and biodiversity preservation, but also generates socio-economic advantages by supporting rural livelihoods and promoting sustainable land management practices (Pagiola, 2008; Sardana & Simpson, 2023).

Zimbabwe adopted the Communal Areas Management Programme for Indigenous Resources (CAMPFIRE) as a pioneering model of community-based natural resource management that integrates biodiversity conservation with rural development. The program emphasizes regulated trophy hunting, landscape maintenance, and biodiversity protection, while channeling revenues back to local communities as direct benefits. By devolving authority over wildlife resources to rural districts, CAMPFIRE generates financial incentives for conservation, mitigates human–wildlife conflict, and promotes sustainable land use. This approach demonstrates how market-based mechanisms can align ecological preservation with economic empowerment, making conservation both practical and beneficial for rural populations (Sardana & Simpson, 2023).

8.2 The Impact of Biodiversity Loss

Asia, the world's largest and most populous continent (Zhu, 2017), is home to some of the most diverse ecosystems on Earth. From the tropical rainforests of Indonesia to the Himalayan mountain ranges and the coral reefs of the Philippines, Asia hosts an extraordinary variety of species. These ecosystems play important roles for humans, including for human health. Not only diverse biologically, but Asia also has diverse cultures that often interact with its rich biodiversity (Mace et al., 2005). However, rapid industrialization, urbanization, and unsustainable resource exploitation have led to severe biodiversity loss (Asian Development Bank, 2006), which might deteriorate their health-related services. Ecosystem services, which are ecological functions beneficial for the human being, can be categorized into three groups, provisioning services, regulating services, and cultural services. These services can either be utilized by humanity through direct extraction, such as medical compound extraction, or non-extractive way, such as recreational value. Here, we focus on the health-related ecosystem services that are provided by Asia's biodiversity.

(a) *Altered Air and Water Purification and Vector Regulation*

How ecosystems provide clean air and water is often disregarded until these resources are polluted and become scarcely available. These services are provided by forests, wetlands, and other ecosystems that filter pollutants. In these ecosystems, organisms such as plants might play important roles in filtering pollutants. Along with the uncontrolled pollution released to the environment, the loss of biodiversity can cause the failure in filtering air and water. The polluted air and water increase the likelihood of the disease (Fuller et al., 2022; Lin et al., 2022). There have been extensive studies exploring how air pollution worsens the symptoms of air-borne diseases (De Lira-Quezada et al., 2024). The severity of the respiratory illness caused by the recent Covid-19 pandemic is linked to the air quality, where people living in a more air-polluted area are likely to have more severe symptoms. In the aquatic environment, some vectors, such as mosquitos and snails, are likely to be more tolerant to the polluted water (Costa et al., 2024). Meanwhile, organisms that biologically control their populations are negatively affected by water pollution (Almeida et al., 2018). Without the biological agents that work on purifying water quality and buffering the pollution from entering the water body, the water-borne disease or water-based vectors might further harm human health.

(b) *The Loss of Food, Nutrition, and Medicinal Resources*

Human health is more than just about disease and pathogens. Human health relies on the nutritious food and medicine (Nordhagen et al., 2022) that often are sourced from biodiversity. Staple crops that humans currently eat, such as lentils, rice, and maize, come from species that have been domesticated and bred to fulfill human nutritional needs (Chen et al., 2014), with a higher nutritional quality than its original varieties. Similar to how biodiversity contributes to fulfilling human nutritional needs as food sources, biodiversity provides medicinal sources. It has been a long-standing history that biodiversity supplies medicinal materials (Filho, 2025), such as herbal medicines that have been used in China for thousands of years (Chen et al., 2014). As the technology developed and new diseases emerged, there is a rising need to discover a new source of medicine that often starts from natural products from certain species (Thomford et al., 2018). Not only terrestrial species, but natural products are also often extracted from marine species, such as corals. The problem arises when these species are lost before their benefits are discovered while the rate of the biodiversity loss outcompetes the rate of researchers attempting to discover the species.

(c) *Deteriorated Mental Health and Physical Well-Being*

When we discuss human health, it is inevitable to also talk about mental health. There has been strong evidence showing that biodiversity, in the forms of green spaces or other natural settings present in urban areas, provides both mental and physical health benefits, including positive effects on mood, healing, heart rate, blood pressure, stress, and concentration (Kondo et al., 2018). For example, the presence of trees in the pedestrian sidewalks and the availability of green spaces might motivate people to take a walk and do physical activity comfortably. Contrarily, the absence of such activities due to the absence of natural infrastructure negatively affects mental health and physical well-being. In the Asian context, cities are growing along with the human population expansion (Zhu, 2017). In addition, the Asian hustle cultures contribute to the high societal pressure (Yuningsih et al., 2023). Compared to other regions, Asia has one of the highest suicidal rates, indicating the worse mental health condition of the region (Hendin et al., 2008). However, it does not mean that Asia's growing population and culture prevent the society from building biodiversity-friendly cities. Singapore, which has been considered one of the greenest city-states in Asia, could be the reference in how biodiversity becomes part of the city itself (Fujii & Rohan, 2019). In addition, locals are benefited by the appropriate public infrastructure that facilitates pedestrian and physical well-being despite the tropical and humid climate. Therefore, incorporating biodiversity in the urban and regional planning is not only important for the environment but also for the human health that heavily relies on it, particularly in Asia, where mental health has become a serious issue.

8.3 Emerging Infectious Diseases

Loss of biodiversity significantly influences the emergence and re-emergence of infectious diseases (EIDs) by altering interactions among wildlife, domestic animals, and humans. In Asia, a region rich in biodiversity yet undergoing rapid ecological changes driven by urbanization, deforestation, and agricultural expansion, these disruptions increase the risk of zoonotic spillover events, where pathogens transfer from animals to humans (Goldstein et al., 2022). This subchapter explores the ecological and socio-economic mechanisms linking biodiversity decline to EIDs in Asia and highlights the role of the One Health approach in addressing these interconnected challenges through integrated prevention and mitigation strategies.

Loss of biodiversity substantially affects disease dynamics by weakening natural ecological regulatory mechanisms that control pathogen transmission. Key drivers include habitat fragmentation, which increases contact between wildlife, livestock, and humans by isolating habitats and pushing species such as fruit bats closer to human settlements. The loss of the "dilution effect" further elevates disease risk, as highly diverse ecosystems usually contain many poor pathogen reservoirs; with declining biodiversity, competent reservoir species dominate, amplifying transmission potential (Keesing & Ostfeld, 2021).

Environmental disturbances also alter host and vector populations, favoring species with greater transmission capacity, such as rodents that thrive in degraded habitats. Concurrently, declines in predator populations disrupt natural population controls, exacerbating disease risk. Additionally, degradation of ecosystem services, including water purification, pest regulation, and pollination, indirectly promotes disease emergence by expanding vector breeding sites (Ellwanger et al., 2022). In Asia, these dynamics are illustrated by large-scale deforestation for oil palm plantations, urban expansion into forests, and persistent wildlife trade networks, all of which exacerbate biodiversity loss and contribute to the rise of EIDs.

Biodiversity loss plays a critical role in driving the emergence of infectious diseases through several biological mechanisms. One widely discussed explanation is the dilution effect hypothesis, which suggests that high biodiversity can suppress pathogen transmission because many hosts are either poor reservoirs or dead ends for pathogens. However, when biodiversity declines, competent reservoirs dominate, thereby elevating disease risk, as observed in Lyme disease and hantaviruses (Keesing & Ostfeld, 2021). In addition, habitat destruction and resource scarcity force wildlife into closer contact with humans and livestock, particularly in agricultural interface zones, increasing the likelihood of zoonotic spillover events, such as the Nipah virus outbreaks in Malaysia (Klim et al., 2023). Furthermore, biodiversity loss also alters vector ecology and wildlife immunity. Land-use changes can create favorable conditions for disease vectors, such as Anopheles mosquitoes, contributing to malaria resurgence. At the same time, environmental stress weakens wildlife immune systems and increases pathogen shedding, as seen in fruit bats during periods of food shortage (Goldstein et al., 2022).

Emerging infectious diseases in Asia vividly illustrate the complex links between biodiversity loss, ecological change, and human health. Several well-documented outbreaks demonstrate how deforestation, agricultural intensification, wildlife trade, and habitat degradation create conditions that facilitate zoonotic spillovers and sustain disease transmission. The following case studies highlight three prominent examples:

(a) Nipah Virus in Malaysia and Bangladesh

Nipah virus was first identified in Malaysia in 1998–1999, associated with large-scale pig farming near fruit bat habitats. Deforestation and El Niño-driven drought reduced natural food sources for bats, prompting them to forage in fruit orchards adjacent to pig farms. Pigs served as amplifying hosts, transmitting the virus to farm workers. In Bangladesh, repeated outbreaks since 2001 have been linked to consumption of raw date palm sap contaminated by bat saliva or urine (Hauser et al., 2021).

(b) Highly Pathogenic Avian Influenza (H5N1)

The persistence of H5N1 in Southeast Asia is influenced by the loss of wetland biodiversity, changes in migratory bird patterns, and high-density poultry farming. Wetlands act as natural filters and biodiversity reservoirs; their degradation increases contact between wild and domestic birds, facilitating viral exchange (Liang et al., 2020).

(c) Severe Acute Respiratory Syndrome (SARS) and COVID-19

Both SARS-CoV (2002–2003) and SARS-CoV-2 (2019–present) are coronaviruses originating from bat reservoirs, with probable intermediate hosts involved. Wildlife trade networks, live animal markets, and habitat encroachment increased opportunities for viral spillovers. Biodiversity loss plays a role by disrupting natural ecological buffers that historically limited human exposure to these viruses (Platto et al., 2021).

8.4 Socioeconomic and Cultural Dimensions

In Asia, biodiversity loss is deeply intertwined with socioeconomic pressures. Poverty, food insecurity, and livelihood needs drive deforestation, hunting, and wildlife trade. Cultural practices such as bushmeat consumption, traditional medicine use of wildlife products, and informal livestock–wildlife interfaces further increase the risks of emerging infectious diseases (EIDs). Globalization adds to these risks by accelerating pathogen spread through trade and travel. Weak health and ecological surveillance systems in rural biodiversity hotspots hinder early detection of outbreaks (McNeil et al., 2022). In addition, conservation policies may face resistance if they conflict with community livelihood needs, underscoring the importance of participatory approaches (Smith, 2022).

Addressing EIDs linked to biodiversity loss in Asia faces several challenges. Weak enforcement of wildlife trade regulations remains a major issue, as illegal trade continues despite international agreements like CITES, driven by limited enforcement, corruption, and persistent market demand. This ongoing trade increases the risk of zoonotic spillover (Klim et al., 2023). Another challenge is limited cross-sector collaboration, with health, agriculture, and environmental sectors often working in silos. The lack of formal mechanisms for data sharing and joint planning reduces the effectiveness of One Health strategies (Dayapera et al., 2024). Furthermore, many national One Health programs are underfunded and inconsistent, restricting long-term monitoring, research, and policy action (Lâm et al., 2025).

Opportunities exist to overcome these barriers. Mainstreaming One Health into national strategies across environment, agriculture, and public health enables integrated planning and coordinated resource use (Dayapera et al., 2024). Strengthening wildlife disease surveillance and protecting biodiversity hotspots are also essential, particularly in high-risk areas such as agricultural frontiers, wildlife markets, and deforestation zones. Conservation efforts support prevention by reducing human–wildlife contact and maintaining ecosystem functions (McNeil et al., 2022). At the same time, regional cooperation through ASEAN and SAARC is critical for harmonized surveillance, rapid information sharing, and coordinated response. Empowering communities with culturally appropriate risk reduction practices further promotes sustainable changes to reduce disease risks (Teerawattananon et al., 2022).

8.5 Conservation and Restoration of Biodiversity for Health

Every year, Asia, especially its tropical regions, is one of the areas experiencing the fastest deforestation in the world. At the same time, six out of 20 countries with the most threatened species are in Asia (IUCN, 2025). Earth's capability to sustain ecosystem services is ruined whenever certain species or populations become extinct. Asia's biodiversity crisis elevates the risks of disease outbreaks, limits the access to nutritious food, and leads to water scarcity in the continent (Leddin, 2024; Meena & Jha, 2023). While previous parts have discussed the threat of biodiversity loss for human health, this part will focus on the solution by highlighting conservation and restoration efforts as part of intervention and solutions for public health issues in One Health context.

(a) *Conservation and Restoration of Biodiversity as the Pillar of One Health in Asia*

Conservation often focuses on the protection of the ecologically important species in the ecosystems, such as apex predators and keystone species. These kinds of species are likely to be a megafauna, such as elephants, tigers, and orangutans. These megafaunas are currently present in tropical areas, including many parts of Asia, which are under extinction threats. The loss of these species, often referred to as a defaunation, is linked to the emergence of zoonotic disease (Siegel, 2021). As these species often sit on the higher trophic levels and play role in top-down control of the population in the lower trophic levels, megafauna defaunation disrupts the ecosystem balance, often causing uncontrolled growth of some populations, including populations of the species that potentially transmit zoonotic diseases (Doughty et al., 2020; Young et al., 2014). The defaunation occurs due to illegal wildlife trade and illegal hunting. In addition, direct consumption of wildlife through bushmeat harvesting, especially those that might carry zoonotic diseases such as wild bats and rodents, can increase the likelihood of the zoonotic disease transmission. Therefore, preventing the illegal wildlife trade and hunting through community-based conservation and law enforcement are some of the keys in conserving ecologically important fauna (Choo et al., 2023; Siegel, 2021).

Conservation of biodiversity is the important ecological foundation in One Health (Gruetzmacher et al., 2021). This approach can be done by reducing overexploitation of terrestrial, freshwater, and marine ecosystems, halt deforestation, and prevent further encroachment into natural habitat. Conservation efforts often include habitat conservation, where the natural ecosystem is protected to improve biodiversity and prevent species extinction (Supriatna, 2018). One strategy is by establishing protected areas (PAs) for important biodiversity and ecosystem services. This is particularly essential in the areas of potential disease emergence. This is an important pillar of One Health, as healthy natural ecosystems could serve as a buffer that prevents pathogen spillover into humans and other animals (Terraube & Fernández-Llamazares, 2020). Balanced ecosystems prevent the dominance of certain species as disease reservoirs and vectors, distributing disease pathogens among diverse hosts. Potential conflicts between domestic and wildlife animals that act as a chain of disease transmission (e.g., bird flu, anthrax) could be minimized if only natural habitat is conserved (Everard et al., 2020; Keesing et al., 2010).

Plant and species conservation are no less crucial than habitat conservation. Plant conservation efforts improve the quality of human physical and mental health (Buxton et al., 2024; Meng et al., 2024). In Asia, traditional healing practices and herbal medicines from native plants are part of the culture and beliefs. Therefore, there is urgency in protecting medicinal plants from threats like climate change and unsustainable trades across the continent (Cahyaningsih et al., 2021; Cunningham et al., 2019). Biodiversity-friendly agriculture practices are required for a sustainable and healthy food system. Plant conservation itself cannot stand alone, as species conservation of natural predators and pollinators are inevitable for food security (Mainka & Trivedi, 2002; Requier et al., 2023).

While most One Health strategies highlight the importance of preserving biodiversity on land, it should be noted that maintaining marine biodiversity is as important as terrestrial ones (Maes & Messing, 2025). The ocean is the largest protein source provider for living organisms on Earth, with more than 3 billion people depending on it as the source of their protein supply and employment (FAO, 2022). Protected marine ecosystems would support coastal food security, as well as improving the community's economic growth through ecotourism (Cusack et al., 2021; Westlund et al., 2017). Furthermore, preserved coral reefs serve as natural barriers, protecting coastal communities from natural hazards such as storms and tsunamis (Lahcene et al., 2024).

One Health highlights the importance of preventive rather than reactive approaches toward epidemics. Ecosystem restoration is one of the most economical strategies compared to the economic impacts of epidemics such as COVID-19, which was estimated to be trillions of US dollars. Forest restoration, particularly with native plant species, that connects fragmented forests could potentially reduce the spillover of zoonotic diseases by reducing the abundance of particular disease reservoirs/vectors and increasing species diversity (Davidson et al., 2024; Prist et al., 2021). On the other hand, although the impact of mangrove and wetland restoration on mosquito-borne diseases is complex, the benefit outbalances its concerns. Restored mangrove and wetland could substantially reduce flooding incidence, improve water quality, and increase carbon-storing capacity. Habitat restoration can act as climate change mitigation, further preventing the impact of climate change on human, animal, and environmental health.

(b) *Biodiversity Conservation and Restoration Policies in Asia*

UNEP has declared a UN Decade of Ecosystem Restoration, starting from 2021 to 2030, which is implemented globally, including in Asia. This initiative targets restoration of 100 million hectares of degraded lands in the region by 2030 (FAO, 2024). The first global treaty that addresses conservation of biodiversity comprehensively is the Convention on Biological Diversity (CBD). In 2022, CBD passed the Kunming-Montreal Global Biodiversity Framework, targeting the restoration of at least 30% of degraded areas in land, inland waters, coastal, and marine ecosystems by 2030 and a decline in the extinction rate and risk of all species by 2050 (Convention on Biological Diversity, 2022). A number of Asian countries have developed national strategies that aligned with the Kunming-Montreal Global Biodiversity Framework. The government of China encourages its provincial governments and companies across the nation to develop their own biodiversity action plan while calling for public participation (China Development Brief, 2024). On the other hand, based on their positive-economy strategies, the Japanese government is promoting long-term ecotourism to boost their rural biodiversity conservation while focusing on long-term satoyama, forests, and other ecosystem conservation (Ministry of the Environment Japan, 2022). Other countries from Southeast Asia such as Indonesia and Malaysia have developed their National Biodiversity Strategy and Action Plan in accordance with the framework. Although this framework did not explicitly address One Health, it aligns with the One Health approach that recognizes environmental health as the basis of the health of all creatures (Bappenas, 2024; Kementerian Sumber Asli dan Alam Sekitar Malaysia, 2022).

Establishment of protected areas (PAs) could be used as the main approach to overcome biodiversity crisis (Watson et al., 2014). However, in developed and developing countries in Asia, PAs are being downsized due to development and economic pressures. Examples of PA downsizing include the Oryx Sanctuary in Oman, which was removed from the World Heritage List as only 10% of its initial size remained after the government of Oman drilled it for oil and natural gas extraction. Moreover, in many countries PAs are not immune to encroachment. Tesso Nilo National Park, a habitat of Sumatran elephants, has lost more than 40 thousand hectares of its area converted into oil palm plantations and settlements illegally (Hasyim, 2025).

(c) *Community-Based Conservation and Restoration in Asia*

Various community-based conservation and restoration initiatives have been implemented in numerous areas in Asia. Such activities often include indigenous people and local communities (IPLCs) with or without government initiatives. An example includes the Alam Sehat Lestari (ASRI) programme, an initiative that integrates conservation and healthcare in the severely degraded forest of Borneo's Gunung Palung National Park (GPNP), the home of threatened orangutans. Since 2007, besides restoring the forest, ASRI provides affordable healthcare and free training for local people who are willing to reduce their forest logging activity. This work successfully cut the number of logging households from 1350 in 2007 to 150 households 10 years after the initiative started. At the same time, it also improves the community's health quality (Webb et al., 2018). In some ASEAN countries, ecotourism and mangrove conservation are integrated efforts aiming to protect the environment while improving the livelihoods of surrounding communities (Blanton et al., 2024).

Ultimately, ecosystem restoration that has been seen as solely beneficial for the environment and the endangered species turns out to be imperative for human health. In the Anthropocene era where humans have altered the environment, conservation and restoration are getting more important.

Competing Interests The author(s) have no competing interests to declare that are relevant to the content of this manuscript.

References

Adams, W. M. (2004). *Against extinction: The story of conservation*. Earthscan.

Almeida, R. M., Han, B. A., Reisinger, A. J., Kagemann, C., & Rosi, E. J. (2018). High mortality in aquatic predators of mosquito larvae caused by exposure to insect repellent. *Biology Letters, 14*(10), 20180526. https://doi.org/10.1098/rsbl.2018.0526

Anderson, S. (2024). *Nations deadlocked over health-biodiversity framework at COP16*. https://healthpolicy-watch.news/nations-deadlocked-over-health-biodiversity-framework-at-cop16/

Anitha, K., Chenchula, S., Surendran, V., Shvetank, B., Ravula, P., Milan, R., & Chikatipalli, R. (2024). Advancing cancer theranostics through biomimetics: A comprehensive review. *Heliyon, 10*(6), e27692. https://doi.org/10.1016/j.heliyon.2024.e27692

Arifanti, V. B., Kauffman, J. B., Hadriyanto, D., Murdiyarso, D., & Diana, R. (2019). Carbon dynamics and land use carbon footprints in mangrove-converted aquaculture: The case of the Mahakam Delta, Indonesia. *Forest Ecology and Management, 432*, 17–29. https://doi.org/10.1016/j.foreco.2018.08.043

Asian Development Bank. (2006). *Urbanization and sustainability in Asia.* Asian Development Bank. https://www.adb.org/sites/default/files/publication/27965/urbanization-sustainability.pdf

Assmuth, T., Chen, X., Degeling, C., Haahtela, T., Irvine, K. N., Keune, H., Kock, R., Rantala, S., Rüegg, S., & Vikström, S. (2020). Integrative concepts and practices of health in transdisciplinary social ecology. *Socio-Ecological Practice Research, 2*(1), 71–90. https://doi.org/10.1007/s42532-019-00038-y

Bappenas. (2024). *Indonesian biodiversity strategy and action plan 2025–2045.* Bappenas. Retrieved July 30, 2025, from https://perpustakaan.bappenas.go.id/e-library/file_upload/koleksi/dokumenbappenas/konten/Upload%20Terbaru/IBSAP%202025-2045.pdf

Barbier, E. B. (2021). Habitat loss and the risk of disease outbreak. *Journal of Environmental Economics and Management, 108*, 102451. https://doi.org/10.1016/j.jeem.2021.102451

Blanton, A., Ewane, E. B., McTavish, F., Watt, M. S., Rogers, K., Daneil, R., Vizcaino, I., Gomez, A. N., Arachchige, P. S. P., King, S. A. L., Galgamuwa, G. A. P., Peñaranda, M. L. P., Al-Musawi, L., Montenegro, J. F., Broadbent, E. N., Zambrano, A. M. A., Hudak, A. T., Swangjang, K., Velasquez-Camacho, L., et al. (2024). Ecotourism and mangrove conservation in Southeast Asia: Current trends and perspectives. *Journal of Environmental Management, 365*, 121529. https://doi.org/10.1016/j.jenvman.2024.121529

Buxton, R. (2024). *The association between mental health and biodiversity*. Ecology & Evolution and Public Health. https://go.nature.com/45mwgn9

Buxton, R. T., Hudgins, E. J., Lavigne, E., Villeneuve, P. J., Prince, S. A., Pearson, A. L., Halsall, T., Robichaud, C., & Bennett, J. R. (2024). Mental health is positively associated with biodiversity in Canadian cities. *Communications Earth & Environment, 5*(1), 310. https://doi.org/10.1038/s43247-024-01482-9

Cahyaningsih, R., Phillips, J., Magos Brehm, J., Gaisberger, H., & Maxted, N. (2021). Climate change impact on medicinal plants in Indonesia. *Global Ecology and Conservation, 30*, e01752. https://doi.org/10.1016/j.gecco.2021.e01752

Carson, R. (1962). *Silent spring*. Houghton Mifflin.

CBD. (2011). *History of the convention*. Convention on Biological Diversity. https://www.cbd.int/history/

CBD. (2024a). *Costa Rica—National Reporting*. Convention on Biological Diversity. https://www.cbd.int/countries/profile?country=cr

CBD. (2024b). *Namibia—National Reporting*. Convention on Biological Diversity. https://www.cbd.int/countries/profile?country=na

CBD. (2024c). *Indonesia—National reporting*. Convention on Biological Diversity. https://www.cbd.int/countries/profile?country=id

Chen, W., Lewith, G., Wang, L., Ren, J., Xiong, W., Lu, F., & Liu, J. (2014). Chinese proprietary herbal medicine listed in 'China National Essential Drug List' for common cold: A systematic literature review. *PLoS ONE, 9*(10), e110560. https://doi.org/10.1371/journal.pone.0110560

Choo, J., Nghiem, L. T. P., Chng, S., Carrasco, L. R., & Benítez-López, A. (2023). Hotspots of zoonotic disease risk from wildlife hunting and trade in the tropics. *Integrative Conservation, 2*(4), 165–175. https://doi.org/10.1002/inc3.34

CIRAD. (2022). *Horizon Europe: CIRAD's scientific excellence has been recognized.* https://www.cirad.fr/en/press-area/press-releases/2022/horizon-europe-cirad

Costa, A., Guerrero, H., Sureau, A., Tassaint, M., & Augusto, R. D. C. (2024). Contaminated freshwater as a Harbinger of tropical disease spread in Europe. *Frontiers in Environmental Science, 12*, 1410821. https://doi.org/10.3389/fenvs.2024.1410821

Convention on Biological Diversity. Kunming-Montreal Global Biodiversity Framework (CBD/COP/DEC/15/4).Montreal: Convention on Biological Diversity; 2022. Available from: https://www.cbd.int/doc/decisions/cop-15/cop-15-dec-04-en.pdf

Cunningham, A. B., Brinckmann, J. A., Yang, X., & He, J. (2019). Introduction to the special issue: Saving plants, saving lives: Trade, sustainable harvest and conservation of traditional medicinals in Asia. *Journal of Ethnopharmacology, 229*, 288–292. https://doi.org/10.1016/j.jep.2018.10.006

Cusack, C., Sethi, S. A., Rice, A. N., Warren, J. D., Fujita, R., Ingles, J., Flores, J., Garchitorena, E., & Mesa, S. V. (2021). Marine ecotourism for small pelagics as a source of alternative income generating activities to fisheries in a tropical community. *Biological Conservation, 261*, 109242. https://doi.org/10.1016/j.biocon.2021.109242

Davidson, G., Speldewinde, P., Manin, B. O., Cook, A., Weinstein, P., & Chua, T. H. (2024). Forest restoration and the zoonotic vector Anopheles balabacensis in Sabah, Malaysia. *EcoHealth, 21*(1), 21–37. https://doi.org/10.1007/s10393-024-01675-w

Davis, C. C., & Choisy, P. (2024). Medicinal plants meet modern biodiversity science. *Current Biology, 34*(4), R158–R173. https://doi.org/10.1016/j.cub.2023.12.038

Dayapera, L. Z. A., Sy, J. C. Y., Valenzuela, S., Eala, S. J. L., Del Rosario, C. M. I. P., Buensuceso, K. N. C., Dy, A. S., Morales, D. A., Gibson, A. G., & Apostol, G. L. C. (2024). One health in the Philippines: A review and situational analysis. *One Health, 18*, 100758. https://doi.org/10.1016/j.onehlt.2024.100758

De Lira-Quezada, C. E., González-Díaz, S. N., Cotera-de Lira, A. G., Macouzet-Sánchez, C., Acuña-Ortega, N., Guzman-Avilán, R. I., & Macías-Weinmann, A. (2024). The association of air pollution in respiratory allergy: Its impact in an industrial city. *World Allergy Organization Journal, 17*(2), 100867. https://doi.org/10.1016/j.waojou.2023.100867

Diamond, J. (1997). *Guns, germs, and steel: The fates of human societies*. W. W. Norton.

Dias, D. A., Urban, S., & Roessner, U. (2012). A historical overview of natural products in drug discovery. *Metabolites, 2*(2), 303–336. https://doi.org/10.3390/metabo2020303

Doughty, C. E., Prys-Jones, T. O., Faurby, S., Abraham, A. J., Hepp, C., Leshyk, V., Fofanov, V. Y., Nieto, N. C., Svenning, J., & Galetti, M. (2020). Megafauna decline have reduced pathogen dispersal which may have increased emergent infectious diseases. *Ecography, 43*(8), 1107–1117. https://doi.org/10.1111/ecog.05209

Ellwanger, J. H., Fearnside, P. M., Ziliotto, M., Valverde-Villegas, J. M., Veiga, A. B. G. D., Vieira, G. F., Bach, E., Cardoso, J. C., Müller, N. F. D., Lopes, G., Caesar, L., Kulmann-Leal, B., Kaminski, V. L., Silveira, E. S., Spilki, F. R., Weber, M. N., Almeida, S. E. D. M., Hora, V. P. D., & Chies, J. A. B. (2022). Synthesizing the connections between environmental disturbances and zoonotic spillover. *Anais da Academia Brasileira de Ciências, 94*(suppl 3), e20211530. https://doi.org/10.1590/0001-3765202220211530

Everard, M., Johnston, P., Santillo, D., & Staddon, C. (2020). The role of ecosystems in mitigation and management of Covid-19 and other zoonoses. *Environmental Science & Policy, 111*, 7–17. https://doi.org/10.1016/j.envsci.2020.05.017

FAO. (2020). *The state of the world's forests 2020: Forests, biodiversity and people*. Food and Agriculture Organization of the United Nations.

FAO. (2022). *The state of world fisheries and aquaculture 2022*. FAO. https://doi.org/10.4060/cc0461en

FAO. (2024). *Result Asia-Pacific—Restoring and sustaining landscapes together Asia*. https://openknowledge.fao.org/items/fa54d767-9643-4ff3-935e-8ff3a29300bf

Filho, V. C. (2025). *Biodiversity as a source of medicines from nature to the market*. Cambridge Scholars Publishers.

Fujii, T., & Rohan, R. (2019). Singapore as a sustainable city: Past, present and the future. *SSRN Electronic Journal*. https://doi.org/10.2139/ssrn.3480894

Fuller, R., Landrigan, P. J., Balakrishnan, K., Bathan, G., Bose-O'Reilly, S., Brauer, M., Caravanos, J., Chiles, T., Cohen, A., Corra, L., Cropper, M., Ferraro, G., Hanna, J., Hanrahan, D., Hu, H., Hunter, D., Janata, G., Kupka, R., Lanphear, B., et al. (2022). Pollution and health: A progress update. *The Lancet Planetary Health, 6*(6), e535–e547. https://doi.org/10.1016/S2542-5196(22)00090-0

Gadgil, M., Berkes, F., & Folke, C. (1993). Indigenous knowledge for biodiversity conservation. *Ambio, 22*(2/3), 151–156.

Gautier, A., Gardon, S., & Déprés, C. (2023). The emergence of the Biodiversity/Health nexus: Making biodiversity a health issue. *Review of Agricultural, Food and Environmental Studies, 104*(1), 27–46. https://doi.org/10.1007/s41130-023-00189-3

Gibb, R., Redding, D. W., Friant, S., & Jones, K. E. (2025). Towards a 'people and nature' paradigm for biodiversity and infectious disease. *Philosophical Transactions of the Royal Society, B: Biological Sciences, 380*(1917), 20230259. https://doi.org/10.1098/rstb.2023.0259

Glowka, L., Burhenne-Guilmin, F., & Synge, H. (1994). *A guide to the convention on biological diversity*. IUCN.

Goldstein, J. E., Budiman, I., Canny, A., & Dwipartidrisa, D. (2022). Pandemics and the human-wildlife interface in Asia: Land use change as a driver of zoonotic viral outbreaks. *Environmental Research Letters, 17*(6), 063009. https://doi.org/10.1088/1748-9326/ac74d4

Gruetzmacher, K., Karesh, W. B., Amuasi, J. H., Arshad, A., Farlow, A., Gabrysch, S., Jetzkowitz, J., Lieberman, S., Palmer, C., Winkler, A. S., & Walzer, C. (2021). The Berlin principles on one health—Bridging global health and conservation. *Science of the Total Environment, 764*, 142919. https://doi.org/10.1016/j.scitotenv.2020.142919

Hammoud, R., Tognin, S., Smythe, M., Gibbons, J., Davidson, N., Bakolis, I., & Mechelli, A. (2024). Smartphone-based ecological momentary assessment reveals an incremental association between natural diversity and mental wellbeing. *Scientific Reports, 14*(1), 7051. https://doi.org/10.1038/s41598-024-55940-7

Hasyim, I. (2025, June 20). *Kementerian Kehutanan: Separuh Taman Nasional Tesso Nilo Kini Kebun Sawit Ilegal.* Tempo. https://www.tempo.co/lingkungan/kementerian-kehutanan-separuh-taman-nasional-tesso-nilo-kini-kebun-sawit-ilegal-1755596

Hauser, N., Gushiken, A. C., Narayanan, S., Kottilil, S., & Chua, J. V. (2021). Evolution of Nipah virus infection: Past, present, and future considerations. *Tropical Medicine and Infectious Disease, 6*(1), 24. https://doi.org/10.3390/tropicalmed6010024

Hendin, H., Phillips, M. R., Vijayakumar, L., Pirkis, J., Wang, H., Yip, P., & Wasserman, D. (2008). *Suicide and suicide prevention in Asia.* World Health Organization. https://iris.who.int/bitstream/handle/10665/43929/9789241596893_eng.pdf

Holdgate, M. W. (1999). *The green web: A union for world conservation.* Earthscan.

IUCN. (2008). *History of IUCN.* International Union for Conservation of Nature. https://www.iucn.org/about

IUCN. (2025). *Species.* https://iucn.org/our-work/region/asia/our-work/species

Jones, B. T. B. (2010). The evolution of Namibia's communal conservancies. In F. Nelson (Ed.), *Community rights, conservation and contested land* (pp. 106–120). Earthscan.

Keesing, F., & Ostfeld, R. S. (2021). Impacts of biodiversity and biodiversity loss on zoonotic diseases. *Proceedings of the National Academy of Sciences, 118*(17), e2023540118. https://doi.org/10.1073/pnas.2023540118

Keesing, F., Belden, L. K., Daszak, P., Dobson, A., Harvell, C. D., Holt, R. D., Hudson, P., Jolles, A., Jones, K. E., Mitchell, C. E., Myers, S. S., Bogich, T., & Ostfeld, R. S. (2010). Impacts of biodiversity on the emergence and transmission of infectious diseases. *Nature, 468*(7324), 647–652. https://doi.org/10.1038/nature09575

Kementerian Sumber Asli dan Alam Sekitar Malaysia. (2022). *National Policy on Biological Diversity (NPBD) 2022–2030.* Retrieved July 30, 2025 from https://www.nres.gov.my/ms-my/pustakamedia/Penerbitan/NPBD%202022-2030%20(Spread%20View).pdf

Klein, A. M., Vaissière, B. E., Cane, J. H., Steffan-Dewenter, I., Cunningham, S. A., Kremen, C., & Tscharntke, T. (2007). Importance of pollinators in changing landscapes for world crops. *Proceedings of the Royal Society B: Biological Sciences, 274*(1608), 303–313. https://doi.org/10.1098/rspb.2006.3721

Klim, H., William, T., Chua, T. H., Rajahram, G. S., Drakeley, C. J., Carroll, M. W., & Fornace, K. M. (2023). Quantifying human-animal contact rates in Malaysian Borneo: Influence of agricultural landscapes on contact with potential zoonotic disease reservoirs. *Frontiers in Epidemiology, 2*, 1057047. https://doi.org/10.3389/fepid.2022.1057047

Kondo, M., Fluehr, J., McKeon, T., & Branas, C. (2018). Urban green space and its impact on human health. *International Journal of Environmental Research and Public Health, 15*(3), 445. https://doi.org/10.3390/ijerph15030445

Lahcene, E., Suppasri, A., Pakoksung, K., & Imamura, F. (2024). The impact of the coral reef system on the tsunami propagation of the 2004 Indian Ocean event in North Male Atoll. *Ocean and Coastal Management, 257*, 107348. https://doi.org/10.1016/j.ocecoaman.2024.107348

Lâm, S., Dang-Xuan, S., Unger, F., Meeyam, T., Pham-Duc, P., Wacharapluesadee, S., & Nguyen-Viet, H. (2025). Operationalizing regional One Health initiatives in Southeast Asia: Ways forward. *One Health, 20*, 101034. https://doi.org/10.1016/j.onehlt.2025.101034

Larson, G., & Fuller, D. Q. (2014). The evolution of animal domestication. *Annual Review of Ecology, Evolution, and Systematics, 45*, 115–136. https://doi.org/10.1146/annurev-ecolsys-110512-135813

Leddin, D. (2024). The impact of climate change, pollution, and biodiversity loss on digestive health and disease. *Gastro Hep Advances, 3*(4), 519–534. https://doi.org/10.1016/j.gastha.2024.01.018

Lemieux, C. J., Lazarescu, C., Reining, C. E., Groulx, M. W., Lem, M., Astell-Burt, T., & Feng, X. (2025). Prescribing nature for human health: An examination of public interest, barriers, and enablers related to nature prescription programming in Canada. *Wellbeing, Space and Society, 8*, 100251. https://doi.org/10.1016/j.wss.2025.100251

Liang, W.-S., He, Y.-C., Wu, H.-D., Li, Y.-T., Shih, T.-H., Kao, G.-S., Guo, H.-Y., & Chao, D.-Y. (2020). Ecological factors associated with persistent circulation of multiple highly pathogenic avian influenza viruses among poultry farms in Taiwan during 2015–17. *PLoS ONE, 15*(8), e0236581. https://doi.org/10.1371/journal.pone.0236581

Lin, L., Yang, H., & Xu, X. (2022). Effects of water pollution on human health and disease heterogeneity: A review. *Frontiers in Environmental Science, 10*, 880246. https://doi.org/10.3389/fenvs.2022.880246

Linhares, Y., Kaganski, A., Agyare, C., Kurnaz, I. A., Neergheen, V., Kolodziejczyk, B., Kędra, M., Wahajuddin, M., El-Youssf, L., Dela Cruz, T. E., Baran, Y., Pešić, M., Shrestha, U., Bakiu, R., Allard, P.-M., Rybtsov, S., Pieri, M., Siciliano, V., & Flores Bueso, Y. (2023). Biodiversity: The overlooked source of human health. *Trends in Molecular Medicine, 29*(3), 173–187. https://doi.org/10.1016/j.molmed.2022.12.002

Ma, K., & Wu, L. (2025). Perceived biodiversity of public greenspace and mental well-being. *Environmental Research, 269*, 120878. https://doi.org/10.1016/j.envres.2025.120878

Mace, G., Masundire, H., & Baillie, J. (2005). *Ecosystems and human well-being: Current state and trends*. https://www.millenniumassessment.org/documents/document.273.aspx.pdf

Maes, T., & Messing, D. (2025). Food for thought: Marine pollution's impact on One Health and food security in African SIDS. *Regional Studies in Marine Science, 85*, 104136. https://doi.org/10.1016/j.rsma.2025.104136

Mainka, S., & Trivedi, M. (with World Conservation Union). (2002). *Links between biodiversity conservation, livelihoods and food security: The sustainable use of wild species for meat*. IUCN.

Marselle, M. R., Hartig, T., Cox, D. T. C., De Bell, S., Knapp, S., Lindley, S., Triguero-Mas, M., Böhning-Gaese, K., Braubach, M., Cook, P. A., De Vries, S., Heintz-Buschart, A., Hofmann, M., Irvine, K. N., Kabisch, N., Kolek, F., Kraemer, R., Markevych, I., Martens, D., et al. (2021). Pathways linking biodiversity to human health: A conceptual framework. *Environment International, 150*, 106420. https://doi.org/10.1016/j.envint.2021.106420

McCormick, J. (1991). *Reclaiming paradise: The global environmental movement*. Indiana University Press.

McNeil, C., Verlander, S., Divi, N., & Smolinski, M. (2022). The landscape of participatory surveillance systems across the one health spectrum: Systematic review. *JMIR Public Health and Surveillance, 8*(8), e38551. https://doi.org/10.2196/38551

Meena, P., & Jha, V. (2023). Environmental change, changing biodiversity, and infections–Lessons for kidney health community. *Kidney International Reports, 8*(9), 1714–1729. https://doi.org/10.1016/j.ekir.2023.07.002

Meng, L., Li, S., & Zhang, X. (2024). Exploring biodiversity's impact on mental well-being through the social-ecological lens: Emphasizing the role of biodiversity characteristics and nature relatedness. *Environmental Impact Assessment Review, 105*, 107454. https://doi.org/10.1016/j.eiar.2024.107454

Ministry of the Environment, Japan. (2022). *Satoyama in Japan*. Retrieved August 8, 2025, from https://www.env.go.jp/nature/satoyama/pdf/satoyama2022E.pdf

Mitsch, W. J., & Gosselink, J. G. (2015). *Wetlands* (5th ed.). Wiley.

Moeliono, M., Thuy, P. T., Bong, I. W., Wong, G. Y., & Brockhaus, M. (2017). Social forestry—Why and for whom? A comparison of policies in Vietnam and Indonesia. *Forest and Society, 1*(2), 1–20. https://doi.org/10.24259/fs.v1i2.2484

NACSO (Namibian Association of CBNRM Support Organisations). (2013). *The state of community conservation in Namibia: Annual report 2013*. NACSO.

Neergheen-Bhujun, V., Awan, A. T., Baran, Y., Bunnefeld, N., Chan, K., Dela Cruz, T. E., Egamberdieva, D., Elsässer, S., Johnson, M. V., Komai, S., Konevega, A. L., Malone, J. H., Mason, P., Nguon, R., Piper, R., Shrestha, U. B., Pešić, M., & Kagansky, A. (2017). Biodiversity, drug discovery, and the future of global health: Introducing the biodiversity to biomedicine consortium, a call to action. *Journal of Global Health, 7*(2), 020304. https://doi.org/10.7189/jogh.07.020304

Nordhagen, S., Lambertini, E., DeWaal, C. S., McClafferty, B., & Neufeld, L. M. (2022). Integrating nutrition and food safety in food systems policy and programming. *Global Food Security, 32*, 100593. https://doi.org/10.1016/j.gfs.2021.100593

Omidian, H., Wilson, R. L., & Babanejad, N. (2023). Bioinspired polymers: Transformative applications in biomedicine and regenerative medicine. *Life, 13*(8), 1673. https://doi.org/10.3390/life13081673

Pagiola, S. (2008). Payments for environmental services in Costa Rica. *Ecological Economics, 65*(4), 712–724. https://doi.org/10.1016/j.ecolecon.2007.07.033

Pimm, S. L., Russell, G. J., Gittleman, J. L., & Brooks, T. M. (1995). The future of biodiversity. *Science, 269*(5222), 347–350. https://doi.org/10.1126/science.269.5222.347

Pimm, S. L., Jenkins, C. N., Abell, R., Brooks, T. M., Gittleman, J. L., Joppa, L. N., Raven, P. H., Roberts, C. M., & Sexton, J. O. (2014). The biodiversity of species and their rates of extinction, distribution, and protection. *Science, 344*(6187), 1246752. https://doi.org/10.1126/science.1246752

Platto, S., Zhou, J., Wang, Y., Wang, H., & Carafoli, E. (2021). Biodiversity loss and COVID-19 pandemic: The role of bats in the origin and the spreading of the disease. *Biochemical and Biophysical Research Communications, 538*, 2–13. https://doi.org/10.1016/j.bbrc.2020.10.028

Posey, D. A. (1999). *Cultural and spiritual values of biodiversity*. United Nations Environment Programme & Intermediate Technology Publications.

Potts, S. G., Biesmeijer, J. C., Kremen, C., Neumann, P., Schweiger, O., & Kunin, W. E. (2010). Global pollinator declines: Trends, impacts and drivers. *Trends in Ecology & Evolution, 25*(6), 345–353. https://doi.org/10.1016/j.tree.2010.01.007

Prist, P. R., Prado, A., Tambosi, L. R., Umetsu, F., De Arruda Bueno, A., Pardini, R., & Metzger, J. P. (2021). Moving to healthier landscapes: Forest restoration decreases the abundance of Hantavirus reservoir rodents in tropical forests. *Science of the Total Environment, 752*, 141967. https://doi.org/10.1016/j.scitotenv.2020.141967

Requier, F., Pérez-Méndez, N., Andersson, G. K. S., Blareau, E., Merle, I., & Garibaldi, L. A. (2023). Bee and non-bee pollinator importance for local food security. *Trends in Ecology & Evolution, 38*(2), 196–205. https://doi.org/10.1016/j.tree.2022.10.006

Rozario, K., Oh, R. R. Y., Marselle, M., Schröger, E., Gillerot, L., Ponette, Q., Godbold, D., Haluza, D., Kilpi, K., Müller, D., Roeber, U., Verheyen, K., Muys, B., Müller, S., Shaw, T., & Bonn, A. (2024). The more the merrier? Perceived forest biodiversity promotes short-term mental health and well-being—A multicentre study. *People and Nature, 6*(1), 180–201. https://doi.org/10.1002/pan3.10564

Sabu, C., Rejo, C., Kotta, S., & Pramod, K. (2018). Bioinspired and biomimetic systems for advanced drug and gene delivery. *Journal of Controlled Release, 287*, 142–155. https://doi.org/10.1016/j.jconrel.2018.08.033

Sanchez-Azofeifa, G. A., Pfaff, A., Robalino, J. A., & Boomhower, J. P. (2007). Costa Rica's payment for environmental services program: Intention, implementation, and impact. *Conservation Biology, 21*(5), 1165–1173. https://doi.org/10.1111/j.1523-1739.2007.00751.x

Sardana, K., & Simpson, R. D. (2023). Mainstreaming biodiversity into policy—Do the numbers add-up? *Environmental and Sustainability Indicators, 20*, 100314. https://doi.org/10.1016/j.indic.2023.100314

Scannell, J. W., & Bosley, J. (2016). When quality beats quantity: Decision theory, drug discovery, and the reproducibility crisis. *PLoS ONE, 11*(2), e0147215. https://doi.org/10.1371/journal.pone.0147215

Siegel, D. (Ed.). (2021). *Notes from isolation: Global criminological perspectives on coronavirus pandemic*. Eleven International Publishing.

Smith, W. (2022). Understanding the changing role of global public health in biodiversity conservation. *Ambio, 51*(3), 485–493. https://doi.org/10.1007/s13280-021-01576-0

Soroos, M. S. (1997). *The endangered atmosphere: Preserving a global commons*. University of South Carolina Press.

Strong, M. F. (1973). One year after Stockholm: An ecological approach to management. *Foreign Affairs, 51*(4), 690–707.

Supriatna, J. (2018). *Konservasi Biodiversitas: Teori dan Praktik di Indonesia, Jatna Supriatna*. Yayasan Pustaka Obor Indonesia.

Takacs, D. (1996). *The idea of biodiversity: Philosophies of paradise*. Johns Hopkins University Press.

Teerawattananon, Y., Dabak, S. V., Isaranuwatchai, W., Lertwilairatanapong, T., Shafie, A. A., Suwantika, A. A., Oh, C., Srisasalux, J., & Cheanklin, N. (2022). What can we learn from others to develop a regional centre for infectious diseases in ASEAN? Comment on "Operationalising Regional Cooperation for Infectious Disease Control: A Scoping Review of Regional Disease Control Bodies and Networks". *International Journal of Health Policy and Management, 1*. https://doi.org/10.34172/ijhpm.2022.7281

Terraube, J., & Fernández-Llamazares, Á. (2020). Strengthening protected areas to halt biodiversity loss and mitigate pandemic risks. *Current Opinion in Environmental Sustainability, 46*, 35–38. https://doi.org/10.1016/j.cosust.2020.08.014

Thomford, N. E., Senthebane, D. A., Rowe, A., Munro, D., Seele, P., Maroyi, A., & Dzobo, K. (2018). Natural products for drug discovery in the 21st century: Innovations for novel drug discovery. *International Journal of Molecular Sciences, 19*(6), 1578. https://doi.org/10.3390/ijms19061578

UN. (1992). Convention on biological diversity. *United Nations Treaty Series, 1760*, 79.

UNEP. (2012). *The first 40 years: A narrative (1972–2012)*. United Nations Environment Programme.

Watson, J. E. M., Dudley, N., Segan, D. B., & Hockings, M. (2014). The performance and potential of protected areas. *Nature, 515*(7525), 67–73. https://doi.org/10.1038/nature13947

Webb, K., Jennings, J., & Minovi, D. (2018). A community-based approach integrating conservation, livelihoods, and health care in Indonesian Borneo. *The Lancet Planetary Health, 2*, S26. https://doi.org/10.1016/S2542-5196(18)30111-6

Westlund, L., Charles, A., Garcia, S. M., & Sanders, J. (Eds.). (2017). *Marine protected areas: Interactions with fishery livelihoods and food security*. FAO.

Weston, P. (2024). Biodiversity loss is biggest driver of infectious disease outbreaks, says study. *The Guardian*. https://www.theguardian.com/environment/article/2024/may/09/biodiversity-loss-is-biggest-driver-of-infectious-disease-outbreaks-says-study

WHO. (2022a). *New report highlights the impact of changes in environment on One Health*. https://www.who.int/europe/news/item/01-07-2022-new-report-highlights-the-impact-of-changes-in-environment-on-one-health

WHO. (2022b). *One health joint plan of action (2022–2026): Working together for the health of humans, animals, plants and the environment*. https://www.who.int/publications/i/item/9789240059139

Wilson, E. O. (1988). *Biodiversity*. National Academy Press.

Wood, C. L., McInturff, A., Young, H. S., Kim, D., & Lafferty, K. D. (2017). Human infectious disease burdens decrease with urbanization but not with biodiversity. *Philosophical Transactions of the Royal Society, B: Biological Sciences, 372*(1722), 20160122. https://doi.org/10.1098/rstb.2016.0122

Woodie, A. (2024). *Graphing biodiversity to improve drug discovery*. https://www.hpcwire.com/2025/02/20/graphing-biodiversity-to-improve-drug-discovery/

WWF. (2021). *Our history*. World Wide Fund for Nature. https://www.worldwildlife.org/about/history

Young, H. S., Dirzo, R., Helgen, K. M., McCauley, D. J., Billeter, S. A., Kosoy, M. Y., Osikowicz, L. M., Salkeld, D. J., Young, T. P., & Dittmar, K. (2014). Declines in large wildlife increase landscape-level prevalence of rodent-borne disease in Africa. *Proceedings of the National Academy of Sciences, 111*(19), 7036–7041. https://doi.org/10.1073/pnas.1404958111

Yuningsih, Mardiana, N., Jima, H., & Prasetya, M. D. (2023). The effect of hustle culture on psychological distress with self compassion as moderating variable. In R. Perdana, G. E. Putrawan, B. Saputra, & T. Y. Septiawan (Eds.), *Proceedings of the 3rd Universitas Lampung International Conference on Social Sciences (ULICoSS 2022)* (Vol. 740, pp. 1062–1073). Atlantis Press SARL. https://doi.org/10.2991/978-2-38476-046-6_102

Zeder, M. A. (2008). Domestication and early agriculture in the Mediterranean Basin: Origins, diffusion, and impact. *Proceedings of the National Academy of Sciences, 105*(33), 11597–11604. https://doi.org/10.1073/pnas.0801317105

Zhu, J. (2017). *The urban transition and beyond: Facing new challenges of the mobility and settlement transitions in Asia*. United Nations, Department of Economic and Social Affairs, Population Division. https://www.un.org/development/desa/pd/sites/www.un.org.development.desa.pd/files/unpd_egm_201709_s3_paper-zhu-final-rev1.pdf

Convention on Biological Diversity. Kunming-Montreal Global Biodiversity Framework (CBD/COP/DEC/15/4). Montreal: Convention on Biological Diversity; 2022. Available from: https://www.cbd.int/doc/decisions/cop-15/cop-15-dec-04-en.pdf

Chapter 9
Emerging Infectious Disease

Ratna Dwi Puji Astuti, Annisa Utami Rauf, Thoriq Abi Pramana, and Qotru A. N.

9.1 Introduction

Emerging infectious diseases (EIDs) are newly identified infectious diseases or those that have markedly escalated in incidence and geographic spread, presenting a substantial challenge to global public health, economic stability, and social systems. World Health Organization (WHO) defines EIDs as an infectious disease that has newly appeared in a population or that has been known for some time but is rapidly increasing in incidence or geographic range (Kayingo, 2023). Table 9.1 shows the list of EIDs, which have become global public health concern.

The convergence of ecological, environmental, and socioeconomic factors in the region may contribute to the dynamic of disease emergence, affecting the spread and transmission of myriads of pathogens. Climate change has been known as a

R. D. P. Astuti (✉)
Department of Environmental Health, Faculty of Public Health, Universitas Airlangga, Surabaya, Indonesia
e-mail: ratna.dwi@fkm.unair.ac.id

A. U. Rauf
Department of Health Behavior, Environment, and Social Medicine, Faculty of Medicine, Public Health, and Nursing, Universitas Gadjah Mada, Sleman, Yogyakarta, Indonesia
e-mail: annisaur@ugm.ac.id

T. A. Pramana · Qotru A. N.
Master of Public Health Program, Faculty of Medicine, Public Health, and Nursing, Universitas Gadjah Mada, Yogyakarta, Indonesia
e-mail: thoriqabipramana@mail.ugm.ac.id; qotru.alnaday@mail.ugm.ac.id

© The Author(s), under exclusive license to Springer Nature Singapore Pte Ltd. 2026

A. U. Rauf, T. Wibawa (eds.), *The One Health Concept in Asian Contexts*,
https://doi.org/10.1007/978-981-95-9880-9_9

Table 9.1 Global emerging infectious diseases (EIDs)

Agent	Type of microbes	Transmission or route	Disease in human
Human Immunodeficiency virus	Virus	Sexual contact, injection of body fluids	AIDS
MERS-COV	Virus	Droplets and aerosols	Middle Eastern respiratory syndrome
Ebola Virus	Virus	Direct contact with body fluid	Ebola hemorrhagic disease
SARS-COV	Virus	Droplets and aerosols	Severe acute respiratory syndrome
SARS-COV-2	Virus	Droplets and aerosols	COVID19
H5N1 Virus	Virus	Droplets and aerosols	Avian Influenza
West nile virus	Virus	Vector (mosquitos)	West Nile Fever
Marburg virus and Ravn virus	Virus	Direct contact	Marburg hemorrhagic fever
Hendra virus	Virus	Direct contact	Flu-like illness
Escherichia coli O157:H7	Bacteria	Fecal-oral route	Gastrointestinal infection
Cryptosporidium	Protozoa	Fecal-oral route	Gastrointestinal infection
Hanta virus	Virus	Vector (rodents)	Hantavirus pulmonary disease
Yersinia Pestis	Bacteria	Vector (rodents)	Plague
Streptococcus aureus	Bacteria	Contact contagion	Skin infection
Lassa virus	Virus	Ingestion and direct contact	Lassa fever
Clostridium difficile	Bacteria	Fecal-oral route	Pseudomembranous colitis
Whitewater arroyo virus	Virus	Inhalation	Hemorrhagic fever
Candida auris	Fungi	Direct and indirect contact	Severe infection leading to death
Blastomyces dermatitidis	Fungi	Inhalation	Atypical and disseminated blastomycosis
Rasamsonia argillacea	Fungi	Unknown	Chronic granulomatous disease, hematologic malignancies, and colonization in cystic fibrosis patients.
Sporothrix brasiliensis	Fungi	Cat-transmitted	Sporotrichosis
Schistosoma mansoni	Protozoa	Contact-contaminated water	Schistosomiasis
Trichophyton indotineae	Fungi	Sexual contact	Recalcitrant dematophytoses,

(continued)

Table 9.1 (continued)

Agent	Type of microbes	Transmission or route	Disease in human
Schistosoma haematobium	Protozoa	Contact-contaminated water	Schistosomiasis
Aspergillus Fumigatus	Fungi	Airborne	Aspergilosis
Schistosoma japonicum	Protozoa	Contact-contaminated water	Schistosomiasis
Norovirus	Virus	Ingestion	Severe diarrhea, gastroenteritis
Nipah Virus	Virus	Direct contact	Severe encephalitis and respiratory disease
Vibrio Cholerae	Bacteria	Fecal-oral route	Cholera

References: Kayingo (2023) and Ristori et al. (2024)

critical driver influencing the geographical distribution and incidence of infectious disease, especially those transmitted by vectors like mice, mosquitoes, and ticks (Bouzid et al., 2014; Lyth et al., 2005). For instance, modification in climate variables such as temperature and precipitation will alter the habitats of vectors, which are responsible for diseases like malaria and dengue, prompting warnings about potential outbreaks in regions historically considered safe.

Recent outbreaks such as pandemic COVID-19 and severe acute respiratory syndrome (SARS) have also underscored the critical roles of both public health infrastructure and environmental dynamics in disease emergence and dissemination across the Asian region. Moreover, there are zoonotic diseases that can be influenced by complex socio-environmental dynamics such as urbanization, agricultural intensification, and climate change. Despite the emphasis on infectious diseases stemming from animal reservoirs, the importance of human factors should not be overlooked. Human factors that may influence the spread of pathogens are rapid population growth, international trade, and travel.

The EIDs in Asia are a complex issue intimately connected to environmental changes, socioeconomic factors, and disparities in healthcare. Some findings highlight the relevance of a comprehensive approach that combines robust surveillance, health system strengthening, and community engagement to combat existing and future challenges associated with EIDs. As the landscape of infectious diseases evolves, proactive efforts in Asia will be critical in safeguarding public health and enhancing global health security. Figure 9.1 is the history of EIDs pandemic in Asia region.

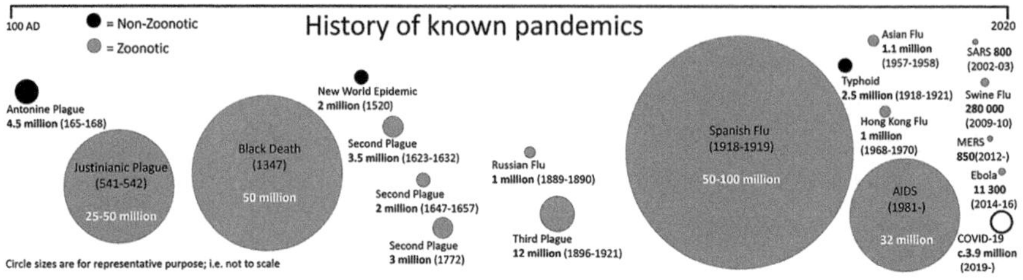

Fig. 9.1 History of known pandemic. (Mishra et al., 2022, licensed under CC-BY 4.0)

9.2 Factors Contributing to the Emergence of EIDs

Recently, numerous outbreaks of EIDs have had a significant impact such as West African Ebola Virus Disease between 2013 and 2016, which led to over 11,000 fatalities. Similarly, the emergence of SARS-COV in 2003, MERS-COV in 2012, SARS-COV-2 in 2019, and avian influenza has triggered widespread outbreaks, with a billion people infected by viruses, and a million deaths worldwide (Anwar et al., 2024; Hui & Zumla, 2019; Jacob et al., 2020, p. 202; Zhang et al., 2020). Spanish influenza pandemic in 1918 caused more than 25 million deaths (Wu et al., 2022). Other than that, arboviruses also constitute a significant and growing public health concern. These viruses, spread and transmitted to humans by arthropod vectors such as mosquitoes, ticks, and fleas, have shown expanding geographic distribution due to factors including global trade, human migration, biodiversity loss, and climate change.

About 60% of global EIDs are of zoonotic origin, and 70% of the diseases originated from wildlife (Krause, 1994). Several EIDs' emergence has been relevant to human activities that place people in expanded contact with wildlife carrying various unfamiliar microbes. Those unfamiliar microbes may lead to pathogen spillover (Jones et al., 2008; Krause, 1994; Morse, 1995). In the context of the contemporary globalization era, the rise of EIDs has been intensified by heightened levels of global trade and human mobility.

A wide range of interconnected factors operating at the environment–human–animal interface collectively contributes to the emergence of EIDs. Changes in ecosystems, human behavior and development, animal populations, and environmental conditions interact in complex ways to create opportunities for novel pathogens to arise and spread. Once these diseases emerge, they can have profound and far-reaching adverse consequences, affecting animal health, disrupting environmental balance, and posing serious threats to human health and well-being.

(a) *Socioeconomic Factor*

A large human population enables the introduction, spread, and maintenance of disease pathogens among its members. For instance, the number of susceptible individuals required for the measles virus to maintain its presence in the area is 200,000 or more (Ka-Wai Hui, 2006). A prior study from Fu and Zhu (2024) using econometric model showed that the influx of human populations will have both direct and indirect effects on infectious diseases. The direct influence is associated with an elevated risk of infectious diseases. The indirect influence of intensified air pollution is expected to affect the incidence rate of infectious diseases (Fu & Zhu, 2024). The influence of population influx is also evident in the diversity. For instance, when comparing the central and western regions of China, the eastern area shows a markedly higher risk of infectious diseases compared to the western area. External factors impact the connection between infectious diseases and population influx, with elements like medical and educational resources and personal income serving to reduce the risk associated with infectious diseases stemming from population influx. Rising population density will facilitate the proliferation of EIDs via mechanisms such as human-to-human transmission and various ecological factors, including heightened agricultural demand, altered land use, and intensified livestock production. A previous study indicated that megacities with high population density may serve as incubators for new zoonotic diseases and epidemics, as the dense population facilitates rapid transmission of disease (Neiderud, 2015).

Urbanization is also drivers for EID transmission and spread in Asia. Urbanization refers to the movement and settling of people in urban regions. Urbanization is correlated to the changes in social structures, extended and changing social networks, and increased personal mobility. The resurgence of dengue in Southeast Asia is associated with the development of peri-urban areas where inadequate water and sanitation facilities, along with the accumulation of social debris such as discarded tires, create breeding sites for Aedes mosquitoes (Mackenzie et al., 2004). Reduced birth and mortality rates, as observed in Thailand, may contribute to a decrease in the transmission of certain diseases (Cummings et al., 2009).

Increasing people's mobility is correlated to the transmission of EIDs. The significant influx of economic and political refugees, along with the regular migration of hill tribe populations and their livestock, poses considerable challenges to cross-border disease management in the Mekong Basin subregion. Consequently, the impoverished migrant will reside in unsanitary and congested conditions, exacerbating the risk of EID transmission (Delacollette et al., 2009; Dondorp et al., 2010). The increase in natural migration and animal trade across borders will also elevate the risk of EIDs. The increasing demand for food, coupled with rapid population growth in Asia, is driving a rise in livestock production. The correlation between increased poultry density and avian influenza cases in humans in Asia is evident. The expansion of pig farming raises concerns regarding the transmission of Nipah virus, Japanese encephalitis, and influenza viruses (Coker et al., 2011).

(b) *Environmental Factor*

Ecological alterations, particularly those resulting from economic or agricultural advancement, are among the most recognized contributors to EIDs. They are particularly prevalent as contributors to disease outbreaks with elevated case fatality rates, such as zoonotic diseases. Agricultural intensification and ecological changes are key drivers of the EIDs, as they impact ecological structures at both community and landscape levels. Alterations in landscapes modify host population dynamics, resulting in increased interaction between human societies and wildlife reservoirs, hence enhancing risk of EIDs and pathogen spillover (Faust et al., 2018; Jones et al., 2013).

Environmental factors may facilitate interaction between humans and unknown hosts for infection or ecological reservoirs, either by enhancing proximity, or, more commonly, by altering conditions to promote population of pathogens or their natural hosts. For instance, the hantavirus. It will spread during rice harvest, when the population of mice will increase in that season. Humans and mice will contact each other frequently in that season. Another example is the Junin virus, the pathogen responsible for Argentine hemorrhagic fever (AHF), which is transmitted via mice. A rodent that was the virus's natural host was favored by the alteration of grassland to maize cultivation, and the number of human cases rose in direct proportion to the increase of maize agriculture (Jones et al., 2013). Alteration of land is closely correlated with an increase in EIDs cases (Faust et al., 2018; Jones et al., 2013). A later study stated that while the relationship between land use changes and pathogen transmission is evident, identifying specific mechanisms remains challenging (Faust et al., 2018). The alteration in land use, whether through urban expansion or agricultural development, disrupts existing ecosystems and changes disease ecology, contributing to the emergence of infectious diseases. As shown in a study by Hahn et al. (2014) alterations in land use and ecosystem configurations significantly influence Nipah virus transmission in Bangladesh (Hahn et al., 2014). The habitat modifications increase spillover likelihood from wildlife reservoirs, amplifying the risk of zoonotic disease becoming endemic in human population. Human-induced changes in land use are main factors for elevated EIDs and modified factors for endemic disease transmission.

A study by Mackenzie et al. (2004) demonstrated that the development of rice fields can enhance the transmission of vector-borne diseases, such as Japanese encephalitis, by serving as breeding sites for vectors and attracting water birds, which are natural reservoirs of the disease (Mackenzie et al., 2004). The presence of various bird species correlates with an increased risk of avian influenza outbreaks in Thailand and Vietnam (Gilbert et al., 2008). Deforestation enhances the interactions among humans, livestock, and wildlife. This will increase the likelihood of pathogens crossing species barriers. Alterations in bat populations and their movements in Malaysia, linked to wildfires, deforestation, the creation of fruit orchards, and the growth of pig farming adjacent to bat habitats, have been suggested as factors influencing the transmission of the Nipah virus in the area (Chua et al., 1999; Lo & Rota, 2008; Patz et al., 2004).

9.3 Surveillance and Early Warning Systems for EIDs

The development of surveillance systems for EIDs in Asia has progressed significantly, though with notable variation among countries. Nations such as Australia and Japan have already established monitoring networks that span both hospital and community levels (Iera et al., 2025; Kajihara et al., 2021), while China has advanced its surveillance capacity through an integrated One Health approach in their policy and community levels (Zhou et al., 2025). This framework encourages cooperation across disciplines and promotes the use of multi-trigger monitoring tools to address the interconnected risks between humans, animals, and the environment. Similarly, Taiwan has implemented an emergency department-based syndromic surveillance system that has improved its pandemic response and early detection of disease outbreaks. Collectively, these efforts underscore the growing recognition that integrating surveillance data from human, animal, and environmental sources enables more comprehensive disease prediction, risk management, and prevention, thereby reinforcing both regional and global health security (Jian et al., 2017).

Although progress has been made, the implementation of robust and unified surveillance and early warning systems across Asia still faces substantial barriers (Ben Jebara, 2004). Many current programs remain fragmented, focusing primarily on individual sectors or addressing immediate health threats without adequately considering long-term or emerging risks. Major constraints include the lack of an overarching framework for integrated disease surveillance, limited mechanisms for sharing and analyzing data, and insufficient tools for detecting real-time epidemiological changes shaped by climate and population dynamics (Liu, 2025; Pham et al., 2025). To overcome these issues, continuous efforts are needed to enhance interdisciplinary research, apply advanced technologies such as artificial intelligence and big data analytics, and build professional capacity to support cross-sector collaboration (Shen et al., 2025).

Low- and middle-income countries in Southeast Asia face heightened risks from EIDs, as most current initiatives remain concentrated on immediate outbreak responses rather than proactive mitigation and preparedness measures (de Sa et al., 2010; Pham et al., 2025). The absence of coordinated and sustained regional actions, along with limited investment in early detection systems, continues to impede the timely identification of zoonotic spillover events and the control of disease spread. As one of the world's major hotspots for EIDs, Southeast Asia contends with intertwined social, environmental, and economic transformations such as rapid urbanization, ecosystem disruption, and agricultural expansion that intensify vulnerability to zoonotic and vector-borne infections (Coker et al., 2011; Moss et al., 2016; Saba Villarroel et al., 2023). These challenges underscore the urgent need to operationalize the One Health framework through stronger collaboration among governments, communities, donors, and international organizations. Furthermore, insufficient population health data, fragmented healthcare infrastructure, and weak surveillance networks across the Asia Pacific region hinder effective risk evaluation and decision-making.

9.4 Global Health Preparedness and Response to EIDs

When the COVID-19 pandemic hit in the beginning of 2020, nations around the world realized the tragic truth: no country was totally prepared. Countries with strong efforts on global health security indices struggled with controlling the epidemic. Emergency rooms packed, testing systems failed, and supply systems for personal protective equipment and ventilators crumbled apart (Priya et al., 2024; Van Nguyen et al., 2020). There were no universally agreed-upon case management methods, standardized mass testing strategies, or pre-made plans to scale up medical services during a crisis. Governments hurried to develop standards for prevention, treatment, and public communication—often in actual time, under heavy political and public scrutiny.

Asia's susceptibility for EIDs is fostered by fast socioeconomic alteration, environmental turbulence, and intense patterns of both human and animal migration. These interactions not only raise the risk of zoonotic spillover but also expedite the transmission of pathogens across territories (Fang et al., 2024). As a global hotspot for zoonotic infections, the region confronts increased hazards to human, animal, and environmental health. In response, countries in Asia and the Pacific have begun to strengthen their health-care systems by investing in surveillance, participatory field research, and forecast disease modeling. Regional partnerships have also gained traction, with states collaborating on preparedness initiatives and knowledge sharing. International collaboration, such as ecological study partnerships between China and the United States, has proven critical for creating more integrated, One Health-focused approaches. Although the region has made significant progress in increasing its ability to recognize and respond to emerging risks, long-term health security and resilience require ongoing investment and cross-sectoral collaboration (Asian Development Bank et al., 2018; Horby et al., 2013; Smiley Evans et al., 2020; Ward & Brookes, 2021).

Preparedness could be defined as the ability of health system to precisely and rapidly identify, prevent, and effectively respond to infectious diseases that pose a threat on a global, national, or regional scale. It includes a wide range of actions such as surveillance, laboratory capacity, a skilled health workers, risk communication, and cross-sectoral collaboration. Infectious diseases transcend boundaries; therefore effective preparedness must operate across multiple levels: global, regional, and national. For example, local discovery of a zoonotic outbreak can minimize regional spread, yet global preparedness structures are required for equal access to vaccinations and countermeasures (Adnyana et al., 2023; Althubyani et al., 2025; Saba Villarroel et al., 2023). The COVID-19 pandemic highlighted the significance of preparedness, revealing significant variations in health system readiness, data exchange, and response coordination. Frameworks such as the International Health Regulations (IHR 2005), the Asia Pacific Strategy for Emerging Diseases (APSED III), and the WHO Pandemic Agreement (WHO CA+) give systematic advice for countries in developing and assessing their preparedness capacities.

Preparedness can be multimodal, including both health-specific capabilities and broader systemic enablers. The Epidemic Preparedness Index (EPI) proposed by Oppenheim et al. (2019) provides a systematic framework for assessing national readiness in five important domains: public health infrastructure, physical infrastructure, institutional capacity, economic resources, and public health communication (Oppenheim et al., 2019). Each sub-index contains quantifiable factors such as surveillance systems, health workforce, water and sanitation, internet availability, political stability, and health financing. This concept highlights that epidemic preparedness is dependent not only on health sector performance but also on the underlying political, infrastructural, and economic conditions that allow for an effective response.

According to APSED III, preparedness strategies should identify susceptible groups, assure the ability to respond to these risks, and increase data collection, analysis, and usage capabilities to identify vulnerable populations. Broader efforts to change health service delivery should also be involved so that vulnerable populations are regularly reached. Ensuring preparedness comprises not just having the ability to respond to emergent threats, but also tailoring that response to the needs of such communities (Gongal et al., 2020). To accomplish this, countries are encouraged to improve data systems to allow for real-time collection, disaggregation, analysis, and utilization of data reflecting socioeconomic and demographic risks. Furthermore, preparedness should be integrated into broader healthcare system reforms that prioritize inclusive service delivery, ensuring that populations at risk are not only included in emergency response plans but also frequently engaged through community-based efforts, mobile health services, and culturally relevant interaction. By focusing preparedness on equity and inclusivity, public health systems can boost resilience and reduce the disproportionate effect of health emergencies on vulnerable groups.

Strengthening preparedness and response to EIDs necessitates a diverse strategy. Primary strategies include creating strategic frameworks that are aligned with national priorities and global guidelines, integrating diverse disease identification and response instruments, and learning from prior epidemics to improve future preparedness. Robust surveillance systems, laboratory capacity, skilled workers, and collaboration with the private sector and communities are all essential elements (Edelstein et al., 2018). Research priorities for boosting preparedness include improving health workers' knowledge and skills, assuring data quality, addressing vaccination reluctance, protecting health workers, and enhancing contact tracing and laboratory infrastructure. To accommodate evolving disease causes, preparedness criteria must be evaluated and updated on a continuous basis. Political commitment along with adequate budget allocation is critical for the successful execution of these measures (Degeling et al., 2015; Lajaunie & Morand, 2024; Lâm et al., 2025; Perez Arredondo, 2022).

9.5 The Role of International Cooperation in Addressing EIDs

The EIDs pose a global hazard that transborder, making international cooperation not only desirable but also necessary. Because infections transcend national borders, outbreaks in one place can quickly turn into pandemics. Dr. Tedros Adhanom Ghebreyesus, Director-General of the World Health Organization, clearly highlighted this requirement during the Second Special Session of the World Health Assembly in November 2021, stating: *"No region, no country, no community, and no individual is safe until we are all safe."* This interrelated vulnerability emphasizes the importance of coordinated surveillance, standardized processes, and fair access to prevention and response resources (WHO, 2021).

International cooperation in EIDs takes several forms, including shared standards, technical support, cooperative monitoring systems, capacity building, and pooling resources. In Asia, a variety of actors contribute to the cooperative landscape. The Quadripartite coalition, which promotes the One Health concept, is comprised of multilateral agencies such as the WHO (via SEARO and WPRO), the Food and Agriculture Organization (FAO), the World Organisation for Animal Health (WOAH), and the United Nations Environment Programme (UNEP) (Couradeau et al., 2025; De La Rocque et al., 2023; Lajaunie & Morand, 2025). ASEAN's Emergency Operations Center (EOC) Network, the ASEAN BioDiaspora Virtual Centre, and the newly established ASEAN Centre for Public Health Emergencies and Emerging Diseases (ACPHEED) are examples of regional procedures. Subregional initiatives, such as the Mekong Basin Disease Surveillance (MBDS) network, promote cross-border cooperation among Thailand, Cambodia, Laos, Vietnam, and Myanmar. Philanthropic groups such as the Gates Foundation, financial bodies like the World Bank and ADB, and bilateral donors such as JICA, USAID, DFAT, GIZ, and the European Union also play important roles (Caballero-Anthony, 2018; Miranda et al., 2021).

According to Durrance-Bagale (2021), while establishing regional bodies for infectious disease control is multifaceted, it may be achievable with strong foundations and dedication to key areas such as organizational systems, diagnostic and detection capacity, workforce development, communication pathways, accreditation processes, funding mechanisms, and sustainability. Success is more conceivable when stakeholders are involved early in the process to maintain local relevance, and employees are supported through capacity-building and mentorship programs, which can boost motivation and reduce attrition (Durrance-Bagale et al., 2021). FAO's, OIE's, and WHO's tripartite coordination structure in the Asia-Pacific area exemplifies successful international cooperation. This method encouraged collaboration between the animal and human health sectors, resulting in the formation of a regional coordination system. Since 2010, it has also conducted eight Asia-Pacific workshops on multisectoral collaboration for zoonotic prevention and control, supporting One Health advocacy and operationalization at the regional and national levels (Gongal et al., 2020).

Multisectoral collaboration is an essential component of the One Health concept. The Pearl River Declaration, which emerged from the Second International Symposium on One Health Research, calls for the formation of a One Health Cooperation Network in the Southeast Asia-Pacific. This network strives to improve regional health security by exchanging expertise, investing in workforce development, and promoting scientific advancements like vaccine research and development. The declaration also underlines the value of sharing epidemic knowledge, risk identification, communication, and response strategies (Alam et al., 2020). Effective surveillance and response systems are critical for recognizing and combating emerging illnesses. A three-step approach has been proposed to achieve comprehensive One Health disease surveillance and response. This method entails simultaneously investigating and managing endemic zoonoses, studying developing illnesses, and improving understanding of variables driving the formation of novel pathogens (Morris & Wang, 2024).

9.6 International Data Sharing and Reporting

The increasing interconnectedness of the world through globalization, international trade, and air travel has significantly accelerated the spread of infectious diseases. Within less than a day, infected travelers can reach almost any location worldwide, increasing the risk of a localized outbreak evolving into a global pandemic. The SARS outbreak in 2003 serves as a striking example of this phenomenon. During that period, international travelers from countries such as Singapore, Canada, and Vietnam contracted the virus while visiting Hong Kong, bringing SARS-CoV to their respective nations and causing secondary transmission chains. In just a month, the infection had spread to nearly 20 countries. Such events emphasize the urgent need for effective international data sharing and transparent reporting to enable rapid detection, coordinated surveillance, and timely response efforts. Without these collaborative mechanisms, delays in information exchange could hinder early containment measures and magnify the public health, social, and economic consequences of EIDs (Mishra et al., 2022).

International data sharing refers to a structured approach aimed at promoting fair and inclusive distribution of public health benefits generated through the exchange of data (Lee & Kim, 2024). This process involves multiple actors, including those who provide the data, individuals or institutions responsible for analyzing and utilizing the data, intermediaries facilitating its dissemination, and beneficiaries who also contribute to the collective health outcomes. Such mechanisms play a critical role in strengthening global preparedness and mitigating the effects of infectious diseases (Edelstein et al., 2018). In practice, this includes the exchange of epidemiological, genomic, and clinical data that enables health authorities to track pathogen evolution, model transmission dynamics, and assess intervention effectiveness across different regions. The approach is critical for predicting outbreaks, determining disease burden, and evaluating interventions (Tornimbene et al., 2025). When implemented systematically, international data sharing not only enhances scientific collaboration but also builds trust among nations, ensuring that both high- and low-resource settings can respond more effectively to global health threats.

One of the most prominent is the International Health Regulations (IHR 2005), which establish a comprehensive legal framework outlining the rights and responsibilities of countries in managing public health events and emergencies that may pose cross-border risks (World Health Organization, 2016). In the animal health sector, the World Organisation for Animal Health's World Animal Health Information System (OIE-WAHIS) compiles and disseminates extensive data provided by national Veterinary Services, covering country-specific reports on outbreaks of World Organisation for Animal Health (WOAH) listed and emerging animal diseases (Morales et al., 2023). Similarly, the Food and Agriculture Organization (FAO) plays a key role in the One Health approach by monitoring and sharing information on animal- and food-related diseases, thus bridging the gap between human, animal, and environmental health (Boutrif, 2014).

Several key international platforms facilitate the timely exchange of disease-related information, enabling rapid detection and coordinated responses to outbreaks. The Global Initiative on Sharing All Influenza Data (GISAID) provides data sharing for seasonal and pandemic influenza preparedness, including influenza, hCoV-19, respiratory syncytial virus (RSV), hMpxV, chikungunya, dengue, and zika (GISAID, 2025). The Global Outbreak Alert and Response Network (GOARN) fosters collaboration among countries and organizations to mobilize resources and expertise during outbreak responses. For the past two decades, the Global Outbreak Response and Alert Network (GOARN) has played a central role in coordinating international responses to disease outbreaks. Recognizing that no single institution possesses all the capabilities needed to manage complex public health emergencies or address every aspect of outbreak response training, GOARN has pursued a capacity-building approach that leverages the distinct expertise of its more than 250 partner organizations (Christensen et al., 2021). These platforms form a critical infrastructure for global health security, ensuring that data flows swiftly from detection to action. Despite its recognized importance, international data sharing continues to face challenges, including reluctance to release data, concerns over privacy and confidentiality, and issues related to obtaining informed consent (Roundtable on Environmental Health Sciences, Research, and Medicine et al., 2016).

In Asia, particularly in the Southeast Asia and Western Pacific regions, antimicrobial resistance (AMR) remains a growing public health challenge despite the development of multiple policies and national action plans. Implementation progress is uneven, reflecting persistent governance and capacity gaps, while effective One Health collaboration across sectors remains limited (Patel et al., 2023; Yu et al., 2026). Given the transboundary nature of AMR in Asia, international data sharing is essential, but it must balance openness with respect for national sovereignty and ensure equity among countries. Mosquito-borne viral diseases continue to pose a substantial public health burden across Southeast and South Asia, driven by high endemicity and increasing regional and global connectivity. Expanded travel and climate-related changes have heightened the risk of virus introduction and spread, underscoring the need for proactive and coordinated regional preparedness beyond the COVID-19 response. Evidence from recent outbreaks highlights the importance of balanced research and surveillance partnerships between high-income and low- and middle-income countries in Asia, particularly where health systems face persistent resource constraints. In this context, effective cross-border data sharing is essential for early warning and control, but it must be grounded in respect for national sovereignty and equitable collaboration to ensure sustainable and trusted regional responses.

Competing Interests The author(s) has no competing interests to declare that are relevant to the content of this manuscript.

References

Adnyana, I. M., Utomo, B., Eljatin, D. S., & Sudaryati, N. L. (2023). One Health approach and zoonotic diseases in Indonesia: Urgency of implementation and challenges. *Narra J, 3*. https://doi.org/10.52225/narra.v3i3.257

Alam, N., Chu, C., Li, Q., Crook, A., Whittaker, M., Aditama, T., Schak, E., Budiman, D., Barber, B., & Lu, J. (2020). The Pearl River Declaration: A timely call for enhancing health security through fostering a regional one health collaboration in the Asia-Pacific. *Globalization and Health, 16*, 79. https://doi.org/10.1186/s12992-020-00606-y

Althubyani, M., Adam, H. D. S., Alalyani, A., Taha, N. E., Taha, K. O., Alharbi, R. A., & Saber, S. (2025). Understanding zoonotic disease spread with a fractional order epidemic model. *Scientific Reports, 15*, 13921. https://doi.org/10.1038/s41598-025-95943-6

Anwar, S., Ahmed, B., & Qadir, M. I. (2024). Arboviruses: Transmission and host resistance. *Critical Reviews in Eukaryotic Gene Expression, 34*, 15–31. https://doi.org/10.1615/CritRevEukaryotGeneExpr.2023049820

Asian Development Bank, Roth, S., Counahan, M., Khetrapal, S., Parry, J., & Servais, G. (2018). *Investing in health security for sustainable development in Asia and the Pacific: Managing health threats through regional and intersectoral cooperation*. Asian Development Bank. https://doi.org/10.22617/WPS189504-2

Ben Jebara, K. (2004). Surveillance, detection and response: Managing diseases at national and international levels: -EN- -FR- -ES-. *Revue scientifique et technique/ Office international des épizooties, 23*, 709–715. https://doi.org/10.20506/rst.23.2.1508

Boutrif, E. (2014). Institutions involved in food safety: Food and Agriculture Organization of the United Nations (FAO). In *Encyclopedia of food safety* (pp. 354–358). Elsevier. https://doi.org/10.1016/B978-0-12-378612-8.00007-X

Bouzid, M., Colón-González, F. J., Lung, T., Lake, I. R., & Hunter, P. R. (2014). Climate change and the emergence of vector-borne diseases in Europe: Case study of dengue fever. *BMC Public Health, 14*, 781. https://doi.org/10.1186/1471-2458-14-781

Caballero-Anthony, M. (2018). Health and human security challenges in Asia: New agendas for strengthening regional health governance. *Australian Journal of International Affairs, 72*, 602–616. https://doi.org/10.1080/10357718.2018.1537356

Christensen, R., Fisher, D., Salmon, S., Drury, P., & Effler, P. (2021). Training for outbreak response through the Global Outbreak Alert and Response Network. *BMC Medicine, 19*, 123. https://doi.org/10.1186/s12916-021-01996-5

Chua, K. B., Goh, K. J., Wong, K. T., Kamarulzaman, A., Tan, P. S. K., Ksiazek, T. G., Zaki, S. R., Paul, G., Lam, S. K., & Tan, C. T. (1999). Fatal encephalitis due to Nipah virus among pig-farmers in Malaysia. *The Lancet, 354*, 1257–1259. https://doi.org/10.1016/S0140-6736(99)04299-3

Coker, R. J., Hunter, B. M., Rudge, J. W., Liverani, M., & Hanvoravongchai, P. (2011). Emerging infectious diseases in Southeast Asia: Regional challenges to control. *The Lancet, 377*, 599–609. https://doi.org/10.1016/S0140-6736(10)62004-1

Couradeau, E., Martiny, J. B. H., Fontaine, F., Brechot, C., Bonneville, M., Callens, K., the Microbiomes for One Health Initiative, Asnicar, F., Baker, B. J., Berg, G., Bonneville, M., Bowler, C., Brechot, C., Callens, K., Couradeau, E., Carmer, A. B., Cattapan, F., Clement, K., Corbin, K. D., Fontaine, F., Hansen, B., Himmelgreen, D., Hirt, H., Lim, S. J., Martiny, J. B. H., Morand, S., Natarajan, O., Philippidis, G. P., Profizi, C., Richie, I. T., Roume, H., Sanseverino, W., Terrill, D., Thomas, S. W., Vermund, S. H., Yadav, H., & Zhao, L. (2025). Incorporating microbiomes into the One Health Joint Plan of Action. *MBio, 16*, e01456–25. https://doi.org/10.1128/mbio.01456-25

Cummings, D. A. T., Iamsirithaworn, S., Lessler, J. T., McDermott, A., Prasanthong, R., Nisalak, A., Jarman, R. G., Burke, D. S., & Gibbons, R. V. (2009). The impact of the demographic transition on dengue in Thailand: Insights from a statistical analysis and mathematical modeling. *PLoS Medicine, 6*, e1000139. https://doi.org/10.1371/journal.pmed.1000139

De La Rocque, S., Errecaborde, K. M. M., Belot, G., Brand, T., Shadomy, S., Von Dobschuetz, S., Aguanno, R., Carron, M., Caya, F., Ding, S., Dhingra, M., Donachie, D., Gongal, G., Hoejskov, P., Ismayilova, G., Lamielle, G., Mahrous, H., Marrana, M., Nzietchueng, S., Oh, Y., Pinto, J., Roche, X., Riviere-Cinnamond, A., Rojo, C., Scheuermann, L., Sinclair, J., Song, J., Skrypnyk, A., Traore, T., & Wongsathapornchai, K. (2023). One health systems strengthening in countries: Tripartite tools and approaches at the human-animal-environment interface. *BMJ Global Health, 8*, e011236. https://doi.org/10.1136/bmjgh-2022-011236

de Sa, J., Mounier-Jack, S., Darapheak, C., Narann, L. K., Phetsouvanh, R., Chanthakoummane, N., Touch, S., Phommasack, B., & Coker, R. (2010). Responding to pandemic influenza in Cambodia and Lao PDR: challenges in moving from strategy to operation. *The Southeast Asian Journal of Tropical Medicine and Public Health, 41*, 1104–1115.

Degeling, C., Johnson, J., Kerridge, I., Wilson, A., Ward, M., Stewart, C., & Gilbert, G. (2015). Implementing a One Health approach to emerging infectious disease: Reflections on the socio-political, ethical and legal dimensions. *BMC Public Health, 15*, 1307. https://doi.org/10.1186/s12889-015-2617-1

Delacollette, C., D'Souza, C., Christophel, E., Thimasarn, K., Abdur, R., Bell, D., Dai, T. C., Gopinath, D., Lu, S., Mendoza, R., Ortega, L., Rastogi, R., Tantinimitkul, C., & Ehrenberg, J. (2009). Malaria trends and challenges in the Greater Mekong Subregion. *The Southeast Asian Journal of Tropical Medicine and Public Health, 40*, 674–691.

Dondorp, A. M., Yeung, S., White, L., Nguon, C., Day, N. P. J., Socheat, D., & Von Seidlein, L. (2010). Artemisinin resistance: current status and scenarios for containment. *Nature Reviews. Microbiology, 8*, 272–280. https://doi.org/10.1038/nrmicro2331

Durrance-Bagale, A., Marzouk, M., Agarwal, S., Ananthakrishnan, A., Gan, S., Hayashi, M., Jacob-Chow, B., Jiayun, K., Tung, L. S., Mkhallalati, H., Newaz, S., Omar, M., Sittimart, M., Ung, M., Yuze, Y., Yang, H. L., & Howard, N. (2021). Operationalising regional cooperation for infectious disease control: A scoping review of regional disease control bodies and networks. *International Journal of Health Policy and Management, 1*. https://doi.org/10.34172/ijhpm.2021.176

Edelstein, M., Lee, L. M., Herten-Crabb, A., Heymann, D. L., & Harper, D. R. (2018). Strengthening global public health surveillance through data and benefit sharing. *Emerging Infectious Diseases, 24*, 1324–1330. https://doi.org/10.3201/eid2407.151830

Fang, C.-T., Ujiie, M., & Yeom, J. S. (2024). East Asia. In *Routledge handbook of infectious diseases* (pp. 158–175). Routledge. https://doi.org/10.4324/9781003531425-14

Faust, C. L., McCallum, H. I., Bloomfield, L. S. P., Gottdenker, N. L., Gillespie, T. R., Torney, C. J., Dobson, A. P., & Plowright, R. K. (2018). Pathogen spillover during land conversion. *Ecology Letters, 21*, 471–483. https://doi.org/10.1111/ele.12904

Fu, H., & Zhu, C. (2024). The impact of population influx on infectious diseases – From the mediating effect of polluted air transmission. *Frontiers in Public Health, 12*, 1344306. https://doi.org/10.3389/fpubh.2024.1344306

Gilbert, M., Xiao, X., Pfeiffer, D. U., Epprecht, M., Boles, S., Czarnecki, C., Chaitaweesub, P., Kalpravidh, W., Minh, P. Q., Otte, M. J., Martin, V., & Slingenbergh, J. (2008). Mapping H5N1 highly pathogenic avian influenza risk in Southeast Asia. *Proceedings. National Academy of Sciences. United States of America, 105*, 4769–4774. https://doi.org/10.1073/pnas.0710581105

GISAID. (2025). *Enabling rapid and open access to epidemic and pandemic virus data* [WWW Document]. https://gisaid.org/

Gongal, G., Ofrin, R., De Balogh, K., Oh, Y., Kugita, H., & Dukpa, K. (2020). Operationalization of One Health and tripartite collaboration in the Asia-Pacific region. *WHO South-East Asia Journal of Public Health, 9*, 21. https://doi.org/10.4103/2224-3151.282991

Hahn, M. B., Gurley, E. S., Epstein, J. H., Islam, M. S., Patz, J. A., Daszak, P., & Luby, S. P. (2014). The role of landscape composition and configuration on Pteropus giganteus roosting ecology and Nipah virus spillover risk in Bangladesh. *The American Society of Tropical Medicine and Hygiene, 90*, 247–255. https://doi.org/10.4269/ajtmh.13-0256

Horby, P. W., Pfeiffer, D., & Oshitani, H. (2013). Prospects for emerging infections in East and Southeast Asia 10 years after severe acute respiratory syndrome. *Emerging Infectious Diseases, 19*. https://doi.org/10.3201/eid1906.121783

Hui, D. S. C., & Zumla, A. (2019). Severe acute respiratory syndrome. *Infectious Disease Clinics of North America, 33*, 869–889. https://doi.org/10.1016/j.idc.2019.07.001

Iera, J., Isonne, C., Seghieri, C., Tavoschi, L., Ceparano, M., Sciurti, A., D'Alisera, A., Sane Schepisi, M., Migliara, G., Marzuillo, C., Villari, P., D'Ancona, F., & Baccolini, V. (2025). Availability and key characteristics of national early warning systems for emerging profiles of antimicrobial resistance in high-income countries: Systematic review. *JMIR Public Health and Surveillance, 11*, e57457. https://doi.org/10.2196/57457

Jacob, S. T., Crozier, I., Fischer, W. A., Hewlett, A., Kraft, C. S., Vega, M.-A. D. L., Soka, M. J., Wahl, V., Griffiths, A., Bollinger, L., & Kuhn, J. H. (2020). Ebola virus disease. *Nature Reviews. Disease Primers, 6*, 13. https://doi.org/10.1038/s41572-020-0147-3

Jian, S.-W., Chen, C.-M., Lee, C.-Y., & Liu, D.-P. (2017). Real-time surveillance of infectious diseases: Taiwan's experience. *Health Security, 15*, 144–153. https://doi.org/10.1089/hs.2016.0107

Jones, K. E., Patel, N. G., Levy, M. A., Storeygard, A., Balk, D., Gittleman, J. L., & Daszak, P. (2008). Global trends in emerging infectious diseases. *Nature, 451*, 990–993. https://doi.org/10.1038/nature06536

Jones, B. A., Grace, D., Kock, R., Alonso, S., Rushton, J., Said, M. Y., McKeever, D., Mutua, F., Young, J., McDermott, J., & Pfeiffer, D. U. (2013). Zoonosis emergence linked to agricultural intensification and environmental change. *Proceedings. National Academy of Sciences. United States of America, 110*, 8399–8404. https://doi.org/10.1073/pnas.1208059110

Kajihara, T., Yahara, K., Hirabayashi, A., Shibayama, K., & Sugai, M. (2021). Japan Nosocomial Infections Surveillance (JANIS): Current status, international collaboration, and future directions for a comprehensive antimicrobial resistance surveillance system. *Japanese Journal of Infectious Diseases, 74*, 87–96. https://doi.org/10.7883/yoken.JJID.2020.499

Ka-Wai Hui, E. (2006). Reasons for the increase in emerging and re-emerging viral infectious diseases. *Microbes and Infection, 8*, 905–916. https://doi.org/10.1016/j.micinf.2005.06.032

Kayingo, G. (2023). Emerging, reemerging infectious diseases and global pandemic preparedness. *Physician Assistant Clinics, 8*, 405–409. https://doi.org/10.1016/j.cpha.2023.02.001

Krause, R. M. (1994). Dynamics of emergence. *Journal of Infectious Diseases, 170*, 265–271. https://doi.org/10.1093/infdis/170.2.265

Lajaunie, C., & Morand, S. (2024). Southeast Asia at the heart of the implementation of the One Health approach. *SSRN Journal*. https://doi.org/10.2139/ssrn.4695021

Lajaunie, C., & Morand, S. (2025). One Health observatories—The example of Southeast Asia. *Encyclopedia, 5*, 121. https://doi.org/10.3390/encyclopedia5030121

Lâm, S., Dang-Xuan, S., Unger, F., Meeyam, T., Pham-Duc, P., Wacharapluesadee, S., & Nguyen-Viet, H. (2025). Operationalizing regional One Health initiatives in Southeast Asia: Ways forward. *One Health, 20*, 101034. https://doi.org/10.1016/j.onehlt.2025.101034

Lee, D., & Kim, K. (2024). A practical approach to multifaceted perspectives for sustainable international collaboration on mosquito-borne diseases in Southeast Asia. *Acta Tropica, 260*, 107481. https://doi.org/10.1016/j.actatropica.2024.107481

Liu, X. (2025). Climate change and sustainable development in Africa: Challenges and how to respond through early warning systems. *Chinese Journal of Urban and Environmental Studies, 13*, 2550005. https://doi.org/10.1142/S2345748125500058

Lo, M. K., & Rota, P. A. (2008). The emergence of Nipah virus, a highly pathogenic paramyxovirus. *Journal of Clinical Virology, 43*, 396–400. https://doi.org/10.1016/j.jcv.2008.08.007

Lyth, A., Holbrook, N. J., & Beggs, P. J. (2005). Climate, urbanisation and vulnerability to vector-borne disease in subtropical coastal Australia: Sustainable policy for a changing environment. *Environmental Hazards, 6*, 189–200. https://doi.org/10.1016/j.hazards.2006.10.001

Mackenzie, J. S., Gubler, D. J., & Petersen, L. R. (2004). Emerging flaviviruses: The spread and resurgence of Japanese encephalitis, West Nile and Dengue viruses. *Nature Medicine, 10*, S98–S109. https://doi.org/10.1038/nm1144

Miranda, A. V., Wiyono, L., Rocha, I. C. N., Cedeño, T. D. D., & Lucero-Prisno, D. E. (2021). Strengthening virology research in the association of Southeast Asian nations: Preparing for future pandemics. *The American Journal of Tropical Medicine and Hygiene, 105*, 1141–1143. https://doi.org/10.4269/ajtmh.21-0589

Mishra, C., Samelius, G., Khanyari, M., Srinivas, P. N., Low, M., Esson, C., Venkatachalam, S., & Johansson, Ö. (2022). Increasing risks for emerging infectious diseases within a rapidly changing High Asia. *Ambio, 51*, 494–507. https://doi.org/10.1007/s13280-021-01599-7

Morales, R., Weber-Vintzel, L., Awada, L., Cãceres, P., Tizzani, P., & Meske, M. (2023). The World Animal Health Information System as a tool to support decision-making and research in animal health: -EN- The World Animal Health Information System as a tool to support decision-making and research in animal health -FR- Le SystÃ¨me mondial d'information zoosanitaire : un outil visant Ã soutenir la prise de décision et la recherche en santé animale -ES- El Sistema Mundial de Información Zoosanitaria como herramienta de apoyo a los procesos decisorios y a la investigación en sanidad animal. *Revue scientifique et technique/ Office international des épizooties, 42*, 242–251. https://doi.org/10.20506/rst.42.3367

Morris, R., & Wang, S. (2024). Building a pathway to One Health surveillance and response in Asian countries. *Science in One Health, 3*, 100067. https://doi.org/10.1016/j.soh.2024.100067

Morse, S. S. (1995). Factors in the emergence of infectious diseases. *Emerging Infectious Diseases, 1*, 7–15. https://doi.org/10.3201/eid0101.950102

Moss, R., Hickson, R. I., McVernon, J., McCaw, J. M., Hort, K., Black, J., Madden, J. R., Tran, N. H., McBryde, E. S., & Geard, N. (2016). Model-informed risk assessment and decision making for an emerging infectious disease in the Asia-Pacific region. *PLoS Neglected Tropical Diseases, 10*, e0005018. https://doi.org/10.1371/journal.pntd.0005018

Neiderud, C.-J. (2015). How urbanization affects the epidemiology of emerging infectious diseases. *Infection Ecology & Epidemiology, 5*, 27060. https://doi.org/10.3402/iee.v5.27060

Oppenheim, B., Gallivan, M., Madhav, N. K., Brown, N., Serhiyenko, V., Wolfe, N. D., & Ayscue, P. (2019). Assessing global preparedness for the next pandemic: Development and application of an Epidemic Preparedness Index. *BMJ Global Health, 4*, e001157. https://doi.org/10.1136/bmjgh-2018-001157

Patel, J., Harant, A., Fernandes, G., Mwamelo, A. J., Hein, W., Dekker, D., & Sridhar, D. (2023). Measuring the global response to antimicrobial resistance, 2020–21: A systematic governance analysis of 114 countries. *The Lancet Infectious Diseases, 23*, 706–718. https://doi.org/10.1016/S1473-3099(22)00796-4

Patz, J. A., Daszak, P., Tabor, G. M., Aguirre, A. A., Pearl, M., Epstein, J., Wolfe, N. D., Kilpatrick, A. M., Foufopoulos, J., Molyneux, D., Bradley, D. J., & Members of the Working Group on Land Use Change Disease Emergence. (2004). Unhealthy landscapes: Policy recommendations on land use change and infectious disease emergence. *Environmental Health Perspectives, 112*, 1092–1098. https://doi.org/10.1289/ehp.6877

Perez Arredondo, A. M. (2022). Research-practice-collaborations addressing One Health and urban transformation. A case study: Commentary on "Research-Practice-Collaborations in International Sustainable Development and Knowledge Production—Reflections from a Political-Economic Perspective". *European Journal of Development Research, 34*, 1745–1756. https://doi.org/10.1057/s41287-022-00553-x

Pham, C. T., Nguyen, H. T., Le, H. H. T. C., Tran, N. Q. L., Do, K. Q., Bui, V., Phung, H., Phung, D., & Chu, C. (2025). Challenges and strategies for the development and implementation of climate-informed early warning systems for vector-borne diseases: A systematic review. *Tropical Medicine & International Health*, tmi.70045. https://doi.org/10.1111/tmi.70045

Priya, S., Iyer, V. R., Kalluri, R. C., Singh, S. K., Raheja, R., Gujarathi, R. H., & Das, S. S. (2024). Healthcare system adaptation strategies in response to pandemics: Case studies from global perspectives. *JoE, 3*. https://doi.org/10.62754/joe.v3i8.6104

Ristori, M. V., Guarrasi, V., Soda, P., Petrosillo, N., Gurrieri, F., Longo, U. G., Ciccozzi, M., Riva, E., & Angeletti, S. (2024). Emerging microorganisms and infectious diseases: One Health approach for health shared vision. *Genes, 15*, 908. https://doi.org/10.3390/genes15070908

Roundtable on Environmental Health Sciences, Research, and Medicine, Board on Population Health and Public Health Practice, Health and Medicine Division, National Academies of Sciences, Engineering, and Medicine. (2016). *Principles and obstacles for sharing data from environmental health research: Workshop summary*. National Academies Press. https://doi.org/10.17226/21703

Saba Villarroel, P. M., Gumpangseth, N., Songhong, T., Yainoy, S., Monteil, A., Leaungwutiwong, P., Missé, D., & Wichit, S. (2023). Emerging and re-emerging zoonotic viral diseases in Southeast Asia: One Health challenge. *Frontiers in Public Health, 11*, 1141483. https://doi.org/10.3389/fpubh.2023.1141483

Shen, Y., Liu, Y., Krafft, T., & Wang, Q. (2025). Progress and challenges in infectious disease surveillance and early warning. *Medicine Plus, 2*, 100071. https://doi.org/10.1016/j.medp.2025.100071

Smiley Evans, T., Shi, Z., Boots, M., Liu, W., Olival, K. J., Xiao, X., Vandewoude, S., Brown, H., Chen, J.-L., Civitello, D. J., Escobar, L., Grohn, Y., Li, H., Lips, K., Liu, Q., Lu, J., Martínez-López, B., Shi, J., Shi, X., Xu, B., Yuan, L., Zhu, G., & Getz, W. M. (2020). Synergistic China–US ecological research is essential for global emerging infectious disease preparedness. *EcoHealth, 17*, 160–173. https://doi.org/10.1007/s10393-020-01471-2

Tornimbene, B., Leiva Rioja, Z. B., Barral-Netto, M., Castillo-Salgado, C., Djordjevic, I., Kraemer, M., McMenamin, M., & Morgan, O. (2025). Data integration and synthesis for pandemic and epidemic intelligence. *BMC Proceedings, 19*, 12. https://doi.org/10.1186/s12919-025-00321-9

Van Nguyen, H., Van Hoang, M., Dao, A. T. M., Nguyen, H. L., Van Nguyen, T., Nguyen, P. T., Khuong, L. Q., Le, P. M., & Gilmour, S. (2020). An adaptive model of health system organization and responses helped Vietnam to successfully halt the Covid-19 pandemic: What lessons can be learned from a resource-constrained country. *Health Planning & Management, 35*, 988–992. https://doi.org/10.1002/hpm.3004

Ward, M. P., & Brookes, V. J. (2021). Rabies in our neighbourhood: Preparedness for an emerging infectious disease. *Pathogens, 10*, 375. https://doi.org/10.3390/pathogens10030375

WHO. (2021). Special session of World Health Assembly 29 November 2021–1 December 2021.

World Health Organization (Ed.). (2016). *International Health Regulations (2005)* (3rd ed.). World Health Organization.

Wu, Q., Li, Q., & Lu, J. (2022). A One Health strategy for emerging infectious diseases based on the COVID-19 outbreak. *Journal of Biosafety and Biosecurity, 4*, 5–11. https://doi.org/10.1016/j.jobb.2021.09.003

Yu, X., Wang, H., Wang, J., Yuan, X., Zhou, X., He, Q., Mokrousov, I., Sun, L., Dong, Y., & Zou, Z. (2026). Using implementation science to bridge the gaps between political commitment and action in antimicrobial resistance governance under the one health approach in the WHO

Southeast Asia and Western Pacific regions. *The Lancet Regional Health—Western Pacific, 66*, 101783. https://doi.org/10.1016/j.lanwpc.2025.101783

Zhang, X.-Y., Huang, H.-J., Zhuang, D.-L., Nasser, M. I., Yang, M.-H., Zhu, P., & Zhao, M.-Y. (2020). Biological, clinical and epidemiological features of COVID-19, SARS and MERS and AutoDock simulation of ACE2. *Infectious Diseases of Poverty, 9*, 99. https://doi.org/10.1186/s40249-020-00691-6

Zhou, C., Wang, S., Wang, C., Qiang, N., Xiu, L., Hu, Q., Wu, W., Zhang, X., Han, L., Feng, X., Zhu, Z., Shi, L., Zhang, P., & Yin, K. (2025). Integrated surveillance and early warning system of emerging infectious diseases in China at community level: Current status, gaps and perspectives. *Science in One Health, 4*, 100102. https://doi.org/10.1016/j.soh.2024.100102

Chapter 10
Tropical Diseases and One Health

Lita Eliana, Neisry Arysta, Linda Andriani, Kharisma Dewi, Febriani Putri, Chaterine Rahel Anggrainy, and Annisa Utami Rauf

10.1 Introduction

Neglected tropical diseases (NTDs) are a group of diseases caused by various pathogens, including viruses, bacteria, parasites, fungi, and toxins, that significantly impact the health, social, and economic well-being of communities. These diseases are common in tropical regions and are estimated to affect more than one billion people (Ito et al., 2019). This is particularly felt by vulnerable populations who are continually exposed to risks, leading to health vulnerabilities, economic stress, and

L. Eliana · N. Arysta
Master of Tropical Medicine Program, Faculty of Medicine, Public Health, and Nursing, Universitas Gadjah Mada, Yogyakarta, Indonesia
e-mail: litaeliana@mail.ugm.ac.id; neisryarysta@mail.ugm.ac.id

L. Andriani
Department of Epidemiology, Population Biostatistics and Health Promotion, Faculty of Public Health, Universitas Airlangga, Surabaya, Indonesia

Sidoarjo Health Office, East Java, Indonesia
e-mail: lindaandriani1234@gmail.com

K. Dewi (✉)
Department of Parasitology, Faculty of Medicine, Public Health, and Nursing, Universitas Gadjah Mada, Yogyakarta, Indonesia
e-mail: kharisma.dewi@mail.ugm.ac.id

F. Putri · C. R. Anggrainy
Master of Public Health Program, Faculty of Medicine, Public Health, and Nursing, Universitas Gadjah Mada, Yogyakarta, Indonesia
e-mail: febrianiputri.f@mail.ugm.ac.id; chaterinerahelanggrainy.c@mail.ugm.ac.id

A. U. Rauf
Department of Health Behavior, Environment and Social Medicine, Faculty of Medicine, Public Health, and Nursing, Universitas Gadjah Mada, Sleman, Yogyakarta, Indonesia
e-mail: annisaur@ugm.ac.id

© The Author(s), under exclusive license to Springer Nature Singapore Pte Ltd. 2026

A. U. Rauf, T. Wibawa (eds.), *The One Health Concept in Asian Contexts*,
https://doi.org/10.1007/978-981-95-9880-9_10

social exclusion due to stigma. As the name suggests, "neglected," NTDs are often overlooked from the global health agenda despite their significant disease burden.

That burden was borne by more than 1,7 billion people worldwide who still live with one or more NTDs each year, and the majority of this burden occurs in Asia, particularly Southeast Asia (Yajima et al., 2023). The transmission of tropical diseases in this region is influenced by dynamic environmental conditions, climate change, economic inequality, and urbanization. Ecosystem changes also create conditions that support the life cycles of vectors and animal reservoirs. Behavioral factors, high mobility, and limited health systems accelerate the spread of disease (Khew et al., 2025). This complexity is intensified by the double burden of infectious and noncommunicable diseases, which is increasing with lifestyle changes. To reduce this burden, NTD management strategies need to focus on efforts to reduce inequality, strengthen community resilience, and promote sustainable development to achieve "better health and sustainability for all."

The One Health approach offers a relevant framework for addressing the complexity of NTDs. This concept balances human, animal, and environmental health and encourages interdisciplinary collaboration to holistically understand the multiple dimensions of disease. At the same time, examining problems from environmental, animal, and human perspectives may reveal previously unseen factors and allow for more precise and comprehensive intervention design. Unlike a one-dimensional approach, the One Health approach provides a more comprehensive picture of tropical disease prevention opportunities (Angkurawaranon et al., 2014; Feng et al., 2023).

The application of One Health strategies to NTD interventions also demonstrates the potential for long-term sustainability. For example, a cofinancing model for the management of *Taenia solium* in Madagascar, which combines human treatment with pig vaccination, has been shown to sustainably reduce disease prevalence (Ramiandrasoa et al., 2020). Strengthening this strategy relies on open communication and effective coordination among stakeholders, both formally and informally. Exploring human, animal, and environmental health as a single, interdependent system, One Health provides a strategic framework for anticipating and managing the health impacts of future variability and ecological disturbances. This approach encourages collaboration across sectors (public health, veterinary medicine, agriculture, environmental science, and climate policy), enabling early detection, coordinated response, and more efficient use of resources (Cao et al., 2017; Gyapong et al., 2025).

10.2 Global Burden of Tropical Diseases in Asia

While remarkable improvements in health outcomes have been achieved over recent decades, such as reduced maternal and child mortality, expanded vaccine coverage, and progress in controlling major infectious diseases, many Asian countries continue to struggle with persistent and emerging health challenges (Asian Development Bank, 2006; Bhatia & Narain, 2010; Megawati Saputra et al., 2023). The region faces a double burden of disease in which longstanding infectious diseases persist alongside a rising prevalence of noncommunicable diseases driven by lifestyle transitions, aging populations, environmental degradation, and widening socioeconomic disparities. Various infectious diseases, including malaria, dengue, tuberculosis, and antimicrobial-resistant pathogens, continue to exert a significant impact on vulnerable populations in low- and middle-income settings (Cummings et al., 2009; Kumar et al., 2020; Wu et al., 2023). Among these, neglected tropical diseases (NTDs) represent a major yet often overlooked contributor to long-term disability, poverty, and limited socioeconomic development across Asia.

The World Health Organization (WHO) and the global community of countries, partners, donors, technical experts, scientific and field implementation teams continue to work toward the ultimate goal of a world free from the burden of NTDs. WHO also manages a diverse portfolio of 20 diseases and disease group whose public health is often overlooked and neglected by relevant authorities or decision-making bodies. Conservative estimates indicate that this NTD accounts for some 14,5 million disability-adjusted life years (DALYs) with significant variation especially among tropical diseases in developed and developing countries (WHO, 2023). NTDs are a group of bacterial, parasitic, viral, and fungal infections that are prevalent in many of the tropical and subtropical developing countries where poverty is rampant. According to a World Bank study, 51% of the population of sub-Saharan Africa, a major focus for NTDs, lives on less than US$1,25 per day, and 73% of the population lives on less than US$2 per day. In the 2010 GBD Study, NTDs accounted for 26,06 million DALYs (95% confidence interval: 20,30, 35,12).

As global attention toward NTDs intensifies, the spectrum of diseases in this classification has expanded from 17 in 2010 to 21 in 2023. In 2020, WHO unveiled its most recent NTD roadmap, articulating clear targets for the control, elimination, or eradication of selected diseases by 2030. Tracking progress toward the targets requires a quantitative basis, and DALYs are a key metric for understanding and evaluating the overall disease burden of NTDs. Unlike incidence, prevalence, or mortality, which focus on specific aspects of a disease's impact, DALYs combine both years of life lost due to premature mortality and years lived with disability (Hassoun & Cosler, 2023). This dual approach allows for a holistic comparison and a more nuanced assessment of the total disease burden, which is particularly valuable for informing public health priorities and resource allocation (Yang et al., 2025). NTDs are disabling, disfiguring, and deadly diseases impacting more than one billion people worldwide. NTDs impair physical and cognitive development, cause adverse pregnancy outcomes, and limit adult productivity in the workforce (Fenwick, 2012).

The global distribution of NTDs is such that the vast majority of cases (seven or more NTDs) are located in Brazil and in some countries in Central and East Africa, and in Yemen, followed by cases (five or more) in India, Bangladesh, and China. Based on the data collected by WHO in 14 of the targeted 20 NTDs, the total worldwide burden is 25.135,59 thousand years lost, as estimated by DALYs in 2015. This enormous burden of the NTDs is mostly shared by *soil-transmitted helminthiasis* (STH) (4443,47 thousand years), *schistosomiasis* (3513,85 thousand years), *dengue fever* (2610,08 thousand years), *lymphatic filariasis* (2070,85 thousand years), *cysticercosis* (a larval tapeworm infection) (1135,57 thousand years), human rabies (1672,17 thousand years), *leishmaniasis* (1356,46 thousand years), *onchocerciasis* (1135,57 thousand years), and foodborne trematodiasis (1066,34 thousand years). These data should be interpreted with caution because data for years of life lost (YLL) were not available for *trichuriasis, hookworm infection, lymphatic filariasis, onchocerciasis*, and *trachoma* for 2015 (Herricks et al., 2017; Mathers et al., 2007).

Schistosomiasis remains endemic in several Asian countries, notably China, the Philippines, and Indonesia (Chen et al., 2024; Feng et al., 2023; Tabilin et al., 2025), where control efforts are challenged by the zoonotic transmission cycle of the parasite. Effective management requires integrated control strategies, combining mass drug administration, improvements in water, sanitation, and hygiene, and veterinary interventions, including the use of animal vaccines. Another important NTD in Asia, Yaws, is a priority disease for elimination in the WHO Southeast Asia Region, with substantial progress achieved in lowering disease prevalence. The infection disproportionately affects marginalized and underserved populations, and elimination efforts focus on mass treatment campaigns and strengthened surveillance to interrupt transmission (WHO, 2023). Healers remain key contributors to mortality and morbidity in the region. Snakebite envenomation is also a major NTD burden in Asia, particularly in South and Southeast Asia. Globally, snakebites cause an estimated 81,000–138,000 deaths and about 400,000 cases of permanent disability each year. Asia accounts for the majority of this burden, with South Asia responsible for approximately 70% of global snakebite deaths and an estimated ~15,900 deaths annually in Southeast Asia. India alone contributes tens of thousands of deaths per year, making it the country with the highest snakebite mortality worldwide. Delayed access to antivenom, limited access to healthcare infrastructure, and reliance on traditional further exacerbate.

Previous study highlights the significant burden of antimicrobial-resistant *Klebsiella pneumoniae* in South and Southeast Asia (Spadar et al., 2022; Wyres et al., 2020), reflecting broader challenges seen across the region in managing infectious diseases. The genomic profiles of isolates reveal extensive multidrug resistance, diverse plasmid replicons, and variable distributions of virulence factors—patterns of pathogens influenced by mobility, environmental change, and uneven healthcare capacity. The findings underscore the need for coordinated, large-scale surveillance across Asian countries to better understand pathogen dissemination and strengthen public health strategies, particularly in settings where infectious disease threats remain persistent and underrecognized.

The global burden of tropical diseases in Asia is substantial, with significant health, social, and economic consequences (Gyapong et al., 2025; Kain et al., 2024; Khew et al., 2025; Ogieuhi et al., 2025; Yajima et al., 2023). The NTDs continue to affect the livelihood of individuals in countries in the Southeast Asia and Western Pacific region, with an estimated 1.7 billion of the world's population suffering from one or more NTDs annually (Khew et al., 2025). The burden of NTDs in the Southeast Asia Region (SEAR) is particularly high, with all 11 countries in the region being affected, bearing 54% of the global burden (Yajima et al.,

2023). The economic impact of NTDs is significant, causing billions of dollars lost in revenue from reduced labor productivity in developing countries alone (Khew et al., 2025). The burden of NTDs and malaria is projected to increase over the next 20 years, particularly in Middle and Low-middle Socio-Demographic Index (SDI) regions, with Western sub-Saharan Africa remaining the most affected region (Lin et al., 2025).

10.3 Factors Contributing to The Transmission of Tropical Diseases

Tropical diseases are often overlooked due to their predominance in low socioeconomic communities, characterized by inadequate sanitation and housing conditions, as well as in communities with constrained access to healthcare services (Uzoka et al., 2021). A correlation has been demonstrated between environmental determinants and the transmission of tropical diseases, including malaria, dengue, helminthiasis, and diarrheal diseases. Malaria is among the most prevalent tropical diseases, with an estimated 3,2 billion individuals globally susceptible to infection (Budiman, 2022; Uzoka et al., 2021). The transmission of tropical diseases is influenced by a multitude of factors, including, but not limited to, pathogenic agents, as well as complex interactions between environmental, social, economic, and biological factors.

More than 1 billion people suffer from NTDs, which cause around 170.000 deaths each year, particularly among impoverished and vulnerable populations in tropical regions such as Asia. In 2017, the WHO updated its list of NTDs to include seven helminth infections: soil-transmitted helminthiases (STH), *schistosomiasis* (SCH), foodborne trematodiases (FBT), *lymphatic filariasis* (LF), *taeniasis/cysticercosis*, guinea-worm disease, and onchocerciasis. The first five of these, along with several other parasitic diseases, remain endemic across East and Southeast Asia, particularly within the ten ASEAN member countries. Despite significant economic progress, ASEAN continues to face a substantial but often overlooked burden of poverty and NTDs. Nearly 200 million people, mostly in Indonesia, the Philippines, Myanmar, Vietnam, and Cambodia, live in extreme poverty, many of whom are affected by at least one NTD. These diseases also persist in upper-middle-income countries like Malaysia and Thailand, particularly among indigenous populations. Major intestinal helminthiases (STH, SCH, and LF) affect about 100 million people in the region, while over 10 million suffer from fluke infections, *schistosomiasis*, or *lymphatic filariasis* (Hotez, 2020; Sripa et al., 2022).

Japanese encephalitis (JE) is the most common preventable mosquito-borne encephalitis in Asia. Despite being vaccine-preventable in humans, controlling *Japanese encephalitis virus* (JEV) remains challenging due to the lack of effective veterinary vaccines (Endy & Nisalak, 2002; Mambully et al., 2025). Pigs act as major amplifying hosts in the zoonotic cycle, and ineffective prevention in these animals makes disease control difficult. In Asia, JEV transmission involves *Culex* mosquitoes, particularly *Culex tritaeniorhynchus*, with water birds as natural reservoirs and pigs as amplifying hosts, while humans are dead-end hosts (Ghosh & Basu, 2009). Human infections often begin with mild symptoms but can progress to severe disease, with mortality rates reaching 30% and a high risk of long-term neurological sequelae. JE outbreaks have been recorded since the 1870s, with a major epidemic in Japan in 1924. The virus is believed to have originated from an ancestral strain in the Indonesia–Malaysia region before spreading throughout Asia, including China, Japan, Korea, India, and Vietnam (Chen, 2012). Climate change, population growth, and environmental changes have expanded the distribution of vectors and reservoir species, increasing transmission risk across the region.

The JEV genome resembles other flaviviruses, consisting of ~11 kb of positive-sense RNA encoding three structural (C, M, E) and seven nonstructural proteins (Le Flohic et al., 2013; Sumiyoshi et al., 1987). The envelope (E) protein is key to infectivity and immunity and is widely used for phylogenetic analysis. Based on this gene, JEV is classified into five genotypes (GI–GV), which circulate across Asia and have recently been identified beyond the continent (Mohammed et al., 2011). In addition to *Japanese encephalitis*, which is a major vector-borne viral disease, Asia bears a substantial burden of other tropical diseases. These conditions, though diverse in their etiologies and clinical manifestations, share common features of chronicity, disability, and disproportionate impact on vulnerable and impoverished populations across the region. As rapid demographic, environmental, and climatic changes unfold, the epidemiology of the diseases continues to shift, reinforcing their significance in the broader landscape of tropical disease burden in Asia.

10.3.1 Environmental Factors

Environmental determinants play a crucial role in shaping the transmission dynamics of tropical diseases in Asia. Global climate change affects the habitat of vectors or reservoirs by increasing rainfall frequency or causing droughts, which leads to the expansion or contraction of their habitats. These environmental factors can strengthen or weaken biological interactions (Feng et al., 2023). About half of India's population still defecates outside due to poor water and sanitation infrastructure (Rajshekhar et al., 2003). Changes in water quality, often driven by climate variability, can alter the biological, physical, and chemical characteristics of water sources, increasing the risk of waterborne diseases such as diarrheal illness, gastroenteritis, cryptosporidiosis, giardiasis, and cholera (El Baz & Kahime, 2022; Kahime et al., 2019). River flow patterns, particularly those influenced by monsoon rainfall and flooding, create favorable conditions for pathogens such as *Vibrio cholerae* and *Leptospira interrogans* while also expanding breeding habitats for mosquito vectors. Stagnant water resulting from altered hydrological systems further enhances vector proliferation and disease transmission (Chandra & Mukherjee, 2022; Verma et al., 2025). Leptospirosis is an emerging zoonotic disease in many regions of Asia and Latin America and shows a clear seasonal pattern linked to the monsoon. The causative organisms, *Leptospira interrogans* and related species, are excreted in the urine of infected rodents and livestock, contaminating floodwaters during episodes of intense rainfall (Govan et al., 2025).

Local climate variables, including temperature, humidity, rainfall, and drought, also significantly affect pathogen survival and vector ecology. Rising temperatures can extend transmission seasons and expand the geographic range of vector-borne diseases by accelerating mosquito development, increasing biting rates, and enhancing pathogen replication (Chandra & Mukherjee, 2022; Zain et al., 2024). In South and Southeast Asia, elevated humidity during monsoon periods contributes to higher transmission of respiratory viruses, invasive fungal infections, and dengue (Fernando et al., 2023). Meanwhile, heavy rainfall and flooding promote mosquito breeding and are strongly associated with epidemic peaks of malaria, dengue, and Japanese encephalitis (Chandra & Mukherjee, 2022; Su et al., 2016; Verma et al., 2025). Conversely, drought conditions can degrade water quality, concentrate pathogens in limited water supplies, and compel communities to rely on unsafe sources, thereby increasing waterborne disease risk (El Baz & Kahime, 2022; Schuster-Wallace et al., 2014; Verma et al., 2025).

10.3.2 Socioeconomic Factors

Paragonimus are mammalian and human parasites that cause the lung disease paragonimiasis, a foodborne zoonotic *helminthiasis* (Blair, 2024). Humans become infected by eating undercooked freshwater crustaceans such as crabs or crayfish or by consuming paratenic hosts. More than 50 *Paragonimus* species have been identified worldwide, most of them in Asia (Yoshida et al., 2019). The transmission of paragonimiasis across Asia is strongly shaped by socioeconomic conditions and culturally rooted dietary behaviors. In many South and Southeast Asian countries, such as India, Thailand, Vietnam, and Lao PDR, human infection typically occurs through the consumption of undercooked freshwater crabs (Choi, 1990; Yoshida et al., 2019). These practices are often linked to economic limitations, as crabs serve as an accessible and inexpensive source of protein in low-income rural communities.

Poverty remains a central factor because limited financial capacity restricts access to healthcare services and preventive interventions, allowing infections to remain widespread in underserved communities (Branda et al., 2024a; Paris & White, 2024). Accelerated urbanization in Southeast Asia has also reshaped disease dynamics; population movement, dense living conditions, and expansion into previously rural zones increase opportunities for infectious disease transmission, while urban lifestyles contribute to rising rates of noncommunicable diseases like diabetes and cardiovascular disorders (Angkurawaranon et al., 2014). Poor sanitation further drives parasitic diseases, as inadequate waste disposal and limited hygiene facilities facilitate the spread of schistosomiasis and soil-transmitted helminths (Abou-El-Naga, 2015; Magalhães et al., 2023). Unequal access to health services, especially in remote areas such as rural China and Mongolia, aggravates disease burdens by delaying diagnosis and limiting treatment availability (Cao et al., 2017).

Education and awareness are equally important, with studies showing that healthcare students in Asia are willing to engage in NTD prevention efforts, highlighting the value of strengthened educational programs (Htay et al., 2024). Environmental conditions intersect with socioeconomic factors, with the region's warm, humid climate enabling vector and pathogen survival and climate change expected to shift transmission patterns in unpredictable ways (Douchet et al., 2022; Paris & White, 2024). Land-use changes, including deforestation and agricultural development, also influence disease risks, as early stages of ecosystem disruption often coincide with increased infection levels. Disease-specific trends further reflect these pressures: drug-resistant malaria and tuberculosis have emerged due to factors such as poverty and substandard anti-infective drugs (Paris & White, 2011), and neglected tropical diseases including leprosy, lymphatic filariasis, and visceral leishmaniasis continue to burden the poorest populations despite ongoing elimination programs (Branda et al., 2024a; Narain et al., 2010). Leptospirosis provides another example of this interconnectedness, with its distribution shaped not only by climatic and environmental characteristics but also by socioeconomic vulnerabilities.

The high incidence of neurocysticercosis (NCC) is a result of poor hygiene, which raises the risk of *Taenia solium* egg contamination of food and drink. The prevalence of NCC varies greatly among Indian states, with socioeconomic position, education, food habits, and cleanliness practices all having a significant impact. The reported patient resided in Uttarakhand, one of the states in Northern India where the condition is common. Pork consumption habits, frequent ingestion of raw vegetables, and poorer cleanliness standards may all contribute to higher incidence in northern areas. A similar situation occurred in the case of a Mongolian traveler who visited India. This NCC case was believed to have resulted from eggs released by adult tapeworm(s) that developed after he consumed raw or undercooked pork contaminated with cysticerci during his stay in India (Davaasuren et al., 2017). This condition also occurs in China, the Philippines, Nepal, Cambodia, Myanmar, Malaysia, South Korea, and Bhutan (Chai, 2013; Chua et al., 1999, 2017; Ito et al., 2019; Myadagsuren et al., 2007).

In Indonesia, despite low overall pork consumption, *Taenia solium* transmission persists in specific communities practicing free-roaming pig husbandry, home slaughtering, and consumption of undercooked pork, particularly in Papua, where cysticercosis is highly endemic (Sutisna et al., 2019). In these areas, free-roaming pig husbandry, home slaughtering, and the local practice of consuming inadequately cooked pork contribute to ongoing transmission. The fact that confirmed *T. solium* tapeworm carriers are concentrated in these locations underscores the need for sustained education and behavior-change programs. In Papua, *T. solium cysticercosis* is considered highly endemic (Margono et al., 2006; Salim et al., 2009). Strengthening interventions such as promoting proper cooking of pork, improving hygiene and latrine use, and shifting toward pen-based pig rearing are essential.

Lessons learned from control programs in Bali may serve as a valuable model for implementation in Papua.

10.3.3 Biological and Ecological Factors

A foodborne trematode infection called paragonimiasis, which is brought on by *Paragonimus* species, causes persistent lung inflammation that mimics lung cancer or tuberculosis. In their study of Asian trends, Yoshida et al. (2019) emphasized biological traits that affect infection dynamics and control initiatives (Yoshida et al., 2019). *Leptospira*, a pathogenic spirochete that causes acute fever, is the cause of leptospirosis. Biological reservoirs —rats in urban areas and cattle, pigs, dogs, cats, and wildlife in rural ones—have a significant influence on transmission. Another study highlighted how reservoir variety and pathogen biology increase the spread of disease in underdeveloped nations (Soo et al., 2020).

Over 15 million persons in the Greater Mekong Subregion are afflicted with liver fluke infections caused by *Opisthorchis viverrini* and *Clonorchis sinensis*. They are classified as group 1 carcinogens by WHO-IARC and have life cycles that include both humans and fish hosts. According to Sripa et al. (2022), despite decades of coordinated efforts, biological traits make long-term control difficult (Sripa et al., 2022). Moreover, biologically complex *Taenia* species are responsible for both cysticercosis and taeniasis. According to Ito et al. (2019), molecular diagnostics are necessary to differentiate between species and monitor transmission because *T. asiatica* and *T. saginata* are genetically similar and not entirely reproductively isolated (Ito et al., 2019).

10.3.4 Infrastructure and Health Systems

It is a well-documented fact that many tropical regions are without adequate diagnostic laboratories. This has been demonstrated to result in delays to diagnosis and treatment, thus increasing the risk of transmission. It is imperative to underscore the significance of expeditious diagnostic tests and novel vaccines for tropical diseases, thereby facilitating early detection and prompt treatment. The deployment of insecticide-treated bed nets, house spraying, and environmental management is recognized as pivotal strategies in the realm of vector control. However, challenges such as insecticide resistance and a lack of community participation often pose significant obstacles (Kumar et al., 2020). In Fig. 10.1, the map shows that countries and provinces in red are classified as endemic areas, while those in bold red indicate regions with high endemicity. Areas marked in orange are presumed to be endemic, although supporting data remain insufficient. No data are available for North Korea; however, the country is presumed to be endemic. This suggests that the quality and capacity of a country's health information system strongly influence

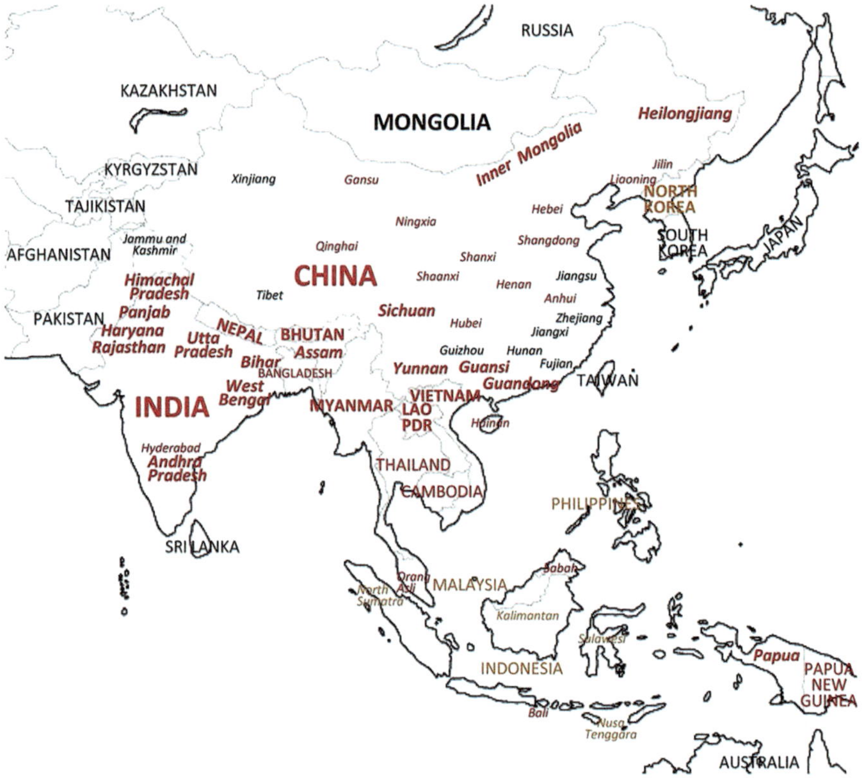

Fig. 10.1 Distribution map of *Taenia solium*—endemic countries and regions across Asia and the Pacific. (Davaasuren et al., 2017)

the accuracy, completeness, and reliability of NTD reporting and surveillance data (Shen et al., 2007).

10.4 One Health Approaches to Addressing Tropical Diseases

One Health is a concept that emphasizes that human health cannot be separated from animal health and the environment. In the context of tropical diseases, this means that the control of malaria, dengue, rabies, or leptospirosis must consider vector factors, animal reservoirs, sanitation conditions, ecosystems, and even climate change (Adisasmito et al., 2023; Manterola et al., 2024; Roy et al., 2025). Several main components in implementing the One Health approach are integrated surveillance and early detection with One Health-based surveillance collecting data from various sectors such as human health, animal health, and environmental conditions. For example, monitoring fever cases in humans is combined with mosquito population surveys, laboratory tests on animal reservoirs, and climate and environmental data. With this integration, the potential for outbreaks can be predicted more quickly. Rabies surveillance systems in Southeast Asia (Thailand, Indonesia, and Vietnam) that combine reports of dog bites, animal vaccination, and human cases have proven effective in reducing cases (Kanankege et al., 2022; Nguyen et al., 2019; Subrata et al., 2022).

Implementing multisectoral prevention and control strategies, such as vaccination, is essential. Rabies programs emphasize dog vaccination, not only the provision of post-exposure vaccination in humans (Subedi et al., 2022). The control of dengue fever and malaria vectors requires environmental management, use of insecticides, and community involvement in eradicating mosquito breeding sites and improving sanitation, while *schistosomiasis* and *leptospirosis* are closely related to access to clean water and waste disposal systems (Chen et al., 2024; Lo Iacono et al., 2017). Conducting collaborative research and innovation on tropical diseases requires a multidisciplinary scientific approach. Molecular studies on mosquitoes, behavioral analysis of animal reservoirs, and social epidemiological studies of communities must be combined to understand transmission dynamics (Branda et al., 2024b; Díaz et al., 2023; Lim et al., 2010).

Policy and cross-sectoral governance, such as World Health Organization (WHO), Food and Agriculture Organization (FAO), World Organization for Animal Health (WOAH), and United Nations Environement Program (UNEP), has promoted the One Health framework at the global level. At the national level, coordination between ministries (health, agriculture, environment, and education) is very necessary. For example, the national rabies elimination strategy in Indonesia involves the Ministry of Health and the Ministry of Agriculture simultaneously. The success of One Health also depends on community involvement. Education about clean living behavior, use of protective equipment, and involvement in vector control are very important. For example, the "3M Plus" program (draining, covering, burying, and local innovation) in dengue control in Indonesia is a real manifestation of community involvement within the One Health framework (Alfalakh, 2023).

In Mongolia and the Philippines, interagency task forces and coordination mechanisms have been instrumental in developing joint operational plans for zoonotic disease control (Batsukh et al., 2012; Dayapera et al., 2024). Strong surveillance systems also underpin the One Health framework by enabling early detection and timely response to outbreaks (Ghosal et al., 2024; Tan, 2025), as seen in Singapore's advanced surveillance tools that enhance interagency coordination and data sharing (Tan, 2025). Capacity building remains essential, with countries needing to strengthen cross-sectoral skills and invest in infrastructure and training to support One Health activities (Afzal, 2022; Dayapera et al., 2024; Munyua et al., 2019). Interministerial collaboration further improves outbreak response by ensuring multisectoral involvement (Deng & Lu, 2022; Gongal, 2012), exemplified by the ASEAN Rabies Elimination Strategy, which highlights the value of regional cooperation (Díaz et al., 2023). By integrating various health-related sectors, One Health provides a more comprehensive understanding of health risks and strengthens prevention and control strategies for tropical diseases (Li et al., 2025), an approach increasingly important as climate change and environmental degradation drive the emergence of new threats (Deng & Lu, 2022; Li et al., 2025). However, implementation challenges persist across Asia due to weak governance, fragmented risk assessment processes, and limited capacity building resources (Afzal, 2022; Dayapera et al., 2024), compounded by the absence of unified strategies and strong political commitment (Li et al., 2025). Sustained financial support is also critical, yet many countries struggle with limited funding and competing priorities. To evaluate progress, countries can adopt monitoring and evaluation frameworks that track interministerial coordination and disease management outcomes (Afzal, 2022; Munyua et al., 2019), allowing regular assessments to identify gaps and ensure continued responsiveness to emerging health threats.

Figure 10.2 shows how the epidemiology of schistosomiasis in the Philippines underscores the importance of a One Health strategy. The center of the figure outlines the simplified *Schistosoma japonicum* life cycle, beginning with cercariae

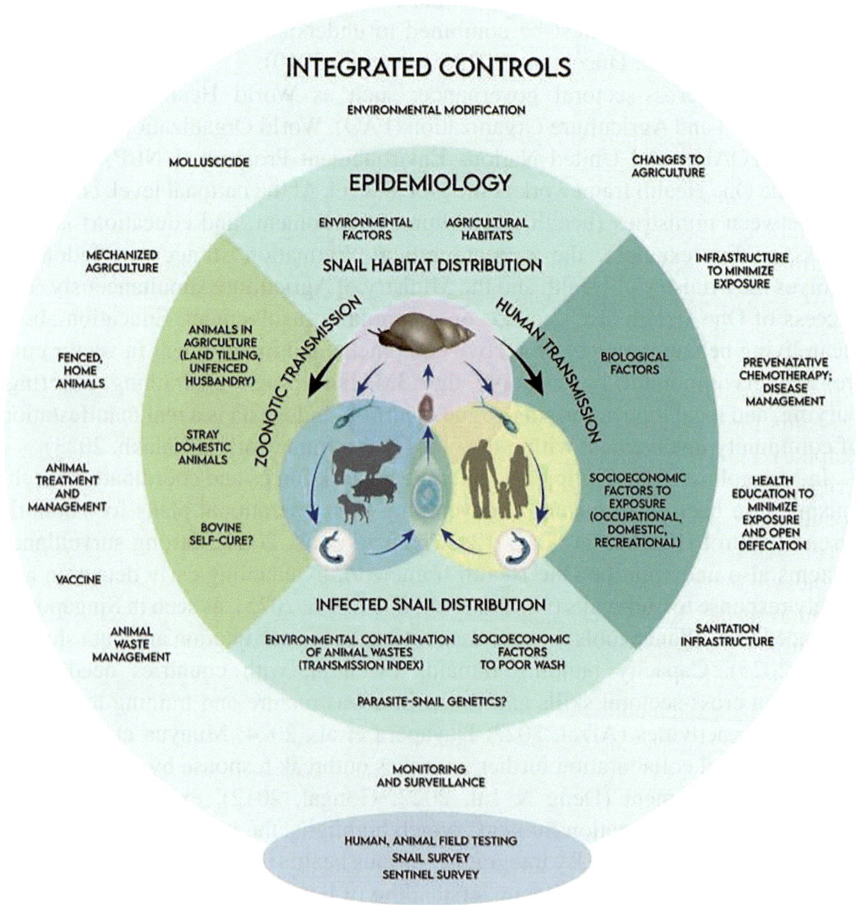

Fig. 10.2 One Health framework for the transmission cycle of *Schistosoma japonicum* and its implications for zoonotic disease control. (Tabilin et al., 2025, licensed under CC-BY 4.0)

released by infected snails that penetrate the skin of human and animal hosts. The parasites mature in the liver, migrate to the mesenteric vessels, and produce eggs that return to the environment through feces. Once in water, the eggs hatch into miracidia, which infect snails and multiply. The next layer highlights the epidemiological factors that drive transmission, and the outer ring presents integrated interventions targeting human, animal, and environmental components, showing how coordinated actions across sectors are essential for effective control.

10.5 Control Strategies of Tropical Diseases in Asia

Challenges in diagnosing and managing tropical diseases in resource-limited settings in Asia include inadequate disease awareness in physicians and the general population, scarcity of diagnostic services, infectious mimics of tropical diseases, and the high cost of therapy. The lack of a centralized healthcare system or universal health insurance, combined with limited access to biologic therapies and the increased risk of opportunistic infections among immunocompromised patients, complicates disease management (Banerjee et al., 2020). The Special Programme for Research and Training in Tropical Diseases (TDR) has issued a strategy to combat tropical diseases and contribute to achieving the health goals of the Sustainable Development Goals (SDGs) in a collaborative and integrated manner (Fang, 2024). Continued research and development are essential to overcome obstacles and ensure better global health outcomes in the face of evolving tropical diseases (Parija & Poddar, 2025).

While local outbreaks do not instantly become global, as seen with COVID-19, which took about 6 months to spread worldwide, the risk of rapid international transmission remains a critical public health concern. This interconnectedness emphasizes the necessity for a collective approach to health (Herricks et al., 2017). Prioritizing One Health is an essential strategy for ensuring economic stability, social equity, and sustainable development globally. The rapid spread of pathogens necessitates agile responses from international organizations. However, the effectiveness of these responses depends on transparency and cooperation among nations. To address such shortcomings, it is imperative to foster stronger partnerships that not only enable rapid and innovative solutions to global health crises but also reinforce mechanisms for accountability and information-sharing, ensuring a more effective and sustainable global health response. These partnerships, often between low-income countries and resource-rich nations, play a crucial role in combating tropical diseases that heavily burden certain regions (Hassoun & Cosler, 2023). However, while international collaboration has been instrumental in eradicating diseases like wild polio in the Africa Region, India provides another example of successful elimination through strong domestic leadership combined with global support. Through sustained government commitment and extensive national immunization campaigns, India achieved polio elimination within its borders (Arndt et al., 2024). This demonstrates that while global partnerships can be essential, building self-sufficient health systems is equally critical for long-term disease eradication.

Although mass drug administration (MDA) programs targeting preventive chemotherapy neglected tropical diseases such as *lymphatic filariasis*, soil-transmitted helminth infections and *schistosomiasis* have been conducted annually for decades; they have not sufficiently improved public awareness of how these diseases are transmitted or how they can be effectively prevented. As a result, risky behaviors persist, and participation in control programs remains suboptimal (Tabilin et al., 2025). In response, the Philippines has adopted new strategies to enhance NTD-related education. A key effort involves embedding NTD-specific training into the pre-service curricula of health-related degree programs including medicine, medical technology, nursing, physical therapy, and midwifery to equip future health workers with the necessary knowledge for proper diagnosis, treatment, prevention, and control of NTDs.

10.6 Conclusion

Tropical diseases, including neglected tropical diseases, remain a major public health challenge in Asia, where the persistent burden of endemic infections coexists with rising noncommunicable diseases. These conditions are caused by a wide range of pathogens, including helminth infections such as schistosomiasis caused by *Schistosoma japonicum* and *lymphatic filariasis* caused by *Wuchereria bancrofti*; protozoan infections such as malaria caused by *Plasmodium falciparum* and *Plasmodium vivax*; bacterial infections such as leptospirosis caused by *Leptospira* interrogans and cholera caused by *Vibrio cholerae*; viral diseases such as dengue caused by dengue virus and Japanese encephalitis caused by Japanese encephalitis virus; and fungal infections such as mycetoma caused by *Madurella mycetomatis*. Socioeconomic disparities, rapid urbanization, environmental changes, inadequate sanitation, limited healthcare access, and emerging antimicrobial resistance collectively fuel continued transmission and poor health outcomes. These diseases disproportionately affect vulnerable populations, leading to chronic disability, reduced productivity, and ongoing economic losses. Addressing this complex burden requires a comprehensive One Health approach that integrates human, animal, and environmental health, strengthened surveillance, improved healthcare systems, multisectoral collaboration, community engagement, and sustained political and financial commitment to support effective control and elimination efforts across the region.

Competing Interests The author(s) have no competing interests to declare that are relevant to the content of this chapter.

References

Abou-El-Naga, I. F. (2015). Demographic, socioeconomic and environmental changes affecting circulation of neglected tropical diseases in Egypt. *Asian Pacific Journal of Tropical Medicine, 8*(11), 881–888. https://doi.org/10.1016/j.apjtm.2015.10.015

Adisasmito, W. B., Almuhairi, S., Barton Behravesh, C., Bilivogui, P., Bukachi, S. A., Casas, N., Becerra, N. C., Charron, D. F., Chaudhary, A., Ciacci Zanella, J. R., Cunningham, A. A., Dar, O., Debnath, N., Dungu, B., Farag, E., Gao, G. F., Hayman, D. T. S., Khaitsa, M., Koopmans, M. P. G., et al. (2023). One Health action for health security and equity. *The Lancet, 401*(10376), 530–533. https://doi.org/10.1016/S0140-6736(23)00086-7

Afzal, S. (2022). Multifactorial complexity and zoonotic aspects of dog-mediated human rabies in Pakistan. *The Pakistan Veterinary Journal, 42*(4), 445–452. https://doi.org/10.29261/pakvetj/2022.081

Alfalakh, A. R. (2023). Pengaruh Faktor Perilaku 3M Plus dengan Kejadian Demam Berdarah Dengue di Indonesia: A meta analysis. *Media Gizi Kesmas, 12*(1), 494–502. https://doi.org/10.20473/mgk.v12i1.2023.494-502

Angkurawaranon, C., Jiraporncharoen, W., Chenthanakij, B., Doyle, P., & Nitsch, D. (2014). Urbanization and non-communicable disease in Southeast Asia: A review of current evidence. *Public Health, 128*(10), 886–895. https://doi.org/10.1016/j.puhe.2014.08.003

Arndt, M. B., Abate, Y. H., Abbasi-Kangevari, M., Abd ElHafeez, S., Abdelmasseh, M., Abd-Elsalam, S., Abdulah, D. M., Abdulkader, R. S., Abidi, H., Abiodun, O., Aboagye, R. G., Abolhassani, H., Abtew, Y. D., Abu-Gharbieh, E., Abu-Rmeileh, N. M., Acuna, J. M., Adamu, K., Adane, D. E., Addo, I. Y., et al. (2024). Global, regional, and national progress towards the 2030 global nutrition targets and forecasts to 2050: A systematic analysis for the Global Burden of Disease Study 2021. *The Lancet, 404*(10471), 2543–2583. https://doi.org/10.1016/S0140-6736(24)01821-X

Asian Development Bank. (2006). *Urbanization and sustainability in Asia.* Asian Development Bank. https://www.adb.org/sites/default/files/publication/27965/urbanization-sustainability.pdf

Banerjee, R., Pal, P., Mak, J. W. Y., & Ng, S. C. (2020). Challenges in the diagnosis and management of inflammatory bowel disease in resource-limited settings in Asia. *The Lancet Gastroenterology & Hepatology, 5*(12), 1076–1088. https://doi.org/10.1016/S2468-1253(20)30299-5

Batsukh, Z., Tsolmon, B., Otgonbaatar, D., Undraa, B., Dolgorkhand, A., & Ariuntuya, O. (2012). One Health in Mongolia. In J. S. Mackenzie, M. Jeggo, P. Daszak, & J. A. Richt (Eds.), *One Health: The human-animal-environment interfaces in emerging infectious diseases* (Vol. 366, pp. 123–137). Springer. https://doi.org/10.1007/978-3-662-45791-7_253

Bhatia, R., & Narain, J. P. (2010). Review paper: The challenge of emerging zoonoses in Asia Pacific. *Asia-Pacific Journal of Public Health, 22*(4), 388–394. https://doi.org/10.1177/1010539510370908

Blair, D. (2024). Paragonimiasis. In R. Toledo & B. Fried (Eds.), *Digenetic Trematodes* (Vol. 1454, pp. 203–238). Springer. https://doi.org/10.1007/978-3-031-60121-7_6

Branda, F., Ali, A. Y., Ceccarelli, G., Albanese, M., Binetti, E., Giovanetti, M., Ciccozzi, M., & Scarpa, F. (2024a). Assessing the burden of neglected tropical diseases in low-income communities: Challenges and solutions. *Viruses, 17*(1), 29. https://doi.org/10.3390/v17010029

Branda, F., Cella, E., Scarpa, F., Slavov, S. N., Bevivino, A., Moretti, R., Degafu, A. L., Pecchia, L., Rizzo, A., Defilippo, F., Moreno, A., Ceccarelli, G., Alcantara, L. C. J., Ferreira, A., Ciccozzi, M., & Giovanetti, M. (2024b). Wolbachia-based approaches to controlling mosquito-borne viral threats: Innovations, AI integration, and future directions in the context of climate change. *Viruses, 16*(12), 1868. https://doi.org/10.3390/v16121868

Budiman. (2022). Environmental factors in tropical diseases in rural children: A systematic review. *Journal of Health Literacy and Qualitative Research, 2*(1), 1–14. https://doi.org/10.61194/jhlqr.v2i1.527

Cao, B., Zhou, F., & Kimura, M. (2017). East Asia. In E. Petersen, L. H. Chen, & P. Schlagenhauf-Lawlor (Eds.), *Infectious diseases* (1st ed., pp. 167–184). Wiley. https://doi.org/10.1002/9781119085751.ch13

Chai, J.-Y. (2013). Human taeniasis in the Republic of Korea: Hidden or gone? *The Korean Journal of Parasitology, 51*(1), 9–17. https://doi.org/10.3347/kjp.2013.51.1.9

Chandra, G., & Mukherjee, D. (2022). Effect of climate change on mosquito population and changing pattern of some diseases transmitted by them. In *Advances in animal experimentation and modeling* (pp. 455–460). Elsevier. https://doi.org/10.1016/B978-0-323-90583-1.00030-1

Chen, S. P. (2012). Molecular phylogenetic and evolutionary analysis of Japanese encephalitis virus in China. *Epidemiology and Infection, 140*(9), 1637–1643. https://doi.org/10.1017/S095026881100255X

Chen, C., He, Z., Zhao, J., Zhu, X., Li, J., Wu, X., Chen, Z., Chen, H., & Jia, G. (2024). Zoonotic outbreak risk prediction with long short-term memory models: A case study with schistosomiasis, echinococcosis, and leptospirosis. *BMC Infectious Diseases, 24*(1), 1062. https://doi.org/10.1186/s12879-024-09892-y

Choi, D. W. (1990). Paragonimus and paragonimiasis in Korea. *The Korean Journal of Parasitology, 28*(Suppl), 79. https://doi.org/10.3347/kjp.1990.28.Suppl.79

Chua, K. B., Goh, K. J., Wong, K. T., Kamarulzaman, A., Tan, P. S. K., Ksiazek, T. G., Zaki, S. R., Paul, G., Lam, S. K., & Tan, C. T. (1999). Fatal encephalitis due to Nipah virus among pig-farmers in Malaysia. *The Lancet, 354*(9186), 1257–1259. https://doi.org/10.1016/S0140-6736(99)04299-3

Chua, T. H., Emmanuel, J., Lee, K. T., Kan, F. K., Tee, K. S., Abidin, Z., Ganeswrie, R., Tan, L. H., Low, E. C., Lim, Y. A. L., & Menon, J. (2017). Taeniasis and neurocysticercosis among Malaysians. *Tropical Biomedicine, 34*(1), 7–13.

Cummings, D. A. T., Iamsirithaworn, S., Lessler, J. T., McDermott, A., Prasanthong, R., Nisalak, A., Jarman, R. G., Burke, D. S., & Gibbons, R. V. (2009). The impact of the demographic transition on dengue in Thailand: Insights from a statistical analysis and mathematical modeling. *PLoS Medicine, 6*(9), e1000139. https://doi.org/10.1371/journal.pmed.1000139

Davaasuren, A., Davaajav, A., Ukhnaa, B., Purvee, A., Unurkhaan, S., Luvsan, A., Logan, J. E., & Ito, A. (2017). Neurocysticercosis: A case study of a Mongolian traveler who visited China and India with an updated review in Asia. *Travel Medicine and Infectious Disease, 20*, 31–36. https://doi.org/10.1016/j.tmaid.2017.04.007

Dayapera, L. Z. A., Sy, J. C. Y., Valenzuela, S., Eala, S. J. L., Del Rosario, C. M. I. P., Buensuceso, K. N. C., Dy, A. S., Morales, D. A., Gibson, A. G., & Apostol, G. L. C. (2024). One health in the Philippines: A review and situational analysis. *One Health, 18*, 100758. https://doi.org/10.1016/j.onehlt.2024.100758

Deng, Q., & Lu, J. (2022). One Health and human health. *Chinese Science Bulletin, 67*(1), 37–46. https://doi.org/10.1360/TB-2021-0520

Díaz, A. V., Walker, M., & Webster, J. P. (2023). Reaching the World Health Organization elimination targets for schistosomiasis: The importance of a One Health perspective. *Philosophical Transactions of the Royal Society, B: Biological Sciences, 378*(1887), 20220274. https://doi.org/10.1098/rstb.2022.0274

Douchet, L., Goarant, C., Mangeas, M., Menkes, C., Hinjoy, S., & Herbreteau, V. (2022). Unraveling the invisible leptospirosis in mainland Southeast Asia and its fate under climate change. *Science of the Total Environment, 832*, 155018. https://doi.org/10.1016/j.scitotenv.2022.155018

El Baz, S., & Kahime, K. (2022). Waterborne diseases arising from climate change: An overview on the possible link. In I. R. Management Association (Ed.), *Research anthology on environmental and societal impacts of climate change* (pp. 64–87). IGI Global). https://doi.org/10.4018/978-1-6684-3686-8.ch004

Endy, T. P., & Nisalak, A. (2002). Japanese encephalitis virus: Ecology and epidemiology. In J. S. Mackenzie, A. D. T. Barrett, & V. Deubel (Eds.), *Japanese encephalitis and West Nile viruses* (Vol. 267, pp. 11–48). Springer. https://doi.org/10.1007/978-3-642-59403-8_2

Fang, J. (2024). [Promoting implementation research and One Health approach to respond the four global health challenges: An interpretation of the Special Programme for Research and Training in Tropical Diseases (TDR) Strategy 2024-2029]. *Zhongguo Xue Xi Chong Bing Fang Zhi Za Zhi = Chinese Journal of Schistosomiasis Control, 36*(1), 13–16. https://doi.org/10.16250/j.32.1374.2023146

Feng, J., Zhang, X., Hu, H., Gong, Y., Luo, Z., Xue, J., Cao, C., Xu, J., & Li, S. (2023). Spatiotemporal distribution of schistosomiasis transmission risk in Jiangling County, Hubei Province, P.R. China. *PLoS Neglected Tropical Diseases, 17*(5), e0011265. https://doi.org/10.1371/journal.pntd.0011265

Fenwick, A. (2012). The global burden of neglected tropical diseases. *Public Health, 126*(3), 233–236. https://doi.org/10.1016/j.puhe.2011.11.015

Fernando, M., Rajapaksha, N. U., & School of Public Health, The University of Queensland, Australia. (2023). How do climate variables affect the transmission of dengue infection in South and Southeast Asia: A scoping review. *Asian Journal of Interdisciplinary Research, 6*(1), 25–41. https://doi.org/10.54392/ajir2314

Ghosal, S., Pradhan, R., Singh, S., Velayudhan, A., Kerketta, S., Parai, D., Choudhary, H. R., Pattnaik, M., Bhattacharya, D., & Pati, S. (2024). One health intervention for the control and elimination of scrub typhus, anthrax, and brucellosis in Southeast Asia: A systematic review. *The Lancet Regional Health—Southeast Asia, 30*, 100503. https://doi.org/10.1016/j.lansea.2024.100503

Ghosh, D., & Basu, A. (2009). Japanese Encephalitis—A pathological and clinical perspective. *PLoS Neglected Tropical Diseases, 3*(9), e437. https://doi.org/10.1371/journal.pntd.0000437

Gongal, G. (2012). One Health approach in the South East Asia region: Opportunities and challenges. In J. S. Mackenzie, M. Jeggo, P. Daszak, & J. A. Richt (Eds.), *One Health: The human-animal-environment interfaces in emerging infectious diseases* (Vol. 366, pp. 113–122). Springer. https://doi.org/10.1007/978-3-662-45791-7_242

Govan, R., Scherrer, R., Fougeron, B., Laporte-Magoni, C., Thibeaux, R., Genthon, P., Fournier-Viger, P., Goarant, C., & Selmaoui-Folcher, N. (2025). Spatio-temporal risk prediction of leptospirosis: A machine-learning-based approach. *PLoS Neglected Tropical Diseases, 19*(1), e0012755. https://doi.org/10.1371/journal.pntd.0012755

Gyapong, J. O., Gohoho, M., Manyeh, A. K., Immurana, M., & Gyapong, M. (2025). Current state and future directions of interventions for neglected tropical diseases. *Nature Human Behaviour, 9*(8), 1557–1570. https://doi.org/10.1038/s41562-025-02219-0

Hassoun, N., & Cosler, L. (2023). Global health impact: A model to alleviate the burden and expand access to treatment of neglected tropical diseases. *The American Journal of Tropical Medicine and Hygiene, 108*(4), 801–806. https://doi.org/10.4269/ajtmh.21-0583

Herricks, J. R., Hotez, P. J., Wanga, V., Coffeng, L. E., Haagsma, J. A., Basáñez, M.-G., Buckle, G., Budke, C. M., Carabin, H., Fèvre, E. M., Fürst, T., Halasa, Y. A., King, C. H., Murdoch, M. E., Ramaiah, K. D., Shepard, D. S., Stolk, W. A., Undurraga, E. A., Stanaway, J. D., et al. (2017). The global burden of disease study 2013: What does it mean for the NTDs? *PLoS Neglected Tropical Diseases, 11*(8), e0005424. https://doi.org/10.1371/journal.pntd.0005424

Hotez, P. J. (2020). The rise or fall of neglected tropical diseases in East Asia Pacific. *Acta Tropica, 202*, 105182. https://doi.org/10.1016/j.actatropica.2019.105182

Htay, M. N. N., Swed, S., Elsayed, Mohamed, E. G., Yasir Arafat, S. M., Marthoenis, M., Marzo, R. R., El-Abasiri, R. A. A., Naing, Z. Y., San, L. P. P., Thantry, A. D. K., Kyaw, T. M., Myint, W. W., Gurusamy, J., Lutfi Abas, A. B., & Moe, S. (2024). Knowledge and awareness of neglected tropical diseases and control strategies among healthcare students in five Asian countries: A cross-sectional study. *Clinical Epidemiology and Global Health, 27*, 101576. https://doi.org/10.1016/j.cegh.2024.101576

Ito, A., Li, T., Wandra, T., Dekumyoy, P., Yanagida, T., Okamoto, M., & Budke, C. M. (2019). Taeniasis and cysticercosis in Asia: A review with emphasis on molecular approaches and local lifestyles. *Acta Tropica, 198*, 105075. https://doi.org/10.1016/j.actatropica.2019.105075

Kahime, K., El Hidan, M. A., El Hiba, O., Sereno, D., & Bounoua, L. (Eds.). (2019). *Handbook of research on global environmental changes and human health*. IGI Global. https://doi.org/10.4018/978-1-5225-7775-1

Kain, M. J. W., Reece, N. L., Parry, C. M., Rajahram, G. S., Paterson, D. L., & Woolley, S. D. (2024). The rapid emergence of hypervirulent Klebsiella Species and *Burkholderia pseudomallei* as major health threats in Southeast Asia: The urgent need for recognition as neglected tropical diseases. *Tropical Medicine and Infectious Disease, 9*(4), 80. https://doi.org/10.3390/tropicalmed9040080

Kanankege, K. S. T., Errecaborde, K. M., Wiratsudakul, A., Wongnak, P., Yoopatthanawong, C., Thanapongtharm, W., Alvarez, J., & Perez, A. (2022). Identifying high-risk areas for dog-mediated rabies using Bayesian spatial regression. *One Health, 15*, 100411. https://doi.org/10.1016/j.onehlt.2022.100411

Khew, C., Akbar, R., & Mohd-Assaad, N. (2025). Progress and challenges for the application of machine learning for neglected tropical diseases. *F1000Research, 12*, 287. https://doi.org/10.12688/f1000research.129064.3

Kumar, R., Farzeen, M., Hafeez, A., Achakzai, B. K., Vankwani, M., Lal, M., Iqbal, R., & Somrongthong, R. (2020). Effectiveness of a health education intervention on the use of long-lasting insecticidal nets for the prevention of malaria in pregnant women of Pakistan: A quasi-experimental study. *Malaria Journal, 19*(1), 232. https://doi.org/10.1186/s12936-020-03298-2

Le Flohic, G., Porphyre, V., Barbazan, P., & Gonzalez, J.-P. (2013). Review of climate, landscape, and viral genetics as drivers of the Japanese Encephalitis Virus ecology. *PLoS Neglected Tropical Diseases, 7*(9), e2208. https://doi.org/10.1371/journal.pntd.0002208

Li, X., Zhang, Y., Zhang, Q., Liu, J., Zhu, Z., Feng, X., Han, L., & Zhang, X. (2025). Strategy and mechanism of One Health governance: Case study of China. *Science in One Health, 4*, 100098. https://doi.org/10.1016/j.soh.2024.100098

Lim, Y. A. L., Jex, A. R., Smith, H. V., & Gasser, R. B. (2010). Cryptosporidiosis in Southeast Asia. In *Advances in parasitology* (Vol. 71, pp. 1–31). Elsevier. https://doi.org/10.1016/S0065-308X(10)71003-4

Lin, Y., Long, Q., Sun, J., Li, J., Li, Y., Liu, J., Zhang, Y., Wang, Y., & Jiang, S. (2025). Global trends, health inequalities, and projections in the burden of neglected tropical diseases and malaria from 1990 to 2021. *Scientific Reports, 15*(1), 20958. https://doi.org/10.1038/s41598-025-05530-y

Lo Iacono, G., Armstrong, B., Fleming, L. E., Elson, R., Kovats, S., Vardoulakis, S., & Nichols, G. L. (2017). Challenges in developing methods for quantifying the effects of weather and climate on water-associated diseases: A systematic review. *PLoS Neglected Tropical Diseases, 11*(6), e0005659. https://doi.org/10.1371/journal.pntd.0005659

Magalhães, A. R., Codeço, C. T., Svenning, J.-C., Escobar, L. E., Van De Vuurst, P., & Gonçalves-Souza, T. (2023). Neglected tropical diseases risk correlates with poverty and early ecosystem destruction. *Infectious Diseases of Poverty, 12*(1), 32. https://doi.org/10.1186/s40249-023-01084-1

Mambully, S., Ramesh, V., Rani, S., Khatoon, M. A. J., Patil, A. V., Palavesam, A., Sengupta, P. P., Patil, S. S., & Kp, S. (2025). Genotype patterns and evolutionary rates: Uncovering Japanese encephalitis virus spread across Asia's climate regions. *Acta Tropica, 267*, 107676. https://doi.org/10.1016/j.actatropica.2025.107676

Manterola, C., Rivadeneira, J., Leal, P., Rojas-Pincheira, C., & Altamirano, A. (2024). Una Sola Salud. Un Enfoque Multisectorial y Transdisciplinario. *International Journal of Morphology, 42*(3), 779–786. https://doi.org/10.4067/s0717-95022024000300779

Margono, S. S., Wandra, T., Swasono, M. F., Murni, S., Craig, P. S., & Ito, A. (2006). Taeniasis/cysticercosis in Papua (Irian Jaya), Indonesia. *Parasitology International, 55*, S143–S148. https://doi.org/10.1016/j.parint.2005.11.051

Mathers, C. D., Ezzati, M., & Lopez, A. D. (2007). Measuring the burden of neglected tropical diseases: The global burden of disease framework. *PLoS Neglected Tropical Diseases, 1*(2), e114. https://doi.org/10.1371/journal.pntd.0000114

Megawati Saputra, I. L., Suwarno, S., Husein, W. F., Suseno, P. P., Prayoga, I. M. A., Vos, A., Arthawan, I. M., Schoonman, L., Weaver, J., & Zainuddin, N. (2023). Immunogenicity of oral rabies vaccine strain SPBN GASGAS in local dogs in Bali, Indonesia. *Viruses, 15*(6), 1405. https://doi.org/10.3390/v15061405

Mohammed, M. A. F., Galbraith, S. E., Radford, A. D., Dove, W., Takasaki, T., Kurane, I., & Solomon, T. (2011). Molecular phylogenetic and evolutionary analyses of Muar strain of Japanese encephalitis virus reveal it is the missing fifth genotype. *Infection, Genetics and Evolution, 11*(5), 855–862. https://doi.org/10.1016/j.meegid.2011.01.020

Munyua, P. M., Njenga, M. K., Osoro, E. M., Onyango, C. O., Bitek, A. O., Mwatondo, A., Muturi, M. K., Musee, N., Bigogo, G., Otiang, E., Ade, F., Lowther, S. A., Breiman, R. F., Neatherlin, J., Montgomery, J., & Widdowson, M.-A. (2019). Successes and challenges of the One Health approach in Kenya over the last decade. *BMC Public Health, 19*(S3), 465. https://doi.org/10.1186/s12889-019-6772-7

Myadagsuren, N., Davaajav, A., Wandra, T., Sandar, T., Ichinkhorloo, P., Yamasaki, H., Sako, Y., Nakao, M., Sato, M. O., Nakaya, K., & Ito, A. (2007). Taeniasis in Mongolia, 2002–2006. *The American Journal of Tropical Medicine and Hygiene, 77*(2), 342–346.

Narain, J. P., Dash, A., Parnell, B., Bhattacharya, S., Barua, S., Bhatia, R., & Savioli, L. (2010). Elimination of neglected tropical diseases in the South-East Asia Region of the World Health Organization. *Bulletin of the World Health Organization, 88*(3), 206–210. https://doi.org/10.2471/BLT.09.072322

Nguyen, H. T. T., Nguyen, H. T., Nguyen, T. T. T., Urabe, M. I., Pham, T. N., Dang, A. D., Afriyie, D. O., Tran, D. N., & Otsu, S. (2019). Progress towards rabies control and elimination in Vietnam: -EN- -FR- Progrès accomplis par le Vietnam sur la voie du contrôle et de l'élimination de la rage -ES- Avances hacia el control y la eliminación de la rabia en el Vietnam. *Revue Scientifique et Technique de l'OIE, 38*(1), 199–212. https://doi.org/10.20506/rst.38.1.2953

Ogieuhi, I. J., Ajekiigbe, V. O., Aremu, S. O., Okpujie, V., Bassey, P. U., Babalola, A. E., Gbolagade-Jonathan, P., Anthony, C. S., & Bakare, I. S. (2025). Global partnerships in combating tropical diseases: Assessing the impact of a U.S. withdrawal from the WHO. *Tropical Medicine and Health, 53*(1), 36. https://doi.org/10.1186/s41182-025-00722-8

Parija, S. C., & Poddar, A. (2025). Parasitic diagnosis: A journey from basic microscopy to cutting-edge technology. *Tropical Parasitology, 15*(2), 71–80. https://doi.org/10.4103/tp.tp_61_24

Paris, D. H., & White, N. J. (2011). South-Eastern Asia. In E. Petersen, L. H. Chen, & P. Schlagenhauf (Eds.), *Infectious diseases: A geographic guide* (1st ed., pp. 170–187). Wiley. https://doi.org/10.1002/9781119971641.ch13

Paris, D. H., & White, N. J. (2024). South-East Asia. In I. E. Petersen, L. H. Chen, & P. Schlagenhauf (Eds.), *Routledge handbook of infectious diseases* (3rd ed., pp. 196–212). Routledge. https://doi.org/10.4324/9781003531425-16

Rajshekhar, V., Joshi, D. D., Doanh, N. Q., Van De, N., & Xiaonong, Z. (2003). Taenia solium taeniosis/cysticercosis in Asia: Epidemiology, impact and issues. *Acta Tropica, 87*(1), 53–60. https://doi.org/10.1016/S0001-706X(03)00055-X

Ramiandrasoa, N. S., Ravoniarimbinina, P., Solofoniaina, A. R., Andrianjafy Rakotomanga, I. P., Andrianarisoa, S. H., Molia, S., Labouche, A.-M., Fahrion, A. S., Donadeu, M., Abela-Ridder, B., & Rajaonatahina, D. (2020). Impact of a 3-year mass drug administration pilot project for taeniasis control in Madagascar. *PLoS Neglected Tropical Diseases, 14*(9), e0008653. https://doi.org/10.1371/journal.pntd.0008653

Roy, S., Malla, S., Dekari, D., & Choudhury, T. G. (2025). One Health approach: Human, environment, and animal health. In S. K. Mallik, N. Shahi, & P. K. Pandey (Eds.), *Management of fish diseases* (pp. 281–297). Springer Nature. https://doi.org/10.1007/978-981-96-0270-4_12

Salim, L., Ang, A., Handali, S., Cysticercosis Working Group in Papua, & Tsang, V. C. W. (2009). Seroepidemiologic survey of cysticercosis-taeniasis in four central highland districts of Papua, Indonesia. *The American Journal of Tropical Medicine and Hygiene, 80*(3), 384–388.

Schuster-Wallace, C., Dickin, S., & Metcalfe, C. (2014). Waterborne and foodborne diseases, climate change impacts on health. In B. Freedman (Ed.), *Global environmental change* (pp. 615–622). Springer). https://doi.org/10.1007/978-94-007-5784-4_102

Shen, C., Li, S., Zheng, S., Choi, M.-H., Bae, Y. M., & Hong, S.-T. (2007). Tissue parasitic helminthiases are prevalent at Cheongjin, North Korea. *The Korean Journal of Parasitology, 45*(2), 139. https://doi.org/10.3347/kjp.2007.45.2.139

Soo, Z. M. P., Khan, N. A., & Siddiqui, R. (2020). Leptospirosis: Increasing importance in developing countries. *Acta Tropica, 201*, 105183. https://doi.org/10.1016/j.actatropica.2019.105183

Spadar, A., Perdigão, J., Campino, S., & Clark, T. G. (2022). Genomic analysis of hypervirulent *Klebsiella pneumoniae* reveals potential genetic markers for differentiation from classical strains. *Scientific Reports, 12*(1), 13671. https://doi.org/10.1038/s41598-022-17995-2

Sripa, B., Leonardo, L., Hong, S.-J., Ito, A., & Brattig, N. W. (2022). Status and perspective of Asian neglected tropical diseases. *Acta Tropica, 225*, 106212. https://doi.org/10.1016/j.actatropica.2021.106212

Su, H.-J., Chen, M.-J., & Chen, N.-T. (2016). Climate variability and human health in Southeast Asia: A Taiwan study. In R. Akhtar (Ed.), *Climate change and human health scenario in South and Southeast Asia* (pp. 237–242). Springer. https://doi.org/10.1007/978-3-319-23684-1_14

Subedi, D., Chandran, D., Subedi, S., & Acharya, K. P. (2022). Ecological and socioeconomic factors in the occurrence of rabies: A forgotten scenario. *Infectious Disease Reports, 14*(6), 979–986. https://doi.org/10.3390/idr14060097

Subrata, I. M., Harjana, N. P. A., Agustina, K. K., Purnama, S. G., & Kardiwinata, M. P. (2022). Designing a rabies control mobile application for a community-based rabies surveillance system during the COVID-19 pandemic in Bali, Indonesia. *Veterinary World*, 1237–1245. https://doi.org/10.14202/vetworld.2022.1237-1245

Sumiyoshi, H., Mori, C., Fuke, I., Morita, K., Kuhara, S., Kondou, J., Kikuchi, Y., Nagamatu, H., & Igarashi, A. (1987). Complete nucleotide sequence of the Japanese encephalitis virus genome RNA. *Virology, 161*(2), 497–510. https://doi.org/10.1016/0042-6822(87)90144-9

Sutisna, P., Kapti, I. N., Wandra, T., Dharmawan, N. S., Swastika, K., Raka Sudewi, A. A., Susilawathi, N. M., Sudarmaja, I. M., Yanagida, T., Okamoto, M., Yoshida, T., Donadeu, M., Lightowlers, M. W., & Ito, A. (2019). Towards a cysticercosis-free tropical resort island: A historical overview of taeniasis/cysticercosis in Bali. *Acta Tropica, 190*, 273–283. https://doi.org/10.1016/j.actatropica.2018.10.012

Tabilin, E. J., Gray, D. J., Jiz, M. A., Mationg, M. L., Inobaya, M., Avenido-Cervantes, E., Sato, M., Sato, M. O., Sako, Y., Mu, Y., You, H., Kelly, M., Cai, P., & Gordon, C. A. (2025). Schistosomiasis in the Philippines: A comprehensive review of epidemiology and current control. *Tropical Medicine and Infectious Disease, 10*(2), 29. https://doi.org/10.3390/tropicalmed10020029

Tan, H. Y. (2025). Overview of Singapore's One Health Strategy. *Zoonotic Diseases, 5*(1), 2. https://doi.org/10.3390/zoonoticdis5010002

Uzoka, F.-M. E., Akwaowo, C., Nwafor-Okoli, C., Ekpin, V., Nwokoro, C., El Hussein, M., Osuji, J., Aladi, F., Akinnuwesi, B., & Akpelishi, T. F. (2021). Risk factors for some tropical diseases in an African country. *BMC Public Health, 21*(1), 2261. https://doi.org/10.1186/s12889-021-12286-3

Verma, A., Satapathy, P., Venugopal, D., Menon, S. V., Vadia, N., Panigrahi, R., Kumar, S., Lakhanpal, S., Ronald, T., & Sah, S. (2025). Monsoon-driven dynamics of infectious diseases: Climatic determinants, outbreak patterns, and public health implications. *Clinical Infection in Practice, 28*, 100516. https://doi.org/10.1016/j.clinpr.2025.100516

WHO. (2023). *Global report on neglected tropical diseases 2023*. https://www.who.int/teams/control-of-neglected-tropical-diseases/global-report-on-neglected-tropical-diseases-2023

Wu, C., Astbury, C. C., Lee, K. M., Gong, Z., Chen, S., Li, A., Tsasis, P., & Penney, T. (2023). Public awareness of One Health in China. *One Health, 17*, 100603. https://doi.org/10.1016/j.onehlt.2023.100603

Wyres, K. L., Nguyen, T. N. T., Lam, M. M. C., Judd, L. M., Van Vinh Chau, N., Dance, D. A. B., Ip, M., Karkey, A., Ling, C. L., Miliya, T., Newton, P. N., Lan, N. P. H., Sengduangphachanh, A., Turner, P., Veeraraghavan, B., Vinh, P. V., Vongsouvath, M., Thomson, N. R., Baker, S., & Holt, K. E. (2020). Genomic surveillance for hypervirulence and multi-drug resistance in invasive *Klebsiella pneumoniae* from South and Southeast Asia. *Genome Medicine, 12*(1), 11. https://doi.org/10.1186/s13073-019-0706-y

Yajima, A., Lin, Z., Mohamed, A. J., Dash, A. P., & Rijal, S. (2023). Finishing the task of eliminating neglected tropical diseases (NTDs) in WHO South-East Asia Region: Promises kept, challenges, and the way forward. *The Lancet Regional Health—Southeast Asia, 18*, 100302. https://doi.org/10.1016/j.lansea.2023.100302

Yang, G.-J., Ouyang, H.-Q., Zhao, Z.-Y., Li, W.-H., Fall, I. S., Djirmay, A. G., & Zhou, X.-N. (2025). Discrepancies in neglected tropical diseases burden estimates in China: Comparative study of real-world data and Global Burden of Disease 2021 data (2004-2020). *BMJ, 388*, e080969. https://doi.org/10.1136/bmj-2024-080969

Yoshida, A., Doanh, P. N., & Maruyama, H. (2019). Paragonimus and paragonimiasis in Asia: An update. *Acta Tropica, 199*, 105074. https://doi.org/10.1016/j.actatropica.2019.105074

Zain, A., Sadarangani, S. P., Shek, L. P.-C., & Vasoo, S. (2024). Climate change and its impact on infectious diseases in Asia. *Singapore Medical Journal, 65*(4), 211–219. https://doi.org/10.4103/singaporemedj.SMJ-2023-180

Chapter 11
Occupational Health Issues and One Health

Vena Jaladara, Kharisma Dewi, Salsabila A. F., Yudhi Ratna Nugraheni, Marselinus Edwin Widyanto Daniwijaya, and Tri Joko

11.1 Understanding the One Health Approach in Occupational Settings

One Health is commonly associated with zoonotic disease outbreaks, the health of animals, or efforts in environmental protection (AL-Eitan et al., 2023; Pettan-Brewer et al., 2021; Redford et al., 2022). However, it is rare for us to deliberate on the question: Is there a connection between One Health and our day-to-day practices, especially in relation to our work? We have overlooked a crucial dimension: One Health issues are closely linked to our daily lives and have a significant impact

V. Jaladara (✉)
Department of Health Behavior, Environment, and Social Medicine, Faculty of Medicine, Public Health, and Nursing, Universitas Gadjah Mada, Yogyakarta, Indonesia

The Graduate School for the Humanities, Faculty of Arts, University of Groningen, Groningen, Netherlands
e-mail: vena.jaladara@ugm.ac.id

K. Dewi
Department of Parasitology, Faculty of Medicine, Public Health, and Nursing, Universitas Gadjah Mada, Yogyakarta, Indonesia
e-mail: kharisma.dewi@mail.ugm.ac.id

Salsabila A. F.
Department of Health, Faculty of Vocational Studies, Universitas Airlangga, Surabaya, Indonesia
e-mail: salsabila.al.firdausi@vokasi.unair.ac.id

Y. R. Nugraheni
Department of Parasitology, Faculty of Veterinary Medicine, Universitas Gadjah Mada, Yogyakarta, Indonesia

One Health Centre of Excellence, Universitas Gadjah Mada, Yogyakarta, Indonesia
e-mail: yudhi.ratna.n@mail.ugm.ac.id

© The Author(s), under exclusive license to Springer Nature Singapore Pte Ltd. 2026

A. U. Rauf, T. Wibawa (eds.), *The One Health Concept in Asian Contexts*,
https://doi.org/10.1007/978-981-95-9880-9_11

on our health and safety (Cediel Becerra et al., 2021). In fact, the workplace stands as one of the most dynamic domains where the interactions of humans, animals, and the surrounding environment transpire—frequently in a sustained and intensive capacity (Roopnarine et al., 2021; Wilkes et al., 2020). From diverse avian farming initiatives to healthcare institutions, from food manufacturing sites to waste management facilities, the workplace operates as a significant hub where risks develop, gather, and potentially proliferate.

This chapter advocates for researchers and practitioners—especially those involved in occupational health or program execution—to explore and understand how the One Health framework can be employed to improve worker safety across multiple sectors (Roopnarine et al., 2021; Togami et al., 2023). Start by reviewing how we understand the risks linked to the workplace setting. In conventional frameworks, risks are categorized into physical, chemical, and psychosocial. However, the One Health paradigm encourages us to enhance this viewpoint. Have we ever contemplated a rice farmer navigating through inundated fields where rodents disseminate leptospirosis? Or a veterinarian attending to livestock amid a brucellosis epidemic? Or even a sanitation worker in an urban locale managing organic refuse that attracts disease-transmitting vectors? All of the examples highlight that no occupation is protected from the intricate relationships of human, animal, and environmental wellness (Connolly, 2020; Perez Arredondo, 2022; Tidman et al., 2022). In fact, specific job activities can amplify or mitigate these risks.

One Health is not just about pandemics—it is also about daily exposures that are often invisible and neglected. Let's examine the situation during the early months of the COVID-19 pandemic. Healthcare workers stood on the front lines, but so did meatpacking workers, migrant farm laborers, and public transportation staff—many of whom worked in conditions where physical proximity, poor ventilation, or interaction with animals increased exposure risk (Streichert et al., 2022). Similarly, in tropical regions, farmers and plantation workers often face dual threats: biological hazards from wildlife and environmental hazards like extreme heat, flooding, or land degradation. These are not theoretical risks; they are lived experiences. Unfortunately, these cases are rarely framed as One Health issues—although they clearly are.

So, what happens when we start applying One Health principles to occupational health? First, we become more proactive. We do not just wait for diseases to emerge—we anticipate them through surveillance that includes animal populations and ecological trends. Second, we foster collaboration across disciplines. A One

M. E. W. Daniwijaya
Department of Microbiology, Faculty of Medicine, Public Health and Nursing, Universitas Gadjah Mada, Yogyakarta, Indonesia
e-mail: m.edwin.d@ugm.ac.id

T. Joko
Department of Plant Protection, Faculty of Agriculture, Universitas Gadjah Mada, Yogyakarta, Indonesia
e-mail: tjoko@ugm.ac.id

Health approach naturally encourages partnerships between health workers, veterinarians, environmental agencies, and even community leaders. This cross-sectoral dialogue is essential, especially in settings with limited resources. Third, we recognize the workplace as both a point of exposure and a site of prevention. Occupational safety programs that factor in environmental and animal risks can be more holistic, more just, and more sustainable (Gomes et al., 2023; Viegas, 2022).

Implementing One Health in the workplace requires strong commitment and alignment (Mumford et al., 2023). At the policy level, national and local occupational health regulations should begin recognizing environmental and zoonotic dimensions of risk—not just chemical and physical ones. Surveillance systems must be designed to detect unusual patterns that span across species and ecosystems. Training for occupational health practitioners should also include One Health thinking—not as an add-on, but as a core competency. And finally, participatory approaches that involve workers themselves can make interventions more effective and grounded.

One Health is more than just a framework; it is a perspective that encourages connections and proactive interventions (Varela et al., 2023). To safeguard workforce health, it is crucial to understand that it is not simply about personal protective equipment and written regulations. It is crucial to recognize that occupational health exists within a broader web of ecological and biological interrelations. Whether one is a policymaker, practitioner, or educator, it is crucial to use One Health as a framework and a way of thinking in the pursuit of a safe and health-promoting work environment. Ultimately, our efforts are not just about safeguarding the health of individuals in the workplace; they also protect the communities and natural ecosystems surrounding workers. We can no longer separate the safety and health of workers from the well-being of the environment they live in, the animals they care for, or the water they use. One Health underscores the crucial idea that the workplace is not independent of the world around it. One Health is an integral component of promoting public health and safety.

11.2 Case studies and Sectoral Insights

The One Health approach has reshaped how we see the link between occupational health and zoonotic risks in today's fast-changing world (Dignard & Leibler, 2019; Munyaneza et al., 2025). At its core, it recognizes that human, animal, and environmental health are deeply connected. Many of the most pressing health threats, such as emerging infectious diseases, antimicrobial resistance, and environmental degradation, often emerge where people, animals, and their shared habitats. People working in sectors such as veterinary practice, laboratory sciences, agriculture, animal husbandry, slaughterhouses and meat processing, wildlife conservation, companion animal care, and food production face multiple points of risk for exposure to pathogens that can cross species and sometimes have pandemic potential (Kumar et al.,

2013). Integrating occupational health and safety (OHS) as a first line of defense not only protects workers but also helps prevent silent threats from taking hold and escalating into wider outbreaks (Dignard & Leibler, 2019; Hulme et al., 2025).

(a) *Veterinary Sectors*

Veterinary workers are repeatedly at the front line of zoonotic spillover events (Ellwanger & Chies, 2021; Kumar et al., 2013; Stull et al., 2018; Tran & Xie, 2024). Their exposure risk arises through direct animal contact, handling of infected materials, diagnostic sampling, and sometimes lack of biosafety (or of awareness of hazards) (Ellwanger & Chies, 2021). Reported hazards range from rabies, anthrax, brucellosis, leptospirosis, Q fever to drug-resistant pathogens like methicillin-resistant *Staphylococcus aureus* (MRSA), and even chronic occupational stress (Dignard & Leibler, 2019; Kumar et al., 2013). WHO and World Organisation for Animal Health (WOAH) call for routine vaccination (for rabies, tetanus, influenza), personal protective equipment (PPE), and OHS training as core interventions (Ficociello et al., 2023; Maehira & Spencer, 2019). However, many workplaces lack enforceable policies, ongoing audits, and practical training, especially in low-resource or field settings (Maehira & Spencer, 2019; Resnik, 2024).

Livestock-associated methicillin-resistant *Staphylococcus aureus* (LA-MRSA) represents a critical occupational and public health hazard within the One Health interface. In Asia, particularly China, the ST9 lineage predominates among livestock-associated strains and exhibits broad resistance to tylosin, florfenicol, and tetracyclines, reflecting sustained antimicrobial selection pressure (Ji et al., 2025). A potential epidemiological shift toward the more robust ST398 clone may occur under stricter antibiotic regulations, potentially altering resistance dynamics and transmission patterns. LA-MRSA constitutes the biological hazard; primary exposure routes include direct contact with colonized livestock, inhalation of contaminated barn aerosols, and contact with manure or farm environments. Monitoring indicators should include MRSA nasal carriage prevalence among livestock workers, clonal distribution (ST9/ST398), antimicrobial consumption rates (e.g., defined daily doses per 100 animals), and environmental MRSA detection in farm dust or wastewater. Control strategies must follow the hierarchy of controls: elimination through reduction of nontherapeutic antimicrobial use; substitution with vaccines or improved husbandry practices; engineering controls such as enhanced barn ventilation and manure management systems; administrative controls including antimicrobial stewardship programs and routine occupational screening; and appropriate PPE (gloves, masks, protective clothing).

Antimicrobial consumption patterns across Asia further amplify antimicrobial resistance (AMR) risks. While Bhutan reports relatively low antimicrobial consumption due to strong governance and regulatory adherence (Gurung et al., 2023), many Southeast Asian countries face high AMR risks driven by intensive farming and widespread antibiotic use, compounded by limited standardized surveillance systems (Malijan et al., 2022). Antibiotic residues released into manure, wastewater, and aquaculture effluents, particularly in China, contribute to environmental contamination and selective pressure in soil and water ecosystems (Quaik et al.,

2020; Rico & Van Den Brink, 2014). Aquaculture systems in Vietnam and China have similarly been implicated in environmental dissemination of veterinary medicines (Rico & Van Den Brink, 2014). In this context, hazards extend beyond resistant pathogens to include antibiotic residues in environmental matrices. Exposure routes involve occupational handling of manure, contact with contaminated water, and foodborne transmission through animal-derived products. Monitoring indicators should therefore encompass antimicrobial sales data, residue concentrations in soil and water, prevalence of multidrug-resistant *Escherichia coli* and *Salmonella* in animal-derived foods (Dushayeva, 2025), and resistance profiles in high-risk settings such as poultry farms and slaughterhouses in Chitwan, Nepal, where non-typhoidal *Salmonella* demonstrates high prevalence and resistance (Fowler et al., 2021). Control measures include strengthened regulatory enforcement, environmental waste treatment systems, standardized AMR surveillance platforms, and biosecurity enhancements at farm level.

Poultry production systems illustrate how sector-specific disease pressures may intensify antimicrobial use. In Bangladesh, conditions such as visceral gout and coccidiosis are prevalent, often accompanied by high antibiotic usage that accelerates resistance development (Islam et al., 2021). Of global concern is the widespread dissemination of the *mcr-1* gene conferring colistin resistance across Asia and other continents (Petrovic et al., 2024), underscoring the urgency of prudent colistin use in livestock. Here, the hazard is transferable colistin resistance; exposure routes include occupational contact, foodborne transmission, and environmental spread via agricultural runoff.

(b) *Laboratory Sectors*

In laboratory settings, occupational hazards are varied and often interconnected. Core risks include aerosol generation during procedures such as centrifugation or necropsy, sharps-related injuries from needles or broken glass, inadequate training or the absence of robust standard operating procedures (SOPs), equipment or infrastructure failures, and insufficient documentation or incident reporting (Stull et al., 2018). Laboratory-acquired infections (LAIs) remain a substantial source of global occupational risk. However, biosafety frameworks, such as the WHO Laboratory Biosafety Manual (4th Edition), the CDC/NIH Biosafety in Microbiological and Biomedical Laboratories (BMBL), and WOAH standards, provide comprehensive guidance to mitigate these risks, which are internationally recognized (Ficociello et al., 2023; Zavaleta-Monestel et al., 2025). These frameworks emphasize hierarchical control measures, beginning with administrative controls (SOPs, structured training), followed by engineering controls (biological safety cabinets, ventilation systems), appropriate PPE, and well-defined operational procedures (Blacksell et al., 2023; Maehira & Spencer, 2019; Zavaleta-Monestel et al., 2025). They also stress the importance of routine risk assessments, transparent evaluation of practices and pathogen handling, and preparedness of facilities. Effective incident response requires thorough documentation of exposures. Evidence from the CAPTURA project conducted across several Asian countries highlighted the importance of expanding AMR data collection through microbiology laboratories, strengthening local representation, and promoting real-time stakeholder engagement to develop context-specific surveillance strategies (Joh et al., 2023a, b; Malijan et al., 2022). However, persistent gaps remain, particularly in data quality, interoperability, and the continued reliance on paper-based reporting systems, which hinder effective analysis and cross-border data sharing. Resistant pathogens such as MRSA and other multidrug-resistant organisms constitute key biological hazards. Exposure routes include aerosol generation during centrifugation or necropsy, sharps-related injuries, mucosal splashes, and improper specimen handling. Monitoring indicators should include laboratory-acquired infection (LAI) incidence rates, sharps injury frequency, MRSA carriage prevalence among laboratory personnel, antimicrobial susceptibility testing (AST) coverage, and electronic data completeness. Control measures should follow the hierarchy of controls: elimination of unnecessary high-risk procedures, substitution with safer diagnostic alternatives, engineering controls such as certified biosafety cabinets and optimized ventilation systems, administrative controls including robust SOPs, biosafety training, audits, and digital reporting platforms.

Country-specific studies further illustrate the relevance of strengthened laboratory surveillance. In Indonesia, a low prevalence of MRSA nasal carriage among surgical patients suggested that routine mupirocin decolonization may not be universally required (Quaik et al., 2020). In Uganda, MRSA carriage was associated with open wounds and contact with pigs, underscoring occupational and zoonotic exposure pathways (Rico & Van Den Brink, 2014). Among healthcare workers in South Asia, the pooled MRSA prevalence reached 9.23%, with higher estimates reported in Pakistan and Sri Lanka (Dushayeva, 2025). These variations likely reflect differences in infection prevention and control (IPC) practices, surveillance capacity, and antimicrobial stewardship implementation across hospital systems. Despite these insights, laboratory capacity varies widely across low- and middle-income countries, with infrastructure limitations and inconsistent AST implementation leading to fragmented datasets (Joh et al., 2023b; Malijan et al., 2022).

(c) *Human–Animal Interactions and OHS*

In various occupational and cultural settings, close and frequent interactions between humans and animals create significant risks for zoonotic disease transmission and other health hazards. In agricultural contexts, especially in developing countries, routine human–animal–environmental contact, traditional husbandry practices, and informal labor contribute to the risk of zoonotic spillover (Ellwanger & Chies, 2021; Kumar et al., 2013). Activities such as assisting in animal birthing, milking, manure handling, and even sleeping near animals are common pathways of exposure to pathogens like brucellosis and leptospirosis (Ellwanger & Chies, 2021; Fouchier et al., 2004; Kumar et al., 2013; Tran & Xie, 2024). Workers in wildlife-related occupations, including researchers, rangers, and veterinarians, are frequently exposed to high-risk pathogens such as rabies, Ebola, Marburg virus, Kyasanur Forest Disease (KFD), SARS, MERS, monkeypox, and various zoonotic enteric pathogens (Kumar et al., 2013). Their proximity to diseased or deceased wild animals substantially heightens the risk (Tran & Xie, 2024).

Similarly, interactions with companion animals place veterinarians, groomers, shelter staff, and even pet owners at risk of infections such as ringworm, cat-scratch disease, leptospirosis, *methicillin-resistant Staphylococcus aureus* (MRSA), and other skin or enteric conditions. Emerging trends, including raw pet diets, the keeping of exotic animals, and the use of animals in therapy programs, further complicate the risk landscape by introducing new transmission routes and lesser-known pathogens into domestic and clinical environments (Ellwanger & Chies, 2021; Tran & Xie, 2024). Preventing these risks requires a multilayered strategy: routine vaccination of pets and occupationally exposed individuals, education on zoonotic diseases and bite prevention, and strict cleaning and disinfection protocols (Ficociello et al., 2023; Stull et al., 2018). These measures are particularly crucial in high-volume facilities like veterinary clinics, grooming salons, and animal shelters, where close quarters and high animal turnover increase cross-transmission potential.

Beyond infectious diseases, the physical demands of animal-related occupations also pose ergonomic and musculoskeletal risks. Manual, repetitive tasks in poor working conditions commonly result in injury (Munyaneza et al., 2025; Tran & Xie, 2024). MRSA colonization has been observed among workers in pig, poultry, and meat processing industries, with variable prevalence but consistent concern across regions. Comprehensive OHS interventions are vital and include strict adherence to personal protective equipment (PPE) use, regular ergonomic assessments, engineering controls for ventilation and aerosol management, and ongoing health surveillance for workers (Ficociello et al., 2023; Stull et al., 2018). Additional preventive strategies encompass occupational vaccination programs, such as those for seasonal influenza and hepatitis, and rapid response mechanisms for outbreak containment (Ficociello et al., 2023; Fouchier et al., 2004). Previous research has shown that minimizing antibiotic resistance across the human–animal–environment interface is a core principle of the One Health framework and a useful benchmark for strengthening control strategies. It also emphasized the importance of incorporating monitoring and mitigation of occupational health hazards in shrimp farming into One Health-based approaches to reduce waterborne infection risks (Ficociello et al., 2023; Stull et al., 2018). Figure 11.1 presents a One Health conceptual framework derived from earlier studies, emphasizing the reduction of antibiotic resistance at the human, animal, environment interface and the integration of occupational health risk management in shrimp farming.

(d) *One Biosecurity Concept in One Health*

A recent One Health study emphasizes the value of integrating the concept of "One Biosecurity" into the broader framework. This approach explicitly links biosafety, biosecurity, and occupational health, creating a unified strategy to reduce the risks of pathogen spillover, accidental release, and deliberate misuse among human, animal, and environment (Hulme et al., 2025). By embedding security considerations alongside health and safety measures, institutions strengthen their resilience against both natural and human-made biological threats (Blacksell et al., 2023; Hulme et al., 2025). This perspective reinforces the view that surveillance and security are not secondary measures, but essential, inseparable components of effective

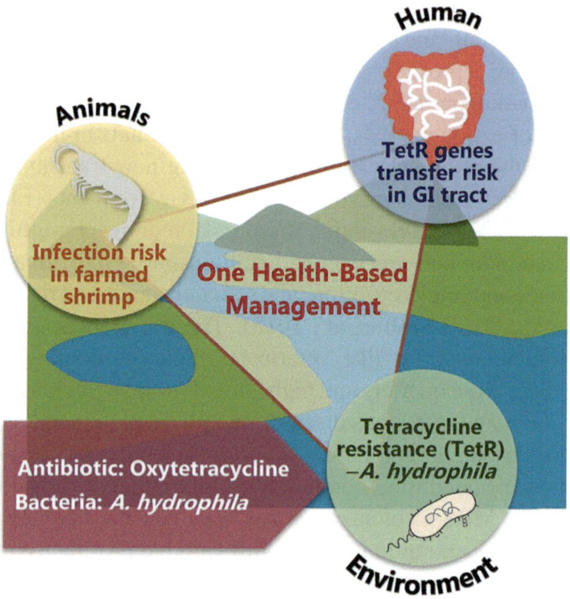

Fig. 11.1 One Health predictive framework for addressing antibiotic resistance and waterborne infection risks. (Lu et al., 2024, licensed under CC-BY 4.0)

occupational health systems, ensuring that prevention, preparedness, and rapid response are fully aligned across human, animal, and environmental health domains.

(e) *Curriculum Integration of Occupational Health and Safety (OHS)*

In a One Health context, strengthening OHS education across veterinary, laboratory, and agricultural sectors is vital to breaking the chain of zoonotic transmission and minimizing occupational hazards. Evidence from multiple case studies shows that embedding OHS into formal curricula, covering both theory (risk assessment, hazard analysis, bloodborne pathogens) and hands-on skills (PPE, incident reporting, hazard identification, and emergency drills), is essential for preparing a resilient workforce (Maehira & Spencer, 2019; Stull et al., 2018). Innovative delivery methods, including digital microlearning, augmented reality (AR)/virtual reality (VR)-based biosafety training, and mobile tools, extend access to training, particularly for migrant and informal workers who may be most vulnerable yet least reached by conventional systems. Ongoing professional development and annual refresher training reinforce these competencies, sustaining high awareness, skill retention, and compliance. By integrating these educational strategies into the One Health approach, institutions can build a workforce that not only safeguards its own health but also acts as a first line of defense against emerging infectious disease threats. Table 11.1 outlines the minimum OHS competencies expected from veterinary students, the assessment modalities, refresher requirements, and credentialing elements necessary to maintain occupational readiness prior to clinical or field placements.

Table 11.1 Minimum occupational health and safety competencies for veterinary training programs

Competency area	Description	Assessment method	Refresher cycle
Risk Assessment & Hazard Identification (DHHS/CDC/NIH, 2020; Williams et al., 2015)	Ability to recognize biological, chemical, physical, and psychosocial hazards in veterinary practice; conduct structured risk assessments; prioritize controls using the hierarchy of controls	Written exam; scenario-based exercises; field practicum evaluation	Annual (or prior to high-risk placement)
PPE Donning & Doffing (DHHS/CDC/NIH, 2020; Williams et al., 2015)	Correct sequencing and technique to prevent self-contamination when putting on and removing PPE; selection of PPE based on exposure risk; respirator fit-checking	Practical skills test; simulation lab with checklist	Annual skills validation
Exposure Management & First Response (Mobo et al., 2010; Williams et al., 2015)	Initial response to sharps injury, mucosal splash, zoonotic exposure, or suspected LAI; immediate containment, reporting, and referral steps	Written exam; scenario-based exercises; field practicum evaluation	Every 12–24 months
Incident & Near-Miss Reporting	Knowledge of mandatory reporting pathways, documentation standards, and reporting timelines for occupational incidents and zoonotic suspicion	Written exam; scenario-based exercises; field practicum evaluation	Annual refresher
Risk Communications & Public Interface (Williams et al., 2015; World Organisation for Animal Health (OIE), 2023)	Communicating occupational and zoonotic risks to peers, clients, farmers, and communities using clear, culturally informed messages	Written exam; scenario-based exercises; field practicum evaluation	Every 2 years
Waste & Carcass Handling Safety (Mobo et al., 2010; Williams et al., 2015)	Safe management of infectious waste, carcasses, and contaminated materials; coordination with veterinary/public health authorities	Field practicum logs; supervisor competency check	Annual refresher
Zoonotic Disease Surveillance Interface (DHHS/CDC/NIH, 2020; Williams et al., 2015)	Understanding surveillance pathways and the role of veterinarians in early detection and notification within One Health systems	Written exam; scenario-based exercises; field practicum evaluation	Every 2–3 years

11.3 Contributions from Key Profession

The environment in the workplace is one of the important factors determining the health of workers (International Labour Organization, 2023). If the workplace conditions are poor, they can pose health risks, including physical, chemical, ergonomic, and biological risks (OSHA, 2016). Biological hazards are a type of hazard that receive less priority in the context of OHS. Practitioners sometimes ignored biological risks in the workplace due to a lack of systematic data, publication bias, and insufficient training (Department of Occupational Safety and Health (DOSH) Ministry of Human Resources (MOHR) Malaysia, 2020; Santos et al., 2020).

The potential biological hazards, particularly in the sectors of healthcare, livestock, food industry, and research laboratories, warrant a collaborative safety approach that provides protection for both humans and the surrounding environment (Bielecka-Oder, 2018). These biological hazards include exposure to microorganisms such as bacteria, viruses, fungi, and parasites. These agents can be found in air, water, soil, animals, and humans and are highly relevant in the context of industry, healthcare facilities, agriculture, and outdoor work. The impacts resulting from these biological hazards can lead to infections, allergies, and even death (Department of Occupational Safety and Health (DOSH) Ministry of Human Resources (MOHR) Malaysia, 2020; Santos et al., 2020). Some infectious diseases can be transmitted from person to person or from animals to humans. Workers may be exposed to various types of contagious diseases, including those transmitted through air, blood, contact, and zoonoses (Ingraham et al., 2021).The complexity of these risks needs a collaborative approach that protects both humans and the surrounding environment.

In Asia, the implementation of One Health with OHS faces significant challenges, especially in developing countries. These challenges include cultural diversity, large population, rapid urbanization, high numbers of informal workers, regulatory discrepancies, and gaps in workers' awareness and training related to safety in the workplace (Gongal, 2012). Low educational levels and limited awareness further reinforce the need for stronger cross-professional integration to ensure more effective and relevant interventions at the local level (Kapilashrami & John, 2023). Moreover, global threats such as pandemics highlight the importance of responsive, multidisciplinary collaboration in building a resilient and adaptive OHS System (Javanmardi et al., 2025).

Safety science plays a role in identifying risks and providing preventive measures to ensure that individuals involved in hazardous work are not adversely affected in terms of safety and health. The collaboration among all parties facilitates early detection, prevention, education, and response to various work-related health threats, thereby strengthening the overall public health system. The following is a description of the main professional contributions involved in this concept:

(a) *Health Care Professionals*

Health professionals play a central role in identifying and managing occupational diseases and communicable diseases with outbreak potential. Community health workers act as frontline actors through education, disease screening, and early interventions about health risks related to the workplace and community (Yasobant et al., 2021). Hospitals serve a curative health role by treating individuals infected with diseases resulting from biological hazards, thereby helping to break the chain of transmission (Dalton et al., 2020).

(b) *Veterinary Professionals*

Veterinarians have an important role in detecting, monitoring, and controlling zoonotic diseases, especially in livestock and agricultural settings. Safety principles can protect them from zoonoses while also creating food products that are safe for public consumption (Mendez et al., 2016). The same level of close monitoring is needed in the field of wildlife veterinary medicine. Wildlife veterinarians are key actors in monitoring diseases that can spill over from wild animals to humans and vice versa. Transmission can occur through multiple pathways, including bushmeat consumption, which involves hunters, hunting dogs, and various other points of contact along the wildlife–human interface (Tran & Xie, 2024). Strong standard operating procedures are therefore essential to prevent zoonotic risks.

(c) *Occupational Health and Safety (OHS) Professional*

Safety professionals are responsible for hazard identification, risk assessment, implementation of appropriate controls, and providing training to workers to create a safe workplace. Data on these risks serve as the basis for developing effective standard operating procedures (SOPs) applicable across sectors.

(d) *Environmental Health Professionals*

Environmental health professionals monitor and control environmental factors, including air quality, water quality, waste management, workplace sanitation, and housing conditions. When environmental conditions fail to meet standards, these professionals collaborate with safety experts to formulate risk mitigation strategies in the workplace.

(e) *Epidemiologists and Policymakers*

Epidemiologists collect, analyze, and interpret disease data to identify relevant patterns and risk factors. The data obtained by these epidemiologists can serve as a foundation for policy-making in designing regulations and occupational health interventions. Regional organizations, such as Association of Southeast Asian Nations (ASEAN) and Southeast Asia One Health University Network (SEAOHUN), support this One Health approach through education, research, and cross-sectoral capacity development (Lâm et al., 2025; WHO, 2022). This collaboration involves interdisciplinary communication networks, joint research, and multidisciplinary case handling in the field (Kamel et al., 2025). This concept of integration can expedite early detection, response to outbreaks, and the development of robust OHS systems while simultaneously strengthening public health resilience.

Table 11.2 summarizes priority occupational sectors within the One Health interface, key hazards, potential exposure pathways, quantifiable indicators for risk

Table 11.2 Occupational hazards, exposure routes, indicators, and controls across key One Health sectors

Sector	Agent/risk type (biological, chemical, physical, psycosocial)	Exposure route	Indicators	Control measures
Veterinary/ Animal Clinics (Fowler et al., 2021; Leggat et al., 2009; Smith et al., 2009)	*Biological:* Rabies, *Brucella* spp., *Leptospira* spp., Q fever, dermatophytosis *Physical:* bites, kicks, musculoskeletal strain *Chemical:* disinfectants, anesthetic gases *Psychosocial:* compassion fatigue, long working hours	Bites and scratches; aerosol inhalation; contact with urine/blood; needle injuries	% staff with rabies vaccination; LAI/10,000 work hours; PPE compliance rate; incidence of bite injuries/year	*Engineering:* animal restraint systems, ventilation, sharps containers *Administrative:* vaccination policy; SOP for animal handling; fatigue management *PPE:* gloves (including cut-resistant, puncture-resistant, and bite-proof), N95 respirator, goggles, face shield, lab coat/gown/ coveralls, waterproof safety boots, masks
Laboratories (DHHS/CDC/ NIH, 2020; Sewell, 2006; Singh, 2009)	*Biological:* influenza A/H5N1, M. tuberculosis, *Salmonella* spp., *Brucella* spp., SARS-CoV-2 *Chemical:* formaldehyde, solvents *Physical:* sharps, noise	Aerosol, droplet, mucosal splash, sharps injury	% certified class II BSCs; LAI rate per 10,000 work hours; corrective maintenance turnaround time; PPE compliance; % biosafety-trained staff	*Engineering:* certified BSCs, HEPA filtration, automatic doors *Administrative:* biosafety training, incident reporting, exposure surveillance *PPE:* gloves, N95 respirator, goggles, face shield, lab coat, waterproof safety boots, masks

(continued)

Table 11.2 (continued)

Sector	Agent/risk type (biological, chemical, physical, psycosocial)	Exposure route	Indicators	Control measures
Poultry Production & Hatcheries (Corbel, 2006)	*Biological:* avian influenza, *Campylobacter*, *Salmonella*, Newcastle disease *Chemical:* disinfectants, fumigants *Physical:* heat stress, repetitive strain	Aerosolized dust; fecal–oral; direct handling; contaminated surfaces	% vaccination uptake against AI; worker respiratory symptom reports; dust concentration mg/m^3; WBGT readings; PPE compliance	*Engineering:* dust extraction, enclosed conveyors, cooling fans *Administrative:* biosecurity zones; rotation schedules to reduce heat stress; vaccination programs *PPE:* gloves (including cut-resistant, puncture-resistant, and bite-proof), N95 respirator, goggles, coveralls, waterproof safety boots, masks
Ruminants/ Dairy & Cattle Farms (Corbel, 2006; Schelling et al., 2007)	*Biological:* brucellosis, leptospirosis, anthrax, Rift Valley fever *Physical:* trampling, crush injuries	Inhalation of aerosols; fecal–oral; percutaneous	% cattle vaccinated; % farm units with certified crush pens; LAI reporting frequency; heat exposure index	*Engineering:* milking parlor shields, crush pens *Administrative:* vaccination schedule compliance; manure handling SOP *PPE:* gloves , N95 respirator, goggles, face shield, coveralls, waterproof safety boots, masks

(continued)

Table 11.2 (continued)

Sector	Agent/risk type (biological, chemical, physical, psycosocial)	Exposure route	Indicators	Control measures
Fisheries & Shrimp Aquaculture (Defoirdt et al., 2011; Pruden et al., 2013)	*Biological: Vibrio* spp., *Leptospira* spp., *Streptococcus iniae* *Chemical:* antimicrobials, disinfectants *Waterborne and AMR:* resistant *Vibrio* spp., residual antibiotics	Dermal contact with contaminated water; shellfish handling injuries	% AMR isolates in pond effluent; antimicrobial usage records; wound infection incidence	*Engineering:* effluent treatment, pond aeration *Administrative:* antimicrobial stewardship; water-testing schedule *PPE:* gloves, N95 respirator, goggles, face shield, coveralls, waterproof safety boots, masks
Waste Management & Sanitation Workers (Cirstea et al., 2025; Rachiotis et al., 2012)	*Biological:* hepatitis A/E, leptospirosis, helminths, hantavirus *Chemical:* cleaning agents, fumes *Physical:* sharps, ergonomic injury	Contact with contaminated waste; sharps injury; aerosol/ dust	Sharps injury rate/1000 workers; % staff vaccinated (Hep A/B); PPE compliance; water quality indicators	*Engineering:* mechanical waste lifters, closed waste containers *Administrative:* vaccination program; sharps protocol; ergonomic training *PPE:* gloves (including cut-resistant, puncture-resistant, and bite-proof), N95 respirator, goggles, face shield, lab coat/gown/ coveralls, waterproof safety boots, masks

(continued)

Table 11.2 (continued)

Sector	Agent/risk type (biological, chemical, physical, psycosocial)	Exposure route	Indicators	Control measures
Healthcare Facilities (Hospital/ Primary Care) (Prüss-Üstün et al., 2005; World Health Organization, 2016)	*Biological:* TB, SARS-CoV-2, MRSA, *Clostridioides difficile*, zoonoses from patients with animal exposure	Airborne, droplet, mucosal splash, needlestick	TB screening positivity rate in HCWs; PPE compliance; AIIR availability; needlestick injuries/1,000 workers	*Engineering:* negative pressure rooms; point-of-care sharps disposal *Administrative:* IPC SOPs; vaccination campaigns; AMR stewardship *PPE:* gloves (including cut-resistant, puncture-resistant, and bite-proof), N95 respirator, goggles, face shield, lab coat/gown/ coveralls, waterproof safety boots, masks

monitoring, and recommended control measures following the hierarchy of controls frameworks.

Effective collaboration requires open communication through scientific forums, seminars, conferences, and workshops. Multidisciplinary networks involving academia, government, practitioners, and nongovernmental organizations for sharing of data, resources, and expertise. For example, addressing complex occupational health cases, such as zoonoses in livestock environments or nosocomial infections, requires collaboration among veterinarians, health workers, occupational health experts, and epidemiologists. Workplace safety policies need to take into account vulnerable workers. Occupational safety policies must also consider vulnerable workers, including those in the informal sector, workers in animal-based industries, underage workers, and female workers. Workers in the informal sector often lack a safety and protection system. Workers in farming and food processing face a high risk of zoonoses due to direct contact with animals. Underage workers and women are particularly susceptible to discrimination and often have limited access to proper health and safety training. The function of safety in the workplace is to respect individuals who are working. It does not view workers as assets whose safety and health are neglected.

11.4 Building an Inclusive Framework: Policies, Partnerships, and Preparedness

When we reflect on how to build better OHS conditions, many of us tie it to compliance measures, workplace assessments, and the application of technical requirements. However, the One Health perspective motivates us to broaden our understanding. Worker protection extends beyond simply preventing accidents and minimizing physical, chemical, and ergonomic dangers; it demands a deep commitment to shielding from risks that arise from the multifaceted connections between humans, creatures, and the ecosystem (He et al., 2022; Marchese & Hovorka, 2022). We need to explore more deeply how the One Health framework can enrich our understanding of OHS.

Every sector is vulnerable to the risks posed by zoonotic and environmental concerns, which affect agriculture, mining operations, and waste disposal. These areas commonly face zoonotic illnesses, ecological risks, and numerous health challenges. Especially, farmers might have an increased likelihood of contracting diseases like leptospirosis and brucellosis (Charypkhan & Rüegg, 2022; Haji Hajikolaei et al., 2022; Mazzanti et al., 2023), while workers in waste management could potentially encounter pathogens including leptospirosis and hantavirus (Riccò et al., 2021). To competently diminish these dangers, it is crucial to establish and apply directives that fuse ecological and zoonotic factors within the realm of OHS.

Several countries have already adopted strategies that integrate One Health concepts. An example can be seen in the Netherlands, which developed an all-encompassing control policy during the Q fever crisis from 2007 to 2010 that integrated public health surveillance, veterinary regulations, and occupational safety standards (Garcia-Vozmediano et al., 2022; Koeijer et al., 2020; Ladbury et al., 2015). This involved compulsory vaccination of livestock, farm biosecurity protocols, and safety regulations for agricultural workers and veterinary professionals (Reukers et al., 2022). Finland, another nation in Europe, likewise incorporates preventive measures against zoonotic diseases into its regulations concerning farmworker safety, requiring farmers to be educated on avoiding cross-contamination between animals and humans to decrease the risk of zoonotic disease transmission (Alves et al., 2023; Li et al., 2023; Tiirinki et al., 2022).

Strong partnerships between government agencies, private industry, academic institutions, and civil society are essential for effective One Health implementation. This cooperation enhances the unification of workplace health tracking insights with community health and ecological evaluation systems, consequently developing a more extensive comprehension of pertinent threats and responses. Significant examples of effective collaborations comprise the “Zoonoses Structure” Partnership in the Netherlands, the One Health Initiative in Uganda, and the intersectoral response team in Canada during the H7N3 avian influenza outbreak.

In the Netherlands, the “Zoonoses Structure” Collaboration integrates public health, veterinary, and occupational safety entities to facilitate real-time data sharing, thereby enhancing the prompt identification of emerging threats (Van Der Giessen et al., 2022). This collaborative framework guarantees that an outbreak in livestock is swiftly identified as a potential workplace risk, instigating precautionary actions for both employees and adjacent communities (Alves et al., 2023; Van Herten et al., 2020). In Uganda, the One Health Platform unites the Ministry of Health, Ministry of Agriculture, Ministry of Water and Environment, along with the Uganda Wildlife Authority (Buregyeya et al., 2020). This platform ensures that OSH efforts in slaughterhouses and markets for live animals are guided by veterinary disease tracking, environmental assessments, and evaluations of public health risks (Medley et al., 2021). During the H7N3 outbreak of avian influenza in British Columbia poultry farms, a team composed of various sectors engaged directly with farmers and processing plant operators in Canada (Mubareka et al., 2023). This partnership led to a decrease in worker infections, enhanced farm biosecurity measures, and expedited the recovery of operations. Preparedness is also a key component of One Health implementation. Countries such as Brazil have provided evidence of this. It is not just about having an emergency plan in place but also about building resilience into day-to-day work systems (Dykstra & Baitchman, 2021; Leandro et al., 2021). This includes scenario planning, simulation exercises, and integrating One Health considerations into emergency response protocols.

By adopting and adapting the One Health framework, a safer, healthier, and more resilient work environment can be created. It is important to fully recognize that safety and health threats know no boundaries between species, sectors, or regions. Several countries, such as the Netherlands, Finland, Uganda and Canada, have demonstrated that integrated policies, strong commitment, and partnerships and preparedness can prevent health crises and their myriad implications (Redford et al., 2022; Viegas, 2022).

Therefore, it can be concluded that One Health is not merely a framework or theory; it should serve as the foundation for a preventative mindset. By integrating environmental and zoonotic risk considerations into workplace safety protocols, building strong partnerships, and building resilience into daily work systems, we can protect against and prevent health crises. We must stop viewing OHS and One Health as separate entities and recognize that they are part of the same system. By working together, we can create a safer, healthier, and more resilient world for all (Box 11.1).

Box 11.1 Local Case: Waste Mismanagement, Rodent Proliferation, and Occupational Leptospirosis in an Urban Province, Indonesia

Context

In a densely populated urban province in Indonesia, ineffective waste management and insufficient collection capacity led to the accumulation of unmanaged household garbage in public areas. The growing volume of waste became a continuous food source for rodents, contributing to an observable rise in the local rat population. During this period, a municipal waste management worker developed acute febrile illness and later died from laboratory-confirmed leptospirosis, a bacterial zoonosis caused by *Leptospira spp.* transmitted through the urine of infected rodents.

A follow-up investigation revealed that the worker was not using adequate personal protective equipment (PPE) and relied solely on waterproof boots

(continued)

Box 11.1 (continued)

without gloves or protective clothing, despite frequent contact with potentially contaminated waste and wastewater. The case highlights how gaps in occupational protection, combined with environmental drivers, increase workers' vulnerability to leptospirosis.

Exposure Routes

- Percutaneous exposure through cuts, abrasions, or microlesions on the hands and forearms while handling waste contaminated with rodent urine.
- Mucosal exposure via splashes to the eyes or mouth during sweeping and loading of wet waste.
- Indirect environmental exposure through contact with contaminated floodwater and puddles accumulating around unmanaged waste sites.
- Respiratory exposure to aerosolized droplets when disturbing waste piles in rodent-infested areas *(less common but plausible under field conditions).*

Control Measures (What Should Have Happened)

- Integrated waste management improvements to reduce waste accumulation and decrease rodent food sources.
- Rodent control and environmental sanitation, including secure waste storage and targeted rat population management.
- Mandatory use of adequate PPE for waste workers: reinforced gloves, waterproof boots, impermeable coveralls, and access to handwashing and decontamination facilities.
- Health surveillance, prophylaxis strategies, and rapid referral pathways for waste workers presenting with febrile illness in endemic areas.
- Community engagement and behavior change communication to reduce improper disposal practices that sustain rodent populations.

Lessons Learned (Occupational Health Safety and One Health Perspective)

- Waste mismanagement and increasing rodent population density form environmental precursors that heighten occupational exposure risks.
- Inadequate PPE use, whether due to lack of access, insufficient training, or weak compliance, can transform routine waste-handling into a high-risk activity, as demonstrated in this fatal case.
- One Health coordination across municipal waste services, public health authorities, and veterinary surveillance programs is necessary to anticipate risk and prevent transmission.
- System-level interventions, improved waste governance, PPE provision, worker training, and early clinical recognition offer more sustainable prevention than individual actions alone.
- Rising rodent sightings, unmanaged waste buildup, and reports of symptomatic workers may function as environmental and occupational indicators, guiding earlier preventive action.

Disclaimer Parts of the language editing process in this chapter were supported by *Microsoft Copilot*, an AI-powered writing assistant designed to enhance clarity and coherence. While Copilot contributed to refining sentence structure and improving readability, the content and interpretations remain the sole responsibility of the author.

Competing Interests The author(s) have no competing interests to declare that are relevant to the content of this chapter.

References

AL-Eitan, L., Sendyani, S., & Alnemri, M. (2023). Applications of the One Health concept: Current status in the Middle East. *Journal of Biosafety and Biosecurity, 5*(1), 21–31. https://doi.org/10.1016/j.jobb.2023.01.001

Alves, F., Artursson, K., Bloch, J., Brisabois, A., Imberechts, H., Jokelainen, P., La Ragione, R., Lindblad, M., Forss, R. L., Marston, D. A., Parvizi, O., Tuominen, L., & Omazic, A. (2023). A multi-country One Health foodborne outbreak simulation exercise: Cross-sectoral cooperation, data sharing and communication. *Frontiers in Public Health, 11*, 1121522. https://doi.org/10.3389/fpubh.2023.1121522

Bielecka-Oder, A. (2018). Safety and security regulations against biological threats. In V. Radosavljevic, I. Banjari, & G. Belojevic (Eds.), *Defence against bioterrorism* (pp. 151–176). Springer. https://doi.org/10.1007/978-94-024-1263-5_12

Blacksell, S. D., Summermatter, K., Masuku, Z. M., Kojima, K., Ross, E., Harper, D. R., & Hamilton, K. (2023). Investment in biosafety and biosecurity: The need for a risk-based approach and systematic reporting of laboratory accidents to mitigate laboratory-acquired infections and pathogen escapes. *The Lancet Microbe, 4*(11), e854–e855. https://doi.org/10.1016/S2666-5247(23)00288-4

Buregyeya, E., Atusingwize, E., Nsamba, P., Musoke, D., Naigaga, I., Kabasa, J. D., Amuguni, H., & Bazeyo, W. (2020). Operationalizing the One Health approach in Uganda: Challenges and opportunities. *Journal of Epidemiology and Global Health, 10*(4), 250. https://doi.org/10.2991/jegh.k.200825.001

Cediel Becerra, N. M., Olaya Medellin, A. M., Tomassone, L., Chiesa, F., & De Meneghi, D. (2021). A survey on One Health approach in Colombia and some Latin American countries: From a fragmented health organization to an integrated health response to global challenges. *Frontiers in Public Health, 9*, 649240. https://doi.org/10.3389/fpubh.2021.649240

Charypkhan, D., & Rüegg, S. R. (2022). One Health evaluation of brucellosis control in Kazakhstan. *PLoS ONE, 17*(11), e0277118. https://doi.org/10.1371/journal.pone.0277118

Cirstea, I., Radu, A.-F., Radu, A., Tit, D. M., & Bungau, G. S. (2025). Healthcare waste toxicity: From human exposure to toxic mechanisms and management strategies. *Journal of Xenobiotics, 15*(5), 155. https://doi.org/10.3390/jox15050155

Connolly, J. (2020). Global crisis leadership for disease-induced threats: One Health and urbanisation. *Global Policy, 11*(3), 283–292. https://doi.org/10.1111/1758-5899.12806

Corbel, M. J. (2006). *Brucellosis in humans and animals*. WHO Press. https://iris.who.int/server/api/core/bitstreams/eb47fd2c-6626-4dd6-bdaf-314b158335fb/content

Dalton, K. R., Rock, C., Carroll, K. C., & Davis, M. F. (2020). One Health in hospitals: How understanding the dynamics of people, animals, and the hospital built-environment can be used to better inform interventions for antimicrobial-resistant gram-positive infections. *Antimicrobial Resistance & Infection Control, 9*(1), 78. https://doi.org/10.1186/s13756-020-00737-2

Defoirdt, T., Sorgeloos, P., & Bossier, P. (2011). Alternatives to antibiotics for the control of bacterial disease in aquaculture. *Current Opinion in Microbiology, 14*(3), 251–258. https://doi.org/10.1016/j.mib.2011.03.004

Department of Occupational Safety and Health (DOSH) Ministry of Human Resources (MOHR) Malaysia. (2020). *Guideliness on Occupational Safety and Health (OSH) risk management for small and medium enterprises in ASEAN member states*. ASEAN.

DHHS/CDC/NIH. (2020). *Biosafety in microbiological and biomedical laboratories*. CDC NIH. https://www.cdc.gov/labs/pdf/SF__19_308133-A_BMBL6_00-BOOK-WEB-final-3.pdf

Dignard, C., & Leibler, J. H. (2019). Recent research on occupational animal exposures and health risks: A narrative review. *Current Environmental Health Reports, 6*(4), 236–246. https://doi.org/10.1007/s40572-019-00253-5

Dushayeva, L. Z. (2025). Antimicrobial resistance in foodborne *Escherichia coli* and Salmonella spp. from animal-origin foods: Transmission pathways, global surveillance gaps, and alternative therapeutic strategies. *Veterinary World*, 3288–3305. https://doi.org/10.14202/vetworld.2025.3288-3305

Dykstra, M. P., & Baitchman, E. J. (2021). A call for One Health in medical education: How the COVID-19 pandemic underscores the need to integrate human, animal, and environmental health. *Academic Medicine, 96*(7), 951–953. https://doi.org/10.1097/ACM.0000000000004072

Ellwanger, J. H., & Chies, J. A. B. (2021). Zoonotic spillover: Understanding basic aspects for better prevention. *Genetics and Molecular Biology, 44*(1 suppl 1), e20200355. https://doi.org/10.1590/1678-4685-gmb-2020-0355

Ficociello, B., Giordano, D., Incoronato, F., Farinella, A., & Pietrangeli, B. (2023). WHO laboratory biosafety manual: A new approach to security. *Annals of Work Exposures and Health, 67*(4), 425–429. https://doi.org/10.1093/annweh/wxac086

Fouchier, R. A. M., Schneeberger, P. M., Rozendaal, F. W., Broekman, J. M., Kemink, S. A. G., Munster, V., Kuiken, T., Rimmelzwaan, G. F., Schutten, M., Van Doornum, G. J. J., Koch, G., Bosman, A., Koopmans, M., & Osterhaus, A. D. M. E. (2004). Avian influenza A virus (H7N7) associated with human conjunctivitis and a fatal case of acute respiratory distress syndrome. *Proceedings of the National Academy of Sciences, 101*(5), 1356–1361. https://doi.org/10.1073/pnas.0308352100

Fowler, P. D., Sharma, S., Pant, D. K., Singh, S., & Wilkins, M. J. (2021). Antimicrobial-resistant non-typhoidal *Salmonella enterica* prevalence among poultry farms and slaughterhouses in Chitwan, Nepal. *Veterinary World, 14*(2), 437–445. https://doi.org/10.14202/vetworld.2021.437-445

Garcia-Vozmediano, A., De Meneghi, D., Sprong, H., Portillo, A., Oteo, J. A., & Tomassone, L. (2022). A One Health evaluation of the surveillance systems on tick-borne diseases in the Netherlands, Spain and Italy. *Veterinary Sciences, 9*(9), 504. https://doi.org/10.3390/vetsci9090504

Gomes, B., Dias, M., Cervantes, R., Pena, P., Santos, J., Vasconcelos Pinto, M., & Viegas, C. (2023). One Health approach to tackle microbial contamination on poultries—A systematic review. *Toxics, 11*(4), 374. https://doi.org/10.3390/toxics11040374

Gongal, G. (2012). One Health approach in the South East Asia region: Opportunities and challenges. In J. S. Mackenzie, M. Jeggo, P. Daszak, & J. A. Richt (Eds.), *One Health: The human-animal-environment interfaces in emerging infectious diseases* (Vol. 366, pp. 113–122). Springer. https://doi.org/10.1007/978-3-662-45791-7_242

Gurung, R. B., Zangmo, K. P., Gilkerson, J. R., Browning, G. F., Ferdinand, A. S., & Coppo, M. J. C. (2023). Antimicrobial consumption in the livestock sector in Bhutan: Volumes, values, rates, and trends for the period 2017–2021. *Antibiotics, 12*(2), 411. https://doi.org/10.3390/antibiotics12020411

Haji Hajikolaei, M. R., Rezaei, S., Ghadrdan Mashhadi, A. R., & Ghorbanpoor, M. (2022). The role of small ruminants in the epidemiology of leptospirosis. *Scientific Reports, 12*(1), 2148. https://doi.org/10.1038/s41598-022-05767-x

He, J., Guo, Z., Yang, P., Cao, C., Xu, J., Zhou, X., & Li, S. (2022). Social insights on the implementation of One Health in zoonosis prevention and control: A scoping review. *Infectious Diseases of Poverty, 11*(1), 48. https://doi.org/10.1186/s40249-022-00976-y

Hulme, P. E., Dechoum, M. S., Essl, F., Martinou, A. F., Pauchard, A., Pyšek, P., Roy, H. E., Sheppard, A. W., Vilà, M., & Wilson, J. R. U. (2025). One Biosecurity is essential to implement One Health. *BioScience, biaf110*. https://doi.org/10.1093/biosci/biaf110

Ingraham, R., Ingraham, R., & Neilson, C. (2021). *Corporate safety supplementary program—Communicable disease safety plan.* https://www.crd.ca/media/file/communicable-disease-safety-plan

International Labour Organization. (2023). *Call for safer and healthier working environment.* https://www.ilo.org/publications/call-safer-and-healthier-working-environments

Islam, M., Singha, S. P., Belgrad, J., Yasir Hasib, F. M., Abu Sayeed, M., Ershadul Haque, M., Ahad, A., & Hoque, M. A. (2021). Common chicken diseases in Kishoreganj, Bangladesh: Estimation through the veterinary hospital-based passive surveillance system. *Advances in Animal and Veterinary Sciences, 9*(11). https://doi.org/10.17582/journal.aavs/2021/9.11.1951.1958

Javanmardi, S., Rappelt, L., Zangenberg, S., Heinke, L., Baumgart, C., Niederer, D., & Freiwald, J. (2025). Effectiveness of workplace health promotion programs for industrial workers: A systematic review. *BMC Public Health, 25*(1), 168. https://doi.org/10.1186/s12889-025-21365-8

Ji, X., Wang, Y., He, T., Krüger-Haker, H., Wang, Y., Wu, C., Schwarz, S., & Sun, C. (2025). Comparative analysis of colonization and survival strategies of regionally predominant LA-MRSA clones ST398 and ST9. *mSystems, 10*(10), e00397–e00325. https://doi.org/10.1128/msystems.00397-25

Joh, H. S., Dolabella, B., Early, E., Stelling, J., Ak, G., Upadhyaya, M. K., Rahman, A., Chuki, P., MacWright, W. R., Ondoa, P., Sarkar, S., Moore, C., Holm, M., Leslie, T., Zellweger, R. M., Paing, G., Kwon, S. Y., Marks, F., & Poudyal, N. (2023a). CAPTURA regional workshop proceedings (28–30 June 2022, Virtual). *Clinical Infectious Diseases, 77*(Supplement_7), S536–S542. https://doi.org/10.1093/cid/ciad568

Joh, H. S., Yeats, C., Shaw, A., Poudyal, N., Gallagher, P., Kim, J.-H., Shaikh, A., Seo, H. J., Chi, K. K., Prifti, K., Cho, A., Sujan, M. J., Eraly, E., Pham, K. D., Shrestha, S., Aboushady, A. T., Pak, G., Jang, G., Park, E. L., et al. (2023b). Methodological approach to identify and expand the volume of Antimicrobial Resistance (AMR) data in the human health sector in low- and middle-income countries in Asia: Implications for local and regional AMR surveillance systems strengthening. *Clinical Infectious Diseases, 77*(Supplement_7), S507–S518. https://doi.org/10.1093/cid/ciad634

Kamel, M., Aleya, S., Almagharbeh, W. T., Aleya, L., & Abdel-Daim, M. M. (2025). The emergence of highly pathogenic avian influenza H5N1 in dairy cattle: Implications for public health, animal health, and pandemic preparedness. *European Journal of Clinical Microbiology & Infectious Diseases, 44*(8), 1817–1833. https://doi.org/10.1007/s10096-025-05147-z

Kapilashrami, A., & John, E. A. (2023). Health beyond borders: Migration and precarity in South Asia. In S. I. Rajan (Ed.), *Migration in South Asia* (pp. 201–213). Springer. https://doi.org/10.1007/978-3-031-34194-6_14

Koeijer, A. A. D., Hagenaars, T. J., Leuken, J. P. G. V., Swart, A. N., & Boender, G. J. (2020). Spatial transmission risk during the 2007-2010 Q fever epidemic in The Netherlands: Analysis of the farm-to-farm and farm-to-resident transmission. *PLoS ONE, 15*(2), e0227491. https://doi.org/10.1371/journal.pone.0227491

Kumar, H., Lokesha, K., Madhavaprasad, C., Shilpa, V., Karabasanavar, N., & Kumar, A. (2013). Occupational zoonoses in zoo and wildlife veterinarians in India: A review. *Veterinary World, 6*(9), 605. https://doi.org/10.5455/vetworld.2013.605-613

Ladbury, G. A. F., Van Leuken, J. P. G., Swart, A., Vellema, P., Schimmer, B., Ter Schegget, R., & Van Der Hoek, W. (2015). Integrating interdisciplinary methodologies for One Health: Goat farm re-implicated as the probable source of an urban Q fever outbreak, the Netherlands, 2009. *BMC Infectious Diseases, 15*(1), 372. https://doi.org/10.1186/s12879-015-1083-9

Lâm, S., Dang-Xuan, S., Unger, F., Meeyam, T., Pham-Duc, P., Wacharapluesadee, S., & Nguyen-Viet, H. (2025). Operationalizing regional One Health initiatives in Southeast Asia: Ways forward. *One Health, 20*, 101034. https://doi.org/10.1016/j.onehlt.2025.101034

Leandro, A. D. S., Lopes, R. D., Martins, C. A., Rivas, A. V., Da Silva, I., Galvão, S. R., & Maciel-de-Freitas, R. (2021). The adoption of the One Health approach to improve surveillance of venomous animal injury, vector-borne and zoonotic diseases in Foz do Iguaçu, Brazil. *PLoS Neglected Tropical Diseases, 15*(2), e0009109. https://doi.org/10.1371/journal.pntd.0009109

Leggat, P. A., Smith, D. R., & Speare, R. (2009). Exposure rate of needlestick and sharps injuries among Australian veterinarians. *Journal of Occupational Medicine and Toxicology, 4*(1), 25. https://doi.org/10.1186/1745-6673-4-25

Li, O. Y., Wang, X., Yang, K., Liu, D., & Shi, H. (2023). The approaching pilot for One Health governance index. *Infectious Diseases of Poverty, 12*(1), 16. https://doi.org/10.1186/s40249-023-01067-2

Lu, T.-H., Chen, C.-Y., Wang, W.-M., & Liao, C.-M. (2024). One Health-based management for sustainably mitigating tetracycline-resistant *Aeromonas hydrophila*-induced health risk. *Environmental Pollution, 349*, 123943. https://doi.org/10.1016/j.envpol.2024.123943

Maehira, Y., & Spencer, R. C. (2019). Harmonization of biosafety and biosecurity standards for high-containment facilities in low- and middle-income countries: An approach from the perspective of occupational safety and health. *Frontiers in Public Health, 7*, 249. https://doi.org/10.3389/fpubh.2019.00249

Malijan, G. M., Howteerakul, N., Ali, N., Siri, S., Kengganpanich, M., Nascimento, R., Booton, R. D., Turner, K. M. E., Cooper, B. S., & Meeyai, A. (2022). A scoping review of antibiotic use practices and drivers of inappropriate antibiotic use in animal farms in WHO Southeast Asia region. *One Health, 15*, 100412. https://doi.org/10.1016/j.onehlt.2022.100412

Marchese, A., & Hovorka, A. (2022). Zoonoses transfer, factory farms and unsustainable human–animal relations. *Sustainability, 14*(19), 12806. https://doi.org/10.3390/su141912806

Mazzanti, M., Scialfa, E., Rivero, M., & Passucci, J. (2023). Epidemiology of Leptospira spp. Infection in a beef cattle area of Argentina. *Frontiers in Veterinary Science, 10*, 1083024. https://doi.org/10.3389/fvets.2023.1083024

Medley, A. M., Gasanani, J., Nyolimati, C. A., McIntyre, E., Ward, S., Okuyo, B., Kabiito, D., Bender, C., Jafari, Z., LaMorde, M., Babigumira, P. A., Nakiire, L., Agwang, C., Merrill, R., Ndumu, D., & Doris, K. (2021). Preventing the cross-border spread of zoonotic diseases: Multisectoral community engagement to characterize animal mobility—Uganda, 2020. *Zoonoses and Public Health, 68*(7), 747–759. https://doi.org/10.1111/zph.12823

Mendez, D. H., Büttner, P., Kelly, J., Nowak, M., & Speare, R. (2016). Difficulties experienced by veterinarians when communicating about emerging zoonotic risks with animal owners: The case of Hendra virus. *BMC Veterinary Research, 13*(1), 56. https://doi.org/10.1186/s12917-017-0970-2

Mobo, B. H. P., Rabinowitz, P. M., Conti, L. A., & Taiwo, O. A. (2010). Occupational health of animal workers. In *Human-animal medicine* (pp. 343–371). Elsevier. https://doi.org/10.1016/B978-1-4160-6837-2.00012-9

Mubareka, S., Amuasi, J., Banerjee, A., Carabin, H., Copper Jack, J., Jardine, C., Jaroszewicz, B., Keefe, G., Kotwa, J., Kutz, S., McGregor, D., Mease, A., Nicholson, L., Nowak, K., Pickering, B., Reed, M. G., Saint-Charles, J., Simonienko, K., Smith, T., et al. (2023). Strengthening a One Health approach to emerging zoonoses. *FACETS, 8*, 1–64. https://doi.org/10.1139/facets-2021-0190

Mumford, E. L., Martinez, D. J., Tyance-Hassell, K., Cook, A., Hansen, G. R., Labonté, R., Mazet, J. A. K., Mumford, E. C., Rizzo, D. M., Togami, E., Vreedzaam, A., & Parrish-Sprowl, J. (2023). Evolution and expansion of the One Health approach to promote sustainable and resilient health and well-being: A call to action. *Frontiers in Public Health, 10*, 1056459. https://doi.org/10.3389/fpubh.2022.1056459

Munyaneza, C., Bizimana, F., Mukumbo, F., Gatesi, S., Sibomana, E., Munyampuhwe, S., & Dutuze, M. F. (2025). Knowledge, attitudes, practices (KAP), and risk factors toward zoonotic diseases among smallholder livestock farmers in Bugesera district of Rwanda. *Frontiers in Public Health, 13*, 1569682. https://doi.org/10.3389/fpubh.2025.1569682

OSHA. (2016). *Safety management—Hazard identification and assessment—Occupational safety and health administration*. https://www.osha.gov/safety-management/hazard-identification

Perez Arredondo, A. M. (2022). Research-practice-collaborations addressing One Health and urban transformation. A case study: Commentary on "Research-Practice-Collaborations in International Sustainable Development and Knowledge Production—Reflections from a

Political-Economic Perspective". *The European Journal of Development Research, 34*(4), 1745–1756. https://doi.org/10.1057/s41287-022-00553-x

Petrovic, D., Lalošević, V., Kozoderović, G., Vračar, V., & Lalošević, D. (2024). Colistin resistance in pigs from Serbia: Bioinformatics insight into mcr-1 gene sequencing. *Acta Scientiae Veterinariae, 52*. https://doi.org/10.22456/1679-9216.142295

Pettan-Brewer, C., Martins, A. F., Abreu, D. P. B. D., Brandão, A. P. D., Barbosa, D. S., Figueroa, D. P., Cediel, N., Kahn, L. H., Brandespim, D. F., Velásquez, J. C. C., Carvalho, A. A. B., Takayanagui, A. M. M., Galhardo, J. A., Maia-Filho, L. F. A., Pimpão, C. T., Vicente, C. R., & Biondo, A. W. (2021). From the approach to the concept: One Health in Latin America-experiences and perspectives in Brazil, Chile, and Colombia. *Frontiers in Public Health, 9*, 687110. https://doi.org/10.3389/fpubh.2021.687110

Pruden, A., Larsson, D. G. J., Amézquita, A., Collignon, P., Brandt, K. K., Graham, D. W., Lazorchak, J. M., Suzuki, S., Silley, P., Snape, J. R., Topp, E., Zhang, T., & Zhu, Y.-G. (2013). Management options for reducing the release of antibiotics and antibiotic resistance genes to the environment. *Environmental Health Perspectives, 121*(8), 878–885. https://doi.org/10.1289/ehp.1206446

Prüss-Üstün, A., Rapiti, E., & Hutin, Y. (2005). Estimation of the global burden of disease attributable to contaminated sharps injuries among health-care workers. *American Journal of Industrial Medicine, 48*(6), 482–490. https://doi.org/10.1002/ajim.20230

Quaik, S., Embrandiri, A., Ravindran, B., Hossain, K., Al-Dhabi, N. A., Arasu, M. V., Ignacimuthu, S., & Ismail, N. (2020). Veterinary antibiotics in animal manure and manure laden soil: Scenario and challenges in Asian countries. *Journal of King Saud University, Science, 32*(2), 1300–1305. https://doi.org/10.1016/j.jksus.2019.11.015

Rachiotis, G., Papagiannis, D., Markas, D., Thanasias, E., Dounias, G., & Hadjichristodoulou, C. (2012). Hepatitis B virus infection and waste collection: Prevalence, risk factors, and infection pathway. *American Journal of Industrial Medicine, 55*(7), 650–655. https://doi.org/10.1002/ajim.22057

Redford, K. H., Da Fonseca, G. A. B., Gascon, C., Rodriguez, C. M., Adams, J., Andelman, S., Barron, D. H., Batmanian, G., Bierbaum, R., Daszak, P., Daugherty, C., Griffin, J., Kemper, K., Lee, A., Long, B., Lovejoy, T. E., McCauley, D., Romanelli, C., Paxton, M., et al. (2022). Healthy planet healthy people. *Conservation Letters, 15*(3), e12864. https://doi.org/10.1111/conl.12864

Resnik, D. B. (2024). Biosafety, biosecurity, and bioethics. *Monash Bioethics Review, 42*(1), 137–167. https://doi.org/10.1007/s40592-024-00204-3

Reukers, D. F. M., De Boer, P. T., Loohuis, A. O., Wever, P. C., Bleeker-Rovers, C. P., Van Gageldonk-Lafeber, A. B., Van Der Hoek, W., & Timen, A. (2022). Targeted screening for chronic Q fever, the Netherlands. *Emerging Infectious Diseases, 28*(7), 1403–1409. https://doi.org/10.3201/eid2807.212273

Riccò, M., Peruzzi, S., Ranzieri, S., & Magnavita, N. (2021). Occupational hantavirus infections in agricultural and forestry workers: A systematic review and metanalysis. *Viruses, 13*(11), 2150. https://doi.org/10.3390/v13112150

Rico, A., & Van Den Brink, P. J. (2014). Probabilistic risk assessment of veterinary medicines applied to four major aquaculture species produced in Asia. *Science of the Total Environment, 468–469*, 630–641. https://doi.org/10.1016/j.scitotenv.2013.08.063

Roopnarine, R., Boeren, E., & Regan, J.-A. (2021). The missing professional perspective: Medical, veterinary, and dual degree public health student perceptions of One Health. *Frontiers in Public Health, 9*, 704791. https://doi.org/10.3389/fpubh.2021.704791

Santos, J., Ramos, C., Vaz-Velho, M., & Vasconcelos Pinto, M. (2020). Occupational exposure to biological agents. In P. M. Arezes & R. L. Boring (Eds.), *Advances in safety management and human performance* (Vol. 1204, pp. 61–67). Springer. https://doi.org/10.1007/978-3-030-50946-0_9

Schelling, E., Bechir, M., Ahmed, M. A., Wyss, K., Randolph, T. F., & Zinsstag, J. (2007). Human and animal vaccination delivery to remote Nomadic families, Chad. *Emerging Infectious Diseases, 13*(3), 373–379. https://doi.org/10.3201/eid1303.060391

Sewell, D. L. (2006). Laboratory-acquired infections: Are microbiologists at risk? *Clinical Microbiology Newsletter, 28*(1), 1–6. https://doi.org/10.1016/j.clinmicnews.2005.12.004

Singh, K. (2009). Laboratory-acquired infections. *Clinical Infectious Diseases, 49*(1), 142–147. https://doi.org/10.1086/599104

Smith, D. R., Leggat, P. A., Speare, R., & Townley-Jones, M. (2009). Examining the dimensions and correlates of workplace stress among Australian veterinarians. *Journal of Occupational Medicine and Toxicology, 4*(1), 32. https://doi.org/10.1186/1745-6673-4-32

Streichert, L. C., Sepe, L. P., Jokelainen, P., Stroud, C. M., Berezowski, J., & Del Rio Vilas, V. J. (2022). Participation in One Health networks and involvement in the COVID-19 pandemic response: A global study. *Frontiers in Public Health, 10*, 830893. https://doi.org/10.3389/fpubh.2022.830893

Stull, J. W., Bjorvik, E., Bub, J., Dvorak, G., Petersen, C., & Troyer, H. L. (2018). 2018 AAHA infection control, prevention, and biosecurity guidelines. *Journal of the American Animal Hospital Association, 54*(6), 297–326. https://doi.org/10.5326/JAAHA-MS-6903

Tidman, R., Thumbi, S., Wallace, R., De Balogh, K., Iwar, V., Dieuzy-Labaye, I., Song, J., Shadomy, S., Qiu, Y., Torres, G., Hutchison, J., Abela-Ridder, B., Bote, K., Beeching, S., Cronin, K., & Trees, A. (2022). United against rabies forum: the One Health concept at work. *Frontiers in Public Health, 10*, 854419. https://doi.org/10.3389/fpubh.2022.854419

Tiirinki, H., Sulander, J., Sinervo, T., Halme, S., & Keskimäki, I. (2022). Integrating health and social services in Finland: Regional approaches and governance models. *International Journal of Integrated Care, 22*(3), 18. https://doi.org/10.5334/ijic.5982

Togami, E., Behravesh, C. B., Dutcher, T. V., Hansen, G. R., King, L. J., Pelican, K. M., & Mazet, J. A. K. (2023). Characterizing the One Health workforce to promote interdisciplinary, multisectoral approaches in global health problem-solving. *PLoS ONE, 18*(5), e0285705. https://doi.org/10.1371/journal.pone.0285705

Tran, T., & Xie, S. (2024). Mitigating wildlife spillover in the clinical setting: How physicians and veterinarians can help prevent future disease outbreaks. *AJPM Focus, 3*(2), 100193. https://doi.org/10.1016/j.focus.2024.100193

Van Der Giessen, J., Vlaanderen, F., Kortbeek, T., Swaan, C., Van Den Kerkhof, H., Broens, E., Rijks, J., Koene, M., De Rosa, M., Uiterwijk, M., Augustijn-Schretlen, M., & Maassen, C. (2022). Signalling and responding to zoonotic threats using a One Health approach: A decade of the Zoonoses Structure in the Netherlands, 2011 to 2021. *Eurosurveillance, 27*(31). https://doi.org/10.2807/1560-7917.ES.2022.27.31.2200039

Van Herten, J., Buikstra, S., Bovenkerk, B., & Stassen, E. (2020). Ethical decision-making in zoonotic disease control: How do one health strategies function in the Netherlands? *Journal of Agricultural and Environmental Ethics, 33*(2), 239–259. https://doi.org/10.1007/s10806-020-09828-x

Varela, K., Goryoka, G., Suwandono, A., Mahero, M., Valeri, L., Pelican, K., & Salyer, S. J. (2023). One health zoonotic disease prioritization and systems mapping: An integration of two One Health tools. *Zoonoses and Public Health, 70*(2), 146–159. https://doi.org/10.1111/zph.13015

Viegas, S. (2022). One Health approach for the SDGs achievement. *European Journal of Public Health, 32*(Supplement_3), ckac129.017. https://doi.org/10.1093/eurpub/ckac129.017

WHO. (2022). Applying a Primary Health Care approach to investments provided by Gavi. *The Vaccine Alliance*. https://extranet.who.int/uhcpartnership/sites/default/files/media_documents/Gavi-Overview.pdf

Wilkes, M., Papageorgiou, S., Kim, T. Y., Baldrias, L. R., Aguilar, E. K., & Tee, M. L. (2020). The emergence of a One Health workforce: At the crossroads of technology innovation and front-line health workers. *Journal of Global Health, 10*(1). https://doi.org/10.7189/JOGH.10.010333

Williams, C. J., Scheftel, J. M., Elchos, B. L., Hopkins, S. G., & Levine, J. F. (2015). Compendium of veterinary standard precautions for zoonotic disease prevention in veterinary personnel: National Association of State Public Health Veterinarians: Veterinary Infection Control Committee 2015. *Journal of the American Veterinary Medical Association, 247*(11), 1252–1277. https://doi.org/10.2460/javma.247.11.1252

World Health Organization. (2016). *Guidelines on core components of infection prevention and control programmes at the national and acute health care facility level.* World Health Organization. https://apps.who.int/iris/handle/10665/251730

World Organisation for Animal Health (OIE). (2023). *Competency guidelines for veterinary para-professionals.* OIE.

Yasobant, S., Bruchhausen, W., Saxena, D., Memon, F. Z., & Falkenberg, T. (2021). Who could be One Health Activist at the community level? A case for India. *Human Resources for Health, 19*(1), 13. https://doi.org/10.1186/s12960-021-00558-3

Zavaleta-Monestel, E., Rojas-Chinchilla, C., Anchía-Alfaro, A., Quesada-Loría, D., García-Montero, J., Arguedas-Chacón, S., & Hanley-Vargas, G. (2025). Tracking the threat, 50 years of laboratory-acquired infections: A systematic review. *Acta Microbiologica Hellenica, 70*(2), 11. https://doi.org/10.3390/amh70020011

Chapter 12
Policy and Governance

Annisa Utami Rauf, Mubasysyir Hasanbasri, Annisa Kharismaningtyas Astuti, Bagas Suryo Bintoro, and Annisa Nur Balqis

12.1 Global Governance and Institutional Leadership in One Health

The One Health approach emphasizes the interdependence of human, animal, and environmental health in addressing complex health challenges (CDC, 2025; WHO, 2023a). Its goal is to achieve a sustainable balance between people, animals, and ecosystems by engaging multiple sectors, disciplines, and communities. This is essential not only for ensuring access to safe food, clean water, energy, and air, but also for mitigating climate change and contributing to sustainable development (Adisasmito et al., 2023). The COVID-19 pandemic further demonstrated the urgency of this integrated perspective. With millions of deaths and severe global economic disruption, the crisis revealed how the absence of cross-sectoral surveillance systems across human, animal, and environmental health amplifies the risks of ecosystem-related infectious diseases (Lefrançois et al., 2023). The pandemic

A. U. Rauf (✉) · B. S. Bintoro
Department of Health Behavior, Environment, and Social Medicine, Faculty of Medicine, Public Health, and Nursing, Universitas Gadjah Mada, Sleman, Yogyakarta, Indonesia
e-mail: annisaur@ugm.ac.id; bagas.suryo.b@ugm.ac.id

M. Hasanbasri
Department of Biostatistics, Epidemiology, and Population Health, Faculty of Medicine, Public Health, and Nursing, Universitas Gadjah Mada, Yogyakarta, Indonesia
e-mail: mhasanbasri@ugm.ac.id

A. K. Astuti · A. N. Balqis
Master of Public Health Program, Faculty of Medicine, Public Health, and Nursing, Universitas Gadjah Mada, Yogyakarta, Indonesia
e-mail: annisakharismaningtyasastuti@mail.ugm.ac.id; annisanuurbalqis533164@mail.ugm.ac.id

© The Author(s), under exclusive license to Springer Nature Singapore Pte Ltd. 2026

A. U. Rauf, T. Wibawa (eds.), *The One Health Concept in Asian Contexts*,
https://doi.org/10.1007/978-981-95-9880-9_12

highlighted the interconnectedness of human, animal, and plant health with the global food system, calling for integrated strategies to avert similar crises.

In response, major international bodies—including the World Health Organization (WHO), the Food and Agriculture Organization (FAO), the World Organization for Animal Health (WOAH), and the United Nations Environment Programme (UNEP)—formed a Quadripartite partnership to strengthen policies and the implementation of One Health across sectors (*One Health Joint Plan of Action, 2022–2026*, 2022). Within this collaboration, each organization carries distinct roles. WHO advances the integration of One Health into the global health framework through its One Health Initiative (OHI), which acts as secretariat for the One Health High Level Expert Panel (OHHLEP), coordinates internal initiatives, and promotes governance, cross-sectoral engagement, and political advocacy in multilateral forums such as the G20, G7, and UNGA (WHO, 2023a, b, 2024b, c). WOAH focuses on strengthening animal health and welfare as a central component of One Health, contributing to the development of global strategies against emerging and re-emerging zoonotic threats through multi-sectoral partnerships (WOAH). FAO and UNEP, together with WHO and WOAH, reinforce this collective effort to build more resilient health systems and safeguard global health security.

International organizations play a central role in advancing the One Health approach by shaping national health priorities through funding allocation, standard-setting, and technical guidance (Revill et al., 2020). Their efforts ensure that resources are channeled to areas with the greatest potential impact on population health, particularly in low- and middle-income countries, where development assistance and coordinated global action enable access to life-saving interventions (Dieleman et al., 2015, pp. 1990–2014; Zinsstag, 2024). Beyond resource distribution, these organizations strengthen collaboration across human, animal, and environmental health sectors by providing platforms for dialogue, fostering multidisciplinary research, and supporting the creation of national and regional One Health strategies (Danasekaran, 2024; Roy et al., 2025). Such actions bridge the gap between politics, science, and society, while also promoting equity by prioritizing vulnerable populations and integrating cultural perspectives into health initiatives. Despite these significant contributions, international organizations face notable challenges in institutionalizing and harmonizing the One Health framework. Barriers such as fragmented governance, uneven integration of agriculture and environmental perspectives, limited citizen engagement, and competition for resources hinder progress (Selter & Salloch, 2023; Verbeek et al., 2023; Yasobant et al., 2024). Furthermore, the absence of systematic funding and the lack of strong economic justifications for integrated programs create additional constraints. To remain effective, these organizations must continuously reform health regulations, address conceptual inconsistencies, and strengthen cross-sectoral coordination (Hassoun & Herlitz, 2019).

12.2 Legal Frameworks and National Strategies

The adoption of the One Health approach across Asia demonstrates a strong reliance on intersectoral coordination as the foundation for effective implementation. In many settings, this has required close collaboration among human health, animal health, agriculture, and environmental sectors to respond to emerging and re-emerging zoonotic threats (Paul et al., 2025). India provides a notable example, where institutionalized collaborative frameworks were created to control outbreaks of avian influenza (Chatterjee et al., 2016). Such initiatives underscore that without legal and organizational structures to mandate cooperation, sustained One Health implementation is difficult to achieve (Woolaston et al., 2022). The majority of One Health (OH) initiatives were implemented at the national level (64%), followed by local (17%) and regional efforts (13%). Regional initiatives typically covered multiple countries within defined areas, such as the Eastern Mediterranean (Mahrous et al., 2020), the European Union (Muñoz Madero et al., 2016), and the Caribbean. In total, these programs were carried out across 33 countries on five continents, with the highest concentration (72.7%) located in Asia and Africa (Shallcross & Davies, 2014). To illustrate the scope of One Health implementations (OHIs) across different administrative scales, their geographical distribution was mapped. Figure 12.1 presents the spread of OHIs at national, local, and regional levels.

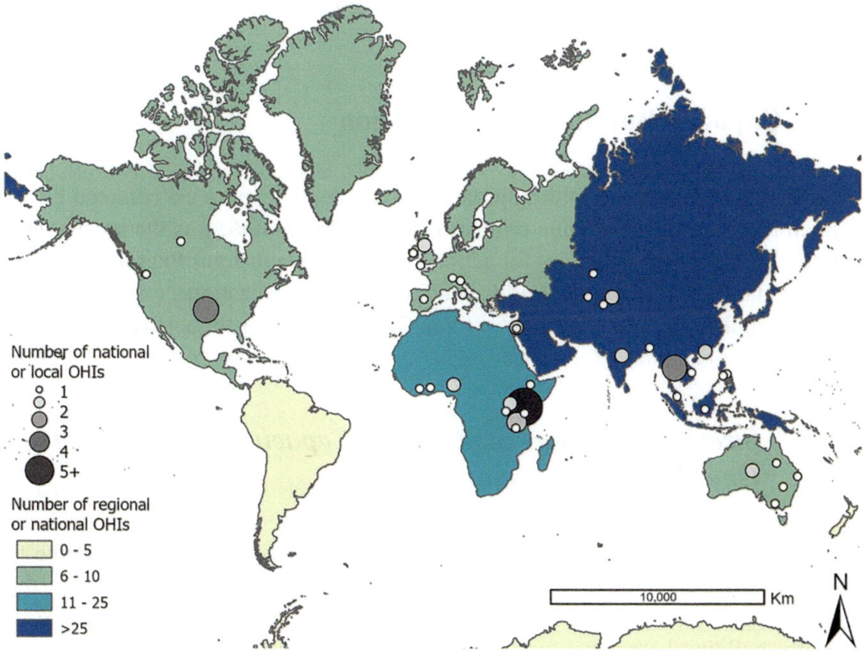

Fig. 12.1 Distribution of One Health initiatives across administrative levels. (Milazzo et al., 2025, licensed under CC-BY 4.0)

Several countries have gone further by embedding One Health into national strategies. Singapore, Hong Kong, Bangladesh, and Thailand, for instance, have formalized action plans that include interministerial coordination and flexible operational linkages between public servants (Beltramo et al., 2024). These frameworks not only enhance responsiveness to zoonotic diseases but also ensure that public health priorities are supported by agricultural and environmental policy. Similarly, China's engagement in Africa shows that One Health is being integrated into epidemic surveillance and response systems as well as broader agendas such as climate change adaptation and disaster risk management, reflecting the scalability of these strategies beyond domestic concerns (Tambo et al., 2017).

Analyzing these patterns highlights a regional convergence toward comprehensive governance of health threats, yet with varying degrees of institutionalization (Chatterjee et al., 2016; Woolaston et al., 2022). High-income economies like Singapore and Hong Kong have established advanced interministerial mechanisms, whereas middle-income countries such as Bangladesh and Thailand focus on operational flexibility and capacity building. India demonstrates the importance of legally anchored frameworks for specific diseases, while China expands One Health into foreign policy and international cooperation. At the regional level, organizations like ASEAN emphasize collective health security by embedding One Health into broader human security frameworks (Caballero-Anthony, 2018). This suggests that while the pathways differ, countries are aligning around the principle that long-term effectiveness depends on strong legal backing, cross-sectoral strategies, and regional cooperation (Meslin & Briggs, 2013; Paul et al., 2025).

12.3 Capacity Building and Education

The success of the One Health approach in Asia depends on a coordinated effort from all levels of society. While policies provide a framework, it is the people who turn those policies into meaningful action. The One Health Joint Plan of Action, a foundational document by the world's leading health organizations, explicitly identifies "strengthening One Health workforces" as a core pillar for action.

12.3.1 Strengthening Key Stakeholder Capacity for Integrated One Health Governance

Effective One Health governance requires building capacity across a wide range of interconnected stakeholders (WHO, 2024a). The government sector remains the central pillar, responsible for policy and national coordination (CISDI, 2024). Capacity building here must target both leadership and technical staff (Hashimy et al., 2023). A systematic review on the topic supports the necessity of addressing these two areas. First, it must target 'governance and leadership' to secure high-level political commitment. Second, it must overcome the 'lack of training and technical capacities' by providing essential skills in areas like zoonotic disease diagnosis and management to health workers (Yopa et al., 2023).

These national efforts are often supported by international organizations. Academic discourse highlights their role in setting standards, providing technical assistance, and fostering cooperation among member states. Through these mechanisms, these organizations are key to strengthening global governance, particularly in areas like public health, by encouraging countries to align their national strategies with international norms (Lie, 2024). Acting as a bridge between policy and the populace are non-governmental organizations (NGOs). These groups play a vital role in "domesticating" complex health concepts at the local government and community level, where these ideas often remain theoretical (Mugisha et al., 2017). Their function involves translating policy into practice by designing and implementing actionable community programs, such as rabies awareness and vaccination campaigns. A key capacity of these groups is their ability to raise awareness and mobilize communities through public health campaigns and educational activities (Besançon et al., 2022). The private sector, including commercial farms, pharmaceutical industries, and veterinary drug shops, is a powerful stakeholder. Engaging this sector is essential for tackling issues like antimicrobial resistance (AMR), for instance, through public-private partnerships. These collaborations aim to secure commitments from industry partners for the judicious use of antimicrobials and the implementation of good waste management practices, which are critical strategies for promoting responsible antimicrobial stewardship (Sihombing et al., 2023).

Many One Health organizations worldwide, such as One Health Lessons, promote education on topics including emerging infectious diseases, zoonoses, antimicrobial resistance, climate change, and food security, often using social media to reach diverse communities (One Health Lesson, 2023). Collaborative programs such as internships, fellowships, and study abroad initiatives like the COVAB-Mississippi State University Tropical Veterinary Medicine and One Health program connect students and professionals across disciplines, providing hands-on, multicultural experiences that integrate human, animal, and environmental health. Encouraging interdisciplinary collaboration and cultural awareness, these initiatives prepare a global workforce capable of addressing complex, context-specific health and environmental challenges through practical, cooperative strategies (Akello, 2025; Cai et al., 2024).

12.3.2 The Role of Academic and Research Sectors

Academic and research sectors play a pivotal role in advancing One Health initiatives by fostering knowledge integration across disciplines and stakeholders to address complex public health challenges. The establishment of the One Health Action Commission (OHAC) in the Asia-Pacific region exemplifies how academic communities contribute to setting research agendas and identifying actions with the greatest potential impact (Hitziger et al., 2021; Zhang et al., 2024). Collaborative efforts are also evident through workshops that convene experts from governments, research institutes, universities, and international organizations in Southeast Asia to strengthen regional One Health initiatives (Lâm et al., 2025). The interdisciplinary research networks in Southeastern Europe and West-Central Asia highlight the importance of cross-border academic partnerships in addressing environmental and occupational health issues, offering valuable lessons for Asia (Coman et al., 2015).

Despite these advances, significant challenges remain in implementing One Health principles within academic and research sectors in Asia. Policymaking often struggles to integrate agriculture and environmental perspectives, leading to fragmented initiatives that limit effectiveness (Beltramo et al., 2024). Ensuring meaningful and equal participation across diverse actors adds another layer of complexity (Dos et al., 2019). Emerging trends, however, suggest a growing commitment to overcoming these barriers. For instance, Singapore has expanded its role in global health education and research, while resources like the One Health Case Studies book document best practices, challenges, and opportunities for advancing One Health globally. These developments demonstrate both the progress made and the evolving role of academia in strengthening One Health approaches in Asia (Cork & Lindenmayer, 2024; Jahncke et al., 2010).

Universities and research institutions are critical in deconstructing the siloed mindset early in a professional's career. Recent educational initiatives, such as the inclusion of a One Health module at the College of Natural Resources (CNR) in Bhutan, are noted as a potential reason for more positive attitudes towards One Health among professionals. This highlights the impact of integrating OH education into university curricula to ensure future professionals have the necessary competencies (Rai et al., 2025). Regional university networks are a powerful driver of changes in this process. Networks like the Southeast Asian One Health University Network (SEAOHUN), a coalition of over 95 universities, play a key role by leveraging education to train the next generation of professionals. Their aim is to foster a systems approach to problem-solving that considers all aspects of the human-animal-ecosystem interface (Lajaunie & Morand, 2024). Beyond teaching, universities are vital for generating the local evidence needed for sound governance. They are key partners in collaborative frameworks that ensure the transfer of knowledge from academia to policymakers (Kehinde et al., 2024). Through biostatistical and epidemiological methods, they can analyze data to identify disease hotspots and risk factors, thereby providing the robust scientific basis needed to design effective, evidence-based interventions (Bruno et al., 2024).

According to Adeyemi (2024), One Health master's programs are generally structured as multidisciplinary and research-oriented degrees (Fig. 12.2). Most programs require mandatory onsite attendance (63%), while others are delivered fully online (23.3%) or in a hybrid format (11.6%). The majority are designed for full-time students, although some offer part-time or blended full-time/part-time options. The typical duration of study is 1–2 years, except for bachelor's levels that follow a standard 4-year structure. In terms of curriculum, all programs include foundational

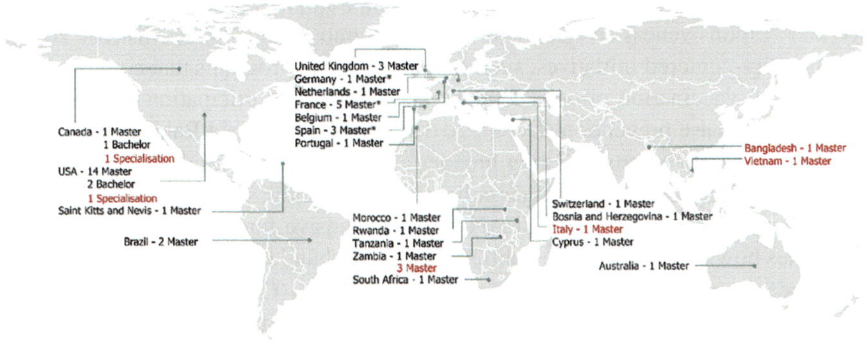

Fig. 12.2 Postgraduate program of One Health across region. (Adeyemi et al., 2024)

modules on One Health principles and concepts, with most also offering epidemiology and biostatistics, core One Health branches (human, animal, and ecosystem health), infectious diseases and zoonoses with surveillance components, and a mandatory internship or research project.

In Asia, several countries—including Bangladesh, Indonesia, Japan, and Vietnam—have developed programs related to One Health, serving as important entry points for advancing One Health studies in the region. At Universitas Gadjah Mada (UGM), for example, the establishment of a One Health program within the Master of Public Health programs, officially launched in 2024, has created new opportunities and academic pathways to tackle complex public health challenges through an integrated approach. In addition, various symposia and guest lectures have been actively organized, featuring speakers from CIRAD, University of Montpellier, Leipzig University, and Yamaguchi University, thereby strengthening international collaboration and academic exchange in the field of One Health.

12.3.3 Empowering the General Public

Influencing the general public within the One Health framework requires strong investments in education, awareness, and governance mechanisms. Education and training initiatives, such as capacity development programs at the Master's level for public health professionals and veterinarians, not only strengthen individual competencies but also foster multidisciplinary networks that are essential for addressing health challenges across human, animal, and environmental sectors (Vink et al., 2012). Beyond individual training, the establishment of sustainable frameworks for collaborative activities, such as zoonotic disease investigation projects and continuing professional development, ensures that these gains are institutionalized and can deliver long-term benefits.

Public engagement also plays a critical role in the success of One Health. National and regional policies that promote interministerial coordination and polycentric governance, involving both state and non-state actors, enhance flexibility and responsiveness to health threats (Beltramo et al., 2024; Mistree, 2022). Community-centered initiatives, such as rabies control programs that combine education with vaccination efforts, demonstrate how local participation directly contributes to disease prevention (Dodet, 2010). Events like World Rabies Day further amplify advocacy efforts, creating broader awareness and commitment among the public. At a regional level, stronger collaboration in health security, disease surveillance, and response, such as ASEAN's comprehensive human security approach, illustrates how empowering the public goes hand in hand with reinforcing collective resilience against pandemics and other emerging threats (Caballero-Anthony, 2018).

Beyond organized institutions, the general public is a fundamental partner in the One Health ecosystem. In Asia, where close human-animal interactions are a part of daily life, empowering individuals and communities with knowledge makes them the first line of defense against health threats. Public education campaigns are essential for addressing critical issues like AMR. A community engagement study in Thailand highlighted the crucial role of local village health volunteers (VHVs) in tackling antimicrobial resistance. Participants identified these volunteers as being best placed to create awareness and share knowledge within their communities. The study documented VHV-led initiatives, such as incorporating AMR as a topic in their monthly meetings and actively seeking further training, demonstrating the power and potential of a grassroots approach in encouraging more responsible antimicrobial use (Poomchaichote et al., 2024). Moreover, an engaged community is a cornerstone of an effective public health system. This concept, often termed 'community engagement,' involves ensuring local communities are sufficiently involved in the planning and implementation of health interventions, which leads to better buy-in and more effective communication (Yopa et al., 2023). The potential for community-based surveillance (CBS), for example, in Indonesia, is highlighted by research in the animal health sector. For instance, CBS implementation for highly pathogenic avian influenza in Indonesia resulted in increased case detection. This aligns with the broader goals of CBS, which include fostering local ownership of and responsibility for health security and building trust through context-appropriate communication (Craig et al., 2025).

A survey in Beijing showed that while only 40% of respondents had heard the term One Health, a much larger proportion recognized its underlying concept, with 83% linking human health to animals and 86% to plants and the environment, with awareness higher among women, younger groups, and those with higher education (Wu et al., 2023). In South Asia, particularly Bangladesh and India, progress in One Health has largely been donor-driven, though challenges such as weak surveillance, uncertain cost-effectiveness, and limited resources remain (Dahal et al., 2017). In Southeast Asia, experts from seven countries highlighted 12 priority actions to strengthen One Health, underscoring the region's vulnerability as an emerging infectious disease hotspot (Lâm et al., 2025). Singapore demonstrates strong interagency coordination and advanced surveillance under its One Health framework, though it still needs broader multi-sectoral engagement and greater public awareness (Tan, 2025). In Thailand, Lao PDR, and Vietnam, farmer awareness of One Health is shaped by socioeconomic factors such as income, gender, age, and household size, with notable differences across countries (Pechdin et al., 2024). More broadly, health communication in Asia is becoming increasingly participatory (Khiun, 2016), with tools like the Living Safely with Bats picture book used to promote awareness of zoonotic disease risks at the community level (Martinez et al., 2022).

12.4 Future Policy of One Health in Asia

The future policy of One Health in Asia is likely to be shaped by the region's persistent vulnerability to zoonotic outbreaks, rapid urbanization, climate change, and growing antimicrobial resistance. To address these challenges, policies will increasingly need to move beyond ad hoc responses toward long-term, institutionalized frameworks that integrate human, animal, and environmental health. Asian governments are expected to prioritize the development of comprehensive national action plans that align with global agendas such as the International Health Regulations (IHR) and the Global Health Security Agenda (GHSA), while tailoring these frameworks to the socioeconomic, cultural, and ecological diversity across the region (Besançon et al., 2022; Caballero-Anthony, 2018; CISDI, 2024; Vermund & Karim, 2009).

At the governance level, future One Health policies must overcome existing fragmentation by establishing polycentric and multisectoral coordination mechanisms. Regional cooperation through organizations such as ASEAN, SAARC, and the Asia-Pacific Economic Cooperation (APEC) will be essential in creating platforms for harmonized surveillance, data sharing, and rapid response (Durrance-Bagale et al., 2022; Rai et al., 2025; Robbiati et al., 2024). Countries with stronger health systems can play a leadership role by providing technical assistance and resources to lower-income neighbors, thereby reducing disparities in preparedness. This cooperative governance model will ensure that health security becomes a shared responsibility across borders rather than remaining a solely national agenda. The way forward for One Health in Asia requires the establishment of robust governance mechanisms supported by comprehensive national strategic action plans, as demonstrated in countries such as Singapore, Hong Kong, Bangladesh, and Thailand (Dahal et al., 2017; Pechdin et al., 2024; Tan, 2025). These strategies serve as a foundation for interministerial coordination, ensuring coherence between health, agriculture, and environmental sectors, while also allowing flexibility for collaboration among public institutions in response to emerging health threats. For example, the International Livestock Research Institute (ILRI) operates in low- and middle-income countries (LMICs) to support smallholder farmers in producing healthy livestock, thereby improving livelihoods, reducing poverty, and ensuring access to nutritious, high-quality protein. However, these livestock systems face major challenges from zoonotic diseases that can spread between animals and humans (https://www.ilri.org). In Fig. 12.3, the ILRI One Health framework illustrates three core

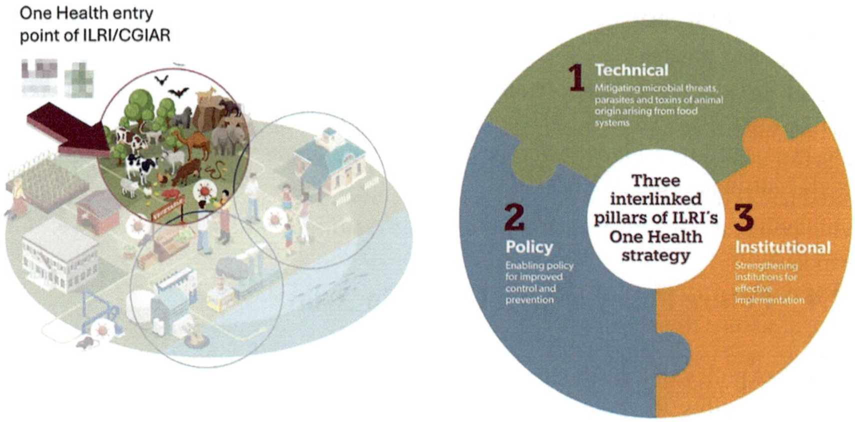

Fig. 12.3 Framework of ILRI One Health approach. (Nguyen-Viet et al., 2025, licensed under CC-BY 4.0)

pillars that integrate science, innovation, and policy to advance One Health approaches in addressing challenges within food systems.

Policy frameworks will also need to emphasize investment in scientific research and technological innovation. Strengthening genomic surveillance, artificial intelligence-driven outbreak prediction, and integrated databases that connect animal, human, and environmental health data will be key areas of focus. Establishing regional centers of excellence for training and research can help build a skilled workforce capable of responding to complex health threats (Lâm et al., 2025; Nambiar, 2020; Parodi et al., 2011). Furthermore, future policies must secure sustainable funding streams by incorporating One Health considerations into national budgets and leveraging international financing mechanisms, such as development banks and climate adaptation funds. For example, governmental sources of funding include the National Institutes of Health (NIH) in the United States, which plays a pivotal role in supporting global health research. Similarly, countries in Asia such as Japan, China, India, and Thailand have established government agencies and funding mechanisms that contribute significantly to advancing research and strengthening health systems (Vermund & Karim, 2009).

Equity and inclusivity are likely to become central principles in the formulation of future policies. Many rural and marginalized communities across Asia remain disproportionately affected by zoonotic diseases due to limited access to healthcare, sanitation, and veterinary services. Ensuring that policies are not only urban-centric but also responsive to rural realities will be essential for achieving meaningful impact (Caballero-Anthony, 2018). Integrating gender-sensitive approaches and recognizing the role of local knowledge and practices will further enhance policy effectiveness and acceptance. The success of future One Health policies in Asia will depend on the ability of governments and stakeholders to institutionalize cross-sectoral collaboration, sustain investment, and foster public trust (Vandermissen & Welburn, 2014).

12.5 Conclusion

The advancement of the One Health approach in Asia reflects a growing recognition that human, animal, and environmental health are inseparable pillars of sustainable development and global health security. Across the region, progress has been shaped by global governance frameworks, national legal reforms, academic leadership, and community engagement, with international partnerships, particularly the Quadripartite collaboration of the World Health Organization, Food and Agriculture Organization, World Organisation for Animal Health, and United Nations Environment Programme, providing strategic direction and normative guidance. Countries such as Singapore, Bangladesh, Thailand, India, and China illustrate diverse yet converging pathways toward institutionalizing One Health within national systems. Nevertheless, persistent structural barriers, including fragmented surveillance systems, inconsistent cross-sectoral coordination, uneven funding mechanisms, and limited public awareness, continue to constrain full implementation. Although educational expansion, regional university networks, and capacity-building initiatives are strengthening the One Health workforce, sustainable impact requires stronger legal anchoring, harmonized data-sharing mechanisms, and long-term political commitment. Moving forward, the effectiveness of One Health in Asia will depend on institutionalizing multisectoral governance, ensuring equitable resource allocation, investing in research and innovation, and fostering meaningful public participation, with strengthened regional cooperation through platforms such as ASEAN playing a critical role in addressing transboundary health threats and building resilient, inclusive, and adaptive health systems.

Competing Interests The author(s) has no competing interests to declare that are relevant to the content of this manuscript.

References

Adeyemi, O. A., Agbabiaka, T. O., & Sujon, H. (2024). Global One Health post-graduate programmes: A review. *One Health Outlook, 6*(1), 7. https://doi.org/10.1186/s42522-024-00097-6

Adisasmito, W. B., Almuhairi, S., Barton Behravesh, C., Bilivogui, P., Bukachi, S. A., Casas, N., Becerra, N. C., Charron, D. F., Chaudhary, A., Ciacci Zanella, J. R., Cunningham, A. A., Dar, O., Debnath, N., Dungu, B., Farag, E., Gao, G. F., Hayman, D. T. S., Khaitsa, M., Koopmans, M. P. G., et al. (2023). One Health action for health security and equity. *The Lancet, 401*(10376), 530–533. https://doi.org/10.1016/S0140-6736(23)00086-7

Akello, W. (2025). Harnessing the power of One Health education to tackle Emerging Infectious Diseases (EIDs) and other global health challenges. *One Health Outlook, 7*(1), 23. https://doi.org/10.1186/s42522-025-00139-7

Beltramo, B., Kolluru, S., Slager, L., Wall, L., Ostwald, K., & Rasali, D. (2024). Comparative analysis of One Health policies in Asia for exploring opportunities for British Columbia in Canada. *International Journal of Environmental Research and Public Health, 22*(1), 34. https://doi.org/10.3390/ijerph22010034

Besançon, S., Sidibé, A., Sow, D. S., Sy, O., Ambard, J., Yudkin, J. S., & Beran, D. (2022). The role of non-governmental organizations in strengthening healthcare systems in low- and middle-income countries: Lessons from Santé Diabète in Mali. *Global Health Action, 15*(1), 2061239. https://doi.org/10.1080/16549716.2022.2061239

Bruno, A., Arnoldi, I., Barzaghi, B., Boffi, M., Casiraghi, M., Colombo, B., Di Gennaro, P., Epis, S., Facciotti, F., Ferrari, N., Fesce, E., Ficetola, G. F., Fumagalli, S., Galimberti, A., Ghisleni, G., Nissim, W. G., Mainardi, L., Manenti, R., Messina, V., et al. (2024). The One Health approach in urban ecosystem rehabilitation: An evidence-based framework for designing sustainable cities. *iScience, 27*(10), 110959. https://doi.org/10.1016/j.isci.2024.110959

Caballero-Anthony, M. (2018). Health and human security challenges in Asia: New agendas for strengthening regional health governance. *Australian Journal of International Affairs, 72*(6), 602–616. https://doi.org/10.1080/10357718.2018.1537356

Cai, C., Jung, Y.-S., Pereira, R. V. V., Brouwer, M. S. M., Song, J., Osburn, B. I., McKenzie, J., Van Der Poel, W. H. M., & Qian, Y. (2024). Advancing One Health education: Integrative pedagogical approaches and their impacts on interdisciplinary learning. *Science in One Health, 3*, 100079. https://doi.org/10.1016/j.soh.2024.100079

CDC. (2025). *One Health history*. One Health. https://www.cdc.gov/one-health/about/one-health-history.html

Chatterjee, P., Kakkar, M., & Chaturvedi, S. (2016). Integrating One Health in national health policies of developing countries: India's lost opportunities. *Infectious Diseases of Poverty, 5*(1), 87. https://doi.org/10.1186/s40249-016-0181-2

CISDI. (2024). *Governance for health: Beyond policy, into impactful delivery* (2nd ed.) CISDI.

Coman, A., Chereches, R. M., Ungureanu, M. I., Marton-Vasarhelyi, E. O., Valentine, M. A., Sabo-Attwood, T., & Gray, G. C. (2015). An assessment of the occupational and environmental health needs in seven Southeastern European and West-Central Asian countries. *Journal of Epidemiology and Global Health, 5*(4), 375. https://doi.org/10.1016/j.jegh.2015.04.004

Cork, S., & Lindenmayer, J. (Eds.). (2024). *One Health case studies: Practical applications of the transdisciplinary approach*. CABI. https://doi.org/10.1079/9781800629523.0000

Craig, A. T., Japri, A. P., & Heryanto, B. (2025). Use of community-based surveillance to enhance emerging infectious disease intelligence generation in Indonesia. *Journal of Global Health, 15*, 04118. https://doi.org/10.7189/jogh.15.04118

Dahal, R., Upadhyay, A., & Ewald, B. (2017). One Health in South Asia and its challenges in implementation from stakeholder perspective. *Veterinary Record, 181*(23), 626–626. https://doi.org/10.1136/vr.104189

Danasekaran, R. (2024). One Health: A holistic approach to tackling global health issues. *Indian Journal of Community Medicine, 49*(2), 260–263. https://doi.org/10.4103/ijcm.ijcm_521_23

Dieleman, J. L., Graves, C., Johnson, E., Templin, T., Birger, M., Hamavid, H., Freeman, M., Leach-Kemon, K., Singh, L., Haakenstad, A., & Murray, C. J. L. (2015). Sources and focus of health development assistance, 1990–2014. *JAMA, 313*(23), 2359. https://doi.org/10.1001/jama.2015.5825

Dodet, B. (2010). Report of the sixth AREB meeting, Manila, The Philippines, 10–12 November 2009. *Vaccine, 28*(19), 3265–3268. https://doi.org/10.1016/j.vaccine.2010.02.093

Dos, S. R. C., Van De Burgwal, L. H. M., & Regeer, B. J. (2019). Overcoming challenges for designing and implementing the One Health approach: A systematic review of the literature. *One Health, 7*, 100085. https://doi.org/10.1016/j.onehlt.2019.100085

Durrance-Bagale, A., Marzouk, M., Ananthakrishnan, A., Nagashima-Hayashi, M., Lam, S. T., Sittimart, M., & Howard, N. (2022). 'Science is only half of it': Expert perspectives on operationalising infectious disease control cooperation in the ASEAN region. *PLOS Global Public Health, 2*(5), e0000424. https://doi.org/10.1371/journal.pgph.0000424

Hashimy, S. Q., Jahromi, A., Hamza, M., & Naaz, I. (2023). Nurturing leadership and capacity building for success: Empowering growth. *International Journal of Rehabilitation and Special Education (IJRSE), 3*(2), 33–46. https://doi.org/10.48165/ijrse.2023.3.2.5

Hassoun, N., & Herlitz, A. (2019). Distributing global health resources: Contemporary issues in political philosophy. *Philosophy Compass, 14*(11), e12632. https://doi.org/10.1111/phc3.12632

Hitziger, M., Berezowski, J., Dürr, S., Falzon, L. C., Léchenne, M., Lushasi, K., Markosyan, T., Mbilo, C., Momanyi, K. N., Özçelik, R., Prejit, N., Zinsstag, J., & Rüegg, S. R. (2021). System thinking and citizen participation is still missing in One Health initiatives—Lessons from fifteen evaluations. *Frontiers in Public Health, 9*, 653398. https://doi.org/10.3389/fpubh.2021.653398

Jahncke, E., Lim, M. K., Seow, A., Chia, K. S., & Wilder-Smith, A. (2010). Global health: Challenges and opportunities for Singapore. *Singapore Medical Journal, 51*(7), 536–541.

Kehinde, J. O., Ngozi, L. E., Stephane, J. C. Z., & Jeremiah, O. (2024). Theoretical perspectives on biostatistics and its multifaceted applications in global health studies. *International Journal of Applied Research in Social Sciences, 6*(11), 2791–2806. https://doi.org/10.51594/ijarss.v6i11.1726

Khiun, L. K. (2016). *Liberalizing, feminizing and popularizing health communications in Asia*. Routledge. https://doi.org/10.4324/9781315592312

Lajaunie, C., & Morand, S. (2024). Southeast Asia at the heart of the implementation of the One Health approach. *SSRN Electronic Journal*. https://doi.org/10.2139/ssrn.4695021

Lâm, S., Dang-Xuan, S., Unger, F., Meeyam, T., Pham-Duc, P., Wacharapluesadee, S., & Nguyen-Viet, H. (2025). Operationalizing regional One Health initiatives in Southeast Asia: Ways forward. *One Health, 20*, 101034. https://doi.org/10.1016/j.onehlt.2025.101034

Lefrançois, T., Malvy, D., Atlani-Duault, L., Benamouzig, D., Druais, P.-L., Yazdanpanah, Y., Delfraissy, J.-F., & Lina, B. (2023). After 2 years of the COVID-19 pandemic, translating One Health into action is urgent. *The Lancet, 401*(10378), 789–794. https://doi.org/10.1016/S0140-6736(22)01840-2

Lie, W. (2024). The role of international organizations in facilitating policy diffusion. *Journal of Political Science and Public Affairs*. https://www.longdom.org/open-access/the-role-of-international-organizations-in-facilitating-policy-diffusion-109765.html

Mahrous, H., Redi, N., Nhu Nguyen, T. M., Al Awaidy, S., Mostafavi, E., & Samhouri, D. (2020). One Health operational framework for action for the Eastern Mediterranean Region, focusing on zoonotic diseases. *Eastern Mediterranean Health Journal, 26*(6), 720–725. https://doi.org/10.26719/emhj.20.017

Martinez, S., Sullivan, A., Hagan, E., Goley, J., Epstein, J. H., Olival, K. J., Saylors, K., Euren, J., Bangura, J., Zikankuba, S., Mouiche, M. M. M., Camara, A. O., Desmond, J., Islam, A., Hughes, T., Wacharplusadee, S., Duong, V., Nga, N. T. T., Bird, B., et al. (2022). Living safely with bats: Lessons in developing and sharing a Global One Health educational resource. *Global Health: Science and Practice, 10*(6), e2200106. https://doi.org/10.9745/GHSP-D-22-00106

Meslin, F.-X., & Briggs, D. J. (2013). Eliminating canine rabies, the principal source of human infection: What will it take? *Antiviral Research, 98*(2), 291–296. https://doi.org/10.1016/j.antiviral.2013.03.011

Milazzo, A., Liu, J., Multani, P., Steele, S., Hoon, E., & Chaber, A.-L. (2025). One Health implementation: A systematic scoping review using the Quadripartite One Health Joint Plan of Action. *One Health, 20*, 101008. https://doi.org/10.1016/j.onehlt.2025.101008

Mistree, D. (2022). Polycentric versus state-led responses to the Covid-19 pandemic. In Š. Ganguly & F. O'Donnell (Eds.), *Routledge handbook of the international relations of South Asia* (1st ed., pp. 425–438). Routledge. https://doi.org/10.4324/9781003246626-36

Mugisha, L., Travis, D., & Pelican, K. (2017). Practical experiences of an NGO implementing One Health initiatives in the Albertine Ecosystem, Hoima, South Western Uganda. *27*(4). https://doi.org/10.11604/pamj.supp.2017.27.4.12573

Muñoz Madero, C., Lopez Navas, A., Padilla León, E., & Sacristán Alvarez, S. (2016). Use of antibiotic with ONE HEALTH perspective: Spanish Strategic Action Plan to reduce the risk of selection and dissemination of antibiotic resistance. *Small Ruminant Research, 142*, 44–47. https://doi.org/10.1016/j.smallrumres.2016.05.016

Nambiar, P. (2020). India to envision One Health movement for confronting emerging health threats: From concept to approach toward institutionalization. *International Journal of One Health, 6*(2), 165–176. https://doi.org/10.14202/IJOH.2020.165-176

Nguyen-Viet, H., Lâm, S., Alonso, S., Unger, F., Moodley, A., Bett, B., Fèvre, E. M., Knight-Jones, T., Mor, S. M., Nguyen, H. T. T., & Grace, D. (2025). Insights and future directions: Applying the One Health approach in international agricultural research for development to address food systems challenges. *One Health, 20*, 101007. https://doi.org/10.1016/j.onehlt.2025.101007

One Health Joint Plan of Action, 2022–2026. (2022). FAO; UNEP; WHO; World Organisation for Animal Health (WOAH) (founded as OIE). https://doi.org/10.4060/cc2289en

One Health Lesson. (2023). *One Health lessons*. https://onehealthlessons.org

Parodi, P., Schmid, G., & Ward, D. (2011). One health in central Asia. A situational analysis informing the future. *Giornale Italiano Di Medicina Tropicale*, 3–4.

Paul, M. M., Pradhan, S., Chettri, A., Khaling, S., & Vanak, A. T. (2025). Putting one health to the test: Operational challenges and critical reflections from the global South. *One Health, 20*, 100963. https://doi.org/10.1016/j.onehlt.2024.100963

Pechdin, W., Sinsamphanh, O., Bui-Thanh, L., Naruepatr, J., Swangsilp, S., Chougule, M., Phrasisombath, K., Ho, T. D. N., & Phan, V.-P. (2024). One Health in agricultural sectors in Thailand, Lao PDR, and Vietnam: Interconnectedness between awareness and socioeconomic factors. *International Journal of Public Health, 69*, 1607088. https://doi.org/10.3389/ijph.2024.1607088

Poomchaichote, T., Kiatying-Angsulee, N., Boonthaworn, K., Naemiratch, B., Ruangkajorn, S., Prapharsavat, R., Thirapantu, C., Sukrung, K., Limmathurotsakul, D., Osterrieder, A., & Cheah, P. Y. (2024). Embedding community and public voices in co-created solutions to mitigate antimicrobial resistance (AMR) in Thailand using the 'Responsive Dialogues' public engagement framework. *Antimicrobial Resistance & Infection Control, 13*(1), 71. https://doi.org/10.1186/s13756-024-01416-2

Rai, B. D., Tenzin, T., Tshering, D., Dahal, N., Tessema, G. A., Fritschi, L., Dodzi, S. N., & Pereira, G. (2025). Knowledge, attitude, and practice of One Health and zoonotic diseases among multisectoral collaborators in Bhutan: Results from a nationwide survey. *PLOS Global Public Health, 5*(1), e0004142. https://doi.org/10.1371/journal.pgph.0004142

Revill, P., Phillips, A., Eaton, J. W., & Hallett, T. B. (2020). Modelling and economic evaluation to inform WHO HIV treatment guidelines. In P. Revill, M. Suhrcke, R. Moreno-Serra, M. Sculpher, & M. Goddard (Eds.), *World scientific series in global health economics and public policy* (Vol. 5, pp. 275–285). WORLD SCIENTIFIC. https://doi.org/10.1142/9789813272378_0011

Robbiati, C., Milano, A., Declich, S., & Dente, M. G. (2024). One Health prevention and preparedness to vector-borne diseases: How should we deal with a multisectoral, multilevel and multigroup governance? *One Health Outlook, 6*(1), 21. https://doi.org/10.1186/s42522-024-00114-8

Roy, S., Malla, S., Dekari, D., & Choudhury, T. G. (2025). One Health approach: Human, environment, and animal health. In S. K. Mallik, N. Shahi, & P. K. Pandey (Eds.), *Management of fish diseases* (pp. 281–297). Springer Nature. https://doi.org/10.1007/978-981-96-0270-4_12

Selter, F., & Salloch, S. (2023). Whose health and which health? Two theoretical flaws in the One Health paradigm. *Bioethics, 37*(7), 674–682. https://doi.org/10.1111/bioe.13192

Shallcross, L. J., & Davies, S. C. (2014). The World Health Assembly resolution on antimicrobial resistance. *Journal of Antimicrobial Chemotherapy, 69*(11), 2883–2885. https://doi.org/10.1093/jac/dku346

Sihombing, B., Bhatia, R., Srivastava, R., Aditama, T. Y., Laxminarayan, R., & Rijal, S. (2023). Response to antimicrobial resistance in South-East Asia Region. *The Lancet Regional Health—Southeast Asia, 18*, 100306. https://doi.org/10.1016/j.lansea.2023.100306

Tambo, E., Tang, S., Ai, L., & Zhou, X.-N. (2017). The value of China-Africa health development initiatives in strengthening "One Health" strategy. *Global Health Journal, 1*(1), 33–46. https://doi.org/10.1016/S2414-6447(19)30062-4

Tan, H. Y. (2025). Overview of Singapore's One Health strategy. *Zoonotic Diseases, 5*(1), 2. https://doi.org/10.3390/zoonoticdis5010002

Vandermissen, A., & Welburn, S. C. (2014). Current initiatives in One Health: Consolidating the One Health Global Network: -EN- Current initiatives in One Health: consolidating the One Health Global Network -FR- Initiatives actuelles « Une seule santé » : la consolidation d'un réseau mondial « Une seule santé » -ES- Iniciativas actuales en materia de «Una sola salud»: consolidación de la red mundial por «Una sola salud». *Revue Scientifique et Technique de l'OIE, 33*(2), 421–432. https://doi.org/10.20506/rst.33.2.2297

Verbeek, L., Rabold, D., Hartig, A., Stephan, S., Deus, E., Otte, I., Beutling, A., Schollmeyer, K., De Coninck, P., Höppner, K., Saal, K., Vogler, T., Hach, L., Steinmetz, E., Benner, T., Derksen, L., Militzer, N., Probst, C., & Teichert, U. (2023). One Health: Eine Sichtweise des informellen ministeriellen Netzwerkes: „Was wäre, wenn der One-Health-Ansatz zum Leitmotiv von Kooperation auf nationaler, europäischer und globaler Ebene würde?". *Bundesgesundheitsblatt—Gesundheitsforschung—Gesundheitsschutz, 66*(6), 593–598. https://doi.org/10.1007/s00103-023-03706-3

Vermund, S. H., & Karim, Q. A. (2009). Governmental support of research. In *Clinical and translational science* (pp. 219–236). Elsevier. https://doi.org/10.1016/B978-0-12-373639-0.00016-9

Vink, W. D., McKenzie, J. S., Cogger, N., Borman, B., & Muellner, P. (2012). Building a foundation for 'One Health': An education strategy for enhancing and sustaining national and regional capacity in endemic and emerging zoonotic disease management. In J. S. Mackenzie, M. Jeggo, P. Daszak, & J. A. Richt (Eds.), *One Health: The human-animal-environment interfaces in emerging infectious diseases* (Vol. 366, pp. 185–205). Springer. https://doi.org/10.1007/978-3-662-45791-7_241

WHO. (2023a). *One Health*. One Health. https://www.who.int/news-room/fact-sheets/detail/one-health

WHO. (2023b). *One Health High-Level Expert Panel Annual Report 2023*. OHHLEP. https://cdn.who.int/media/docs/default-source/one-health/ohhlep/ohhlep-annual-report-2023.pdf?sfvrsn=55fc2b9d_3&download=true

WHO. (2024a). *One Health High-Level Expert Panel (OHHLEP)*. https://www.who.int/groups/one-health-high-level-expert-panel

WHO. (2024b). *One Health initiative*. https://www.who.int/publications/m/item/one-health-initiative

WHO. (2024c). *The WHO One Health Initiative (OHI)*. https://www.who.int/publications/m/item/the-who-one-health-initiative

Woolaston, K., Nay, Z., Baker, M. L., Brockett, C., Bruce, M., Degeling, C., Gilbert, J., Jackson, B., Johnson, H., Peel, A., Sahibzada, S., Oskam, C., & Hewitt, C. L. (2022). An argument for pandemic risk management using a multidisciplinary One Health approach to governance: An Australian case study. *Globalization and Health, 18*(1), 73. https://doi.org/10.1186/s12992-022-00850-4

Wu, C., Astbury, C. C., Lee, K. M., Gong, Z., Chen, S., Li, A., Tsasis, P., & Penney, T. (2023). Public awareness of One Health in China. *One Health, 17*, 100603. https://doi.org/10.1016/j.onehlt.2023.100603

Yasobant, S., Yadav, M., & Saxena, D. (2024). Inequity versus inequality in the One Health: Are we doing justice and to whom? In B. W. K. Son (Ed.), *The landscape of global health inequity* (Vol. 22, pp. 243–255). Springer Nature. https://doi.org/10.1007/978-3-031-60502-4_16

Yopa, D. S., Massom, D. M., Kiki, G. M., Sophie, R. W., Fasine, S., Thiam, O., Zinaba, L., & Ngangue, P. (2023). Barriers and enablers to the implementation of one health strategies in developing countries: A systematic review. *Frontiers in Public Health, 11*, 1252428. https://doi.org/10.3389/fpubh.2023.1252428

Zhang, X.-X., Lederman, Z., Han, L.-F., Schurer, J. M., Xiao, L.-H., Zhang, Z.-B., Chen, Q.-L., Pfeiffer, D., Ward, M. P., Sripa, B., Gabriël, S., Dhama, K., Acharya, K. P., Robertson, L. J., Deem, S. L., Aenishaenslin, C., Dantas-Torres, F., Otranto, D., Grace, D., et al. (2024). Towards an actionable One Health approach. *Infectious Diseases of Poverty, 13*(1), 28. https://doi.org/10.1186/s40249-024-01198-0

Zinsstag, J. (2024). One Health. In F. Darbellay (Ed.), *Elgar encyclopedia of interdisciplinarity and transdisciplinarity* (pp. 357–361). Edward Elgar Publishing. https://doi.org/10.4337/9781035317967.ch78

GPSR Compliance

The European Union's (EU) General Product Safety Regulation (GPSR) is a set of rules that requires consumer products to be safe and our obligations to ensure this.

If you have any concerns about our products, you can contact us on ProductSafety@springernature.com

In case Publisher is established outside the EU, the EU authorized representative is:

Springer Nature Customer Service Center GmbH
Europaplatz 3
69115 Heidelberg, Germany

Batch number: 10726135

Printed by Printforce, the Netherlands